Speech Mapping and Probe Microphone Measurements

Editor-in-Chief for Audiology
Brad A. Stach, PhD

Additional Books by These Authors

Modern Hearing Aids: Pre-Fitting Testing and Selection Considerations

Modern Hearing Aids: Verification, Outcome Measures, and Follow-Up

Essentials of Modern Hearing Aids: Selection, Fitting, and Verification
(coming fall 2017)

Speech Mapping and Probe Microphone Measurements

H. Gustav Mueller, PhD
Todd A. Ricketts, PhD
Ruth Bentler, PhD

Plural Publishing Inc.

PLURAL PUBLISHING INC.

5521 Ruffin Road
San Diego, CA 92123

e-mail: info@pluralpublishing.com
Website: http://www.pluralpublishing.com

FSC www.fsc.org MIX Paper from responsible sources FSC® C011935

Typeset in 10.5/13 Minion Pro by Flanagan's Publishing Services, Inc.
Printed in the United States of America by McNaughton & Gunn, Inc.

Library of Congress Cataloging-in-Publication Data:
Names: Mueller, H. Gustav, author. | Ricketts, Todd, author. | Bentler, Ruth A., author.
Title: Speech mapping and probe microphone measurements / H. Gustav Mueller, Todd A. Ricketts, Ruth Bentler.
Description: San Diego, CA : Plural Publishing, [2017] | Includes bibliographical references and index.
Identifiers: LCCN 2017009204| ISBN 9781944883942 (alk. paper) | ISBN 1944883940 (alk. paper) | ISBN 9781944883942 (e-ISBN) | ISBN 1944883940 (e-ISBN)
Subjects: | MESH: Hearing Aids | Correction of Hearing Impairment--instrumentation | Audiometry, Speech--instrumentation
Classification: LCC RF290 | NLM WV 274 | DDC 617.8--dc23
LC record available at https://lccn.loc.gov/2017009204

Contents

Preface *vii*

1 The Underlying Rationale 1

2 Developing a Gold Standard 37

3 Getting Started 65

4 The Essential Measurements 103

5 Verification and Assessment of Fittings and Features 151

6 Putting It All Together 197

7 Frequently Asked Questions 243

References *269*

Appendices *279*

Index *295*

Preface

Although the notion of measuring the output of a hearing aid in the real ear had been tossed around since the 1940s, it was not until the late 1970s that a "dispenser friendly" system was available. In this case, the term "dispenser friendly," is used somewhat loosely. The late 1970s equipment that we are referring to was first described in a paper that was presented by Earl Harford, Ph.D. in September of 1979 at the International Ear Clinics' Symposium in Minneapolis, Minnesota. At this meeting, Earl reported on his clinical experiences of testing hearing aids in the real ear using a miniature (by 1979 standards) Knowles microphone. The microphone was coupled to an interfacing impedance-matching system (developed by David Preves, Ph.D., who at the time worked at Starkey Laboratories), which could be used with existing hearing aid analyzer systems. Unlike today's *probe tube* microphone systems, this early method of clinical real-ear measurement involved putting the entire microphone (about 4 mm by 5 mm by 2 mm) in the ear canal down by the eardrum of the patient. If you think cerumen is a problem with probe microphone measurements today, you should have seen the condition of this microphone after a day's work!

While this early instrumentation was a bit cumbersome, we quickly learned the advantages that probe microphone measures provided in the fitting of hearing aids. We frequently ran into calibration and equalization problems, not to mention a yelp or two from the patient, but the resulting information was worth the trouble. Word of this new testing technique traveled fast, and a study of the clinical applications was soon underway at Walter Reed Medical Center in Washington, D.C. In the fall of 1980, at the ASHA convention in Detroit, Michigan, the first paper on this topic at a national meeting was presented, authored by Walter Reed audiologists Dan Schwartz, Brian Walden, Gus Mueller, and Rauna Surr.

In the early 1980s, the first computerized *probe tube* microphone system, the Rastronics CCI-10 (developed in Denmark by Steen Rasmussen), entered the U.S. market. This system had a silicone tube attached to the microphone (the transmission of sound through this tube was part of the calibration process), which (thankfully) eliminated the need to place the microphone itself in the ear canal. The Rastronics real-ear analyzer (in prototype form) was first demonstrated at the 1982 ASHA convention in Toronto, Canada. At the time, there was a distribution link with Bernafon hearing aids, and the demonstration was at the Bernafon booth. In October of 1983, the first clinical model, the CCI-10, was shown at the national hearing aid meeting in Denver. The product was bundled with Bernafon hearing aid sales, deals were struck, and within a few months, clinical probe microphone testing was occurring at offices across the United States.

We soon saw several other companies introduce equipment to enter into the probe microphone market. One of the first to join Rastronics in the marketplace was the product line Acoustimed from South Africa, which operated using an Acorn Computer, and unlike other products that used swept tones, the Acoustimed used a click as in the input stimulus. The Bosch company introduced a probe microphone product with the perhaps the most intriguing name—the "Invivo." One product that gained popularity quickly, and provided the most competition for Rastronics was the "IGO" (insertion gain optimizer) from Madsen. And finally, maybe the most over-engineered product of the day was the "Aurora," which was part of Nicolet's Project Phoenix, and was used to fit the digital hearing aid from this project. The probe placement device of the Aurora scared away most clinical audiologists, as it was a large metal apparatus, fitted to the head containing various nobs to adjust the probe up or down, right or left, in or out. The preciseness probably pleased a handful of researchers, but the process was too cumbersome for clinical use, and the appearance was something associated more with brain surgery than assessing the performance of a hearing aid.

A bigger issue than the equipment itself was developing standard terminology and procedures for all the new measures that were now being conducted with hearing aids on the real ear. In 1986, Dave Preves was quoted in the *Hearing Journal*, as stating: "An Acoustical Society of America study group will meet this month [May 1986] to begin discussing the standardization of real-ear measurement terminology." It was a decade later before the first ANSI standard on probe microphone measures, S3.46-1997, was published. Like good wine, standards take time to reach maturity.

While waiting for the phantom standard to emerge, audiologists published papers using the terminology that was rumored to be part of the standard, and was already being tossed around by clinicians. The first complete summary of all these terms, however, was in a 1992 book written by Gus Mueller, David Hawkins, and Jerry Northern, titled *Probe Microphone Measurements.* Two hearing aid companies, Starkey and Siemens, bought thousands of these books, and distributed them widely, free-of-charge among audiologists. The word was finally out to the masses describing what probe microphone measurements were all about.

So, 25 years have passed since that first book on probe microphone measurements —it is now out of print, although some pristine collector's copies can be found on eBay. Interestingly, it was never revised, and no other book dedicated to probe microphone measurements has been published since—until now! There are a few things that haven't changed much in 25 years, but there are a lot more things that have. We have tried to include all of them in our current text.

The three of us are pretty confident, and we think we have the answers to most things (at least regarding to hearing aids), but the one thing we can't explain is why the verification of hearing aid gain and output using real-ear measures has not become routine practice—estimates for the U.S. place the adoption of this testing at no more than 20 to 25%. The equipment is readily available, the procedures are easy to learn, and the time commitment is minimal. The penalty (to the patient) if the audiologist does not do the testing can be huge. For the audiologist, failure to verify is bordering on malpractice. Moreover, there isn't an alternative fitting method. We talk about all this in Chapter 1, hoping to get some of you who are on the fence to become *believers.*

Fitting hearing aids using speech mapping procedures indeed does require more time than simply asking the patient "So how does that sound?" Clinicians often ask—is all that work really worth it? The answer is a resounding "yes." Forgetting for a moment the ethical and possible medical-legal ramifications of fitting hearing aids and *not* providing patients with appropriate audibility, considerable data show that as verification and validation measures increase, so do patient benefit and satisfaction. Research findings also show that in general, patients fitted to a validated prescriptive approach have improved speech understanding, real-world outcomes, and a preference for the prescriptive gain and output. Moreover, large studies such as MarkeTrak VIII clearly indicate that as audiologists add various verification and validation components of Best Practice to their fitting protocol, satisfaction increases accordingly, patient loyalty increases significantly, and follow-up visits for hearing aid adjustments are reduced.

The primary use of speech mapping and probe microphone measures is to verify gain and output on the day of the fitting. To state the obvious, if something is verified, there must be a reference standard. We believe an excellent starting point is the use of a validated prescriptive fitting approach. Today, we have two, well-researched methods, the NAL-NL2 and the DSL v5.0. We provide you with a review of both of these well-established and validated methods.

The core of this book is dedicated to the nuts and bolts of conducting the probe microphone measures. This could be speech mapping for determining a match to target, or it could be an RESR85 measure to assure that the MPO is okay, or it could be the use of special speech signals for programming frequency lowering. For each test and procedure, we provide background information, a clinical step-by-step protocol, and case examples, all geared toward the day-to-day fitting of hearing aids. Just in case we forgot to mention something in these core chapters, we also included a special FAQ chapter, which provides the answers to just about every question that we could think of—most of which, are questions that we have gotten at one of our workshops. Finally, because fitting hearing aids is not only just about real-ear verification, we provide a final chapter on "putting it all together." Here we provide a brief outline of other procedures that supplement probe microphone measures before and after the fitting—the details of which you can find in our other three books.

For those of us who use probe microphone measures routinely, it is difficult to imagine how hearing aids could be fitted without this testing. Certainly, using either the REAR or the REIG is essential for verification of prescriptive targets and determining appropriate audibility of the amplified signals—there is no alternative choice. Along with being critical verification measures, these procedures are also helpful in assessing and adjusting several hearing aid features, and in troubleshooting post-fitting problems. Moreover, conducting these measures can be fascinating and educational, and sharing the results with the patient is a very effective counseling procedure. Clearly, the routine use of probe microphone assessment and making reasoned decisions based on the findings is one of the most important components in the overall fitting of hearing aids. Without this information, we are forced to make choices based on guesses, hunches, or clinical intuition, instead of data. This is certainly not something we want to do if we are truly interested in providing evidence-based services.

The authors wish to acknowledge the generous support of Otometrics during the writing and production of this book.

1 The Underlying Rationale

Wrong does not cease to be wrong because the majority share in it.

—Leo Tolstoy

Every university professor who teaches hearing aid classes knows the story. Five years after her graduation, you run into one of your prized AuD students at a conference. She was, of course, trained to follow Best Practice Documents and always conduct probe microphone verification back at the university. But now she says, "I probably shouldn't tell you this, but I never do probe microphone verification anymore. No one else at my clinic is doing it, so I don't either." The Tolstoy quote above says it best.

We want all of our hearing aid patients to be happy, right, and leave our offices with a smile on their face? Although it is nice to see them smile, this *verification* approach doesn't quite follow evidence-based practice. It has been shown time and time again that a *validated* prescriptive fitting method should be used as a starting point for *verification*. As we discuss later, when we have verification of a validated prescriptive method, we have a good understanding of the trade-offs between audibility, speech understanding, sound quality, comfort, and other factors involved in the fitting of the typical patient. This may not be the end point for all patients, and gain adjustments may be necessary. However, if we start with ear canal sound pressure level (SPL) reference information relative to the individual patient's dynamic range, we then know what effect we are having on audibility when we make changes from a validated method, and the potential impact of those changes. Perhaps it's obvious, but we'll say it anyway, the only way you know if you are fitting to a specific fitting method, is to observe SPL in the ear canal.

We all know of cases in which a patient was fitted without real-ear verification, and several patient-driven adjustments had to be made, and the patient ended up with little or no gain. For instance, we recall one case of a hearing aid wearer—who interestingly also happened to be an audiologist—using new instruments he had fitted to himself through careful listening. After volunteering to be a demonstration patient at one of our probe microphone workshops, he and the rest of the audience discovered that he had simply programmed his hearing aids to match his unaided open-ear canal resonance—the hearing aids had no real-ear gain above 1500 Hz.

Although behavioral measures can be helpful, they are complementary and not a substitute for the objective assessment of hearing aid output in the ear canal. It is important to understand that a *prescriptive fitting* is ultimately based on the desired amplified signal level in the ear canal, not a 2cc-coupler measure (at least not without correcting for differences between the ear and the coupler), a KEMAR measure, or a computer simulation in the fitting software. Therefore, *probe microphone measures* of hearing aid performance *(or individual real-ear corrections to the coupler these provide)* are needed for verification of our chosen prescriptive method.

The importance of these procedures has been emphasized and recommended in every hearing aid-fitting guideline published in the past 20 years. As an example, the following excerpt is taken from the 2006 fitting guidelines of the American Academy of Audiology (AAA) (p. 25):

> The objective of this segment of the fitting process is to ensure that the fitting and verification procedure is viewed as a process rather than an event, which culminates in the optimal fitting for the patient. Verification procedures also serve as a benchmark against which future hearing aid changes can be compared. Specific goals and rationales underlie all hearing aid fittings. Verification procedures should be based on validated hearing aid fitting rationales.

As mentioned earlier, you are using a validated method only when that method's prescribed gain and/or output are referenced to what is required in the ear canal. We mention this again as this concept doesn't seem to be obvious to all clinicians. For example, Mueller (2005b) reported that in a survey of audiologists fitting hearing aids, 78% stated that they routinely were using a validated prescriptive fitting approach (i.e., either the NAL or the DSL). Interestingly, however, of this 78%, only 44% reported routinely using probe microphone measures. Question of the day: How do the remaining 56% know what method they are using, or if they are using any method at all? This is like saying that you drove exactly 60 mph all the way to work, only to admit that the speedometer in your car never moves off zero! You need a speedometer, and you have it—it's your probe microphone equipment.

Mueller and Picou (2010) identified a similar disconnect in their survey findings. From their sample, 79% of audiologists reported using a validated prescriptive fitting approach, and yet only 59% of this group routinely used probe microphone verification. Another peculiar finding from this survey was, that of the respondents who said they used prescriptive methods routinely *and* also reported conducting probe microphone testing routinely, only 37% said that their primary reason for using probe microphone testing was to verify these targets.

Real Ear Versus Probe Microphone Versus Speech Mapping

There are a few different terms that refer to the act of putting a tube in the ear canal and measuring the output from the hearing aid in the real ear. An early term that was used for this was *in situ* measurement, meaning "in position"—a reasonable term, as indeed the hearing aid is measured in the *use position*. In early marketing efforts of probe microphone equipment, however, it was important to make the distinction that the testing was conducted on the *real ear* and not in a 2cc coupler. *In situ* did not have much meaning to most audiologists, so it made more sense to refer to the testing as *real-ear measurements* (REM). The term REM (pronounced *rhem*) is sometimes used today by manufacturers and audiologists.

Whereas testing during the first 20 years of probe microphone assessment mostly involved swept pure tones and composite noise as the input signal, in the past decade, speech shaped signals, or real-speech inputs, have become routine. The use of these signals in combination with plotting the patient's

CLINICAL CONCEPT: You Don't Fit Hearing Aids by PROBE

We often overhear at audiology meetings, perhaps around a cocktail table, one audiologist asking another, "So do you fit your aids by probe?" There seems to be a common belief that probe microphone measures are a way to fit hearing aids. They are not. They are simply a way to *verify* your way of fitting hearing aids. We know of large clinics where the audiologists are required by their supervisor to do probe microphone measures. What audiologists may do is push the magic button that provides a fit to the manufacturer's default fitting, then conduct probe microphone testing for inputs of 55, 65, and 75 dB SPL, and put the results in the patient's chart. Not one hearing aid adjustment involved! Did they *fit by probe*? Some might say they do. Are they fitting by a validated rationale? Not likely, as we describe in detail later in this chapter. Again, the act of conducting probe microphone testing is not a way of fitting hearing aids—the validated rationale is the way—which needs to be verified.

To reiterate this point in another way, we use a weekend construction project as an analogy to the fitting of a hearing aid. Let's say you are going to build a doghouse. You start with a general design (type of roof, door size, etc.—just as you start with selection of a validated fitting rationale). You then go online and find a blueprint for building the doghouse that fits your design (exact dimensions for all the pieces that will need to be assembled—just as you obtain desired gain and output values for your fitting method). Now, while cutting the pieces for this doghouse you might use a tape measure to *verify* that all the pieces fit your blueprint. (Remember the adage, "Measure twice, cut once.") Would you tell your woodworking colleagues that a tape measure is a way to build a doghouse? Not likely. But could you build a sturdy and nice-looking doghouse without using a tape measure? Probably not!

dynamic range in SPL has prompted audiologists to refer to the testing as *speech mapping*. This term was first used in the early 1990s when Bill Cole and his colleagues introduced this feature, trademarked as Speechmap™ on the Audioscan coupler/probe microphone unit from his company, Etymonic Design Incorporated. This equipment did not produce a shaped speech signal all at once, but rather a series of tone pips/bursts whose levels reflected the frequency-specific long-term average speech spectrum (LTASS) levels. Most audiologists today use a speech-shaped/shaped-speech input signal, and if different input levels are used and they are plotted relative to the patient's residual range of hearing, they are conducting speech mapping. That is, if it's not plotted for different input levels, it's not really a "map" of the ear canal output. Of course, you can't do REM or speech mapping without a probe microphone, so that too is a reasonable term, particularly because many probe microphone measurements to not involve using a speech signal.

Which term is correct? Or better, which term will cause the least confusion? We believe there is a clear choice, and that choice is probe microphone measures, for several reasons. First, consider the procedures for conducting aided sound-field testing and functional gain. The last time we checked, these are *real-ear measures* of hearing aid performance. There are government forms that very specifically require the "real-ear measure of hearing aid performance" with the patient wearing one versus two hearing aids. They are referring to aided sound-field testing. If you believe that the term *real ear* relates only to probe microphone measures, this request would be quite puzzling, as there is no probe microphone measure that would assess the summation effects of two instruments.

On a recent audiology Listserv we saw this posting: "I'm going to buy some real-ear equipment, but I can't decide if I should purchase probe microphone or speech mapping?" This posting highlights our second point. Probe microphone testing nearly always *is* speech mapping; speech mapping nearly always *is* a component of the probe microphone assessment of a hearing aid. They are not two different things. Therefore, it is much simpler to call the entire process *probe microphone measures*, as, although it is likely that this will include speech mapping, it is also very possible that some of the testing will not be speech mapping; for example, a swept-tone MPO measure, the measure of the occlusion effect, and so forth.

So, with all that said, in this book we use the term *probe microphone measures* to describe all types of real-ear testing of hearing aid performance.

Compliance with Best Practice Guidelines

The use of probe microphone measures for hearing aid verification has always been assumed when Best Practice guidelines were written. Going back to the recommendations of the 1990 Vanderbilt Report II (see Hawkins et al., 1991), probe microphone assessment has been mentioned as either the preferred method or one of the preferred methods for verification. Over the years, published guidelines from the Independent Hearing Aid Fitting Forum (IHAFF), the ASHA, and the AAA have recommended the use of probe microphone verification. The statement on this topic from the 2006 AAA document is unambiguous: "Prescribed gain (output) from a validated prescriptive method should be verified using a probe microphone approach that is referenced to ear canal SPL."

In case you think this is only a United States recommendation, this International Society of Audiology (2005) excerpt from their document "Good Practice Guidance for Adult Hearing Aid Fittings and Services" states the fitting tolerances that are acceptable internationally.

> Where a fitting rationale contains an acoustical target, each hearing aid fitting should be verified by real-ear measurement using an input stimulus appropriate for the hearing aid under test prior to any fine-tuning. Tolerances to the prescription rationale of ±5 dB at frequencies of 250 Hz, 500 Hz, 1000 Hz, and 2000 Hz and of ±8 dB at 3000 and 4000 Hz should be achieved in all cases. In addition, the slope in each octave should be within ±5 dB/octave of the target. Where it is not desirable or possible to achieve a prescriptive target (e.g., because of feedback issues) or where the measurement is not technically feasible, the clinical record should contain an explicit statement to this effect. (p. 5)

We know, however, that what is supported by research evidence, recommended by opinion leaders, and published in Best

Practice Documents, does not always find its way into routine clinical audiology use. The best example of this might be the persistent use of live-voice speech recognition testing, despite the abundance of literature showing the many shortcomings of this practice (see Hornsby & Mueller, 2013; Mueller, Ricketts, & Bentler, 2014). But what about probe microphone measures? The clinically friendly equipment for this testing has been available for more than 30 years. Are these measures a routine part of the hearing aid fitting protocol for all or most audiologists? This topic has generated a number of surveys, so we do have a pretty good idea of compliance. In the following four surveys, the audiologists responding were actively engaged in the fitting of hearing aids, and *routine use* was defined as using probe microphone measures with at least 50% of adult patients:

- In 1995, Mueller and Strouse reported that the routine use of probe microphone measures was 54% for audiologists (n = 134) and 18% for hearing instrument specialists (HISs; n = 108), with an overall average use rate of 39%.
- In 1999, Mueller again examined use rates for both audiologists and HISs, but this time limited the survey to those who owned or had access to the equipment. When the two professional groups were combined, 42% reported routine use.
- In 2003, a Mueller survey of primarily audiologists (n = 558 audiologists, 49 HISs) showed an overall routine use rate of 37%.
- A few years later, Mueller (2005b) again examined the popularity of these measures, this time among audiologists only. The overall use rate was 34%. It was slightly higher (~40%) for recent graduates (either masters level or AuDs) and for experienced audiologists who had obtained their AuD through distance learning.

The results of these surveys are surprisingly similar, showing, in general, routine use of probe microphone verification of about 35% to 40%. This takes us to the most recent and extensive survey on the topic by Mueller and Picou (2010). This online survey used data only from U.S. practitioners who dispense hearing aids, and included a total of 420 respondents, of which 309 were audiologists (74%) and 111 (26%) were HISs. One of the questions related to the routine use of the equipment on the day of the fitting. The results are shown in Figure 1–1.

If we first look at the left portion of Figure 1–1, we see use rates that are quite similar to what has been found in other surveys: about 45% for audiologists, 36% for HISs, with an overall use rate of 41%. These data are for the total sample, which includes individuals who do not have the equipment. The data on the right portion of the chart are only for those respondents who stated that they have the equipment available. As we would predict, this increases the use of this testing (more so for HISs), but not by nearly the amount that would be expected. Consider that for both groups, about 45% of the audiologists and HISs who have the equipment don't use it routinely. These data are nearly as low as surveys regarding use rates for people who own treadmills! Of course, people completing this survey knew what the correct answer was. Using the findings from some lie detector questions embedded in the survey, Mueller and Picou (2010) concluded that the actual use rate is not even as high as their results indicated—as many as 25% of respondents said that they were doing probe microphone measures that don't even exist.

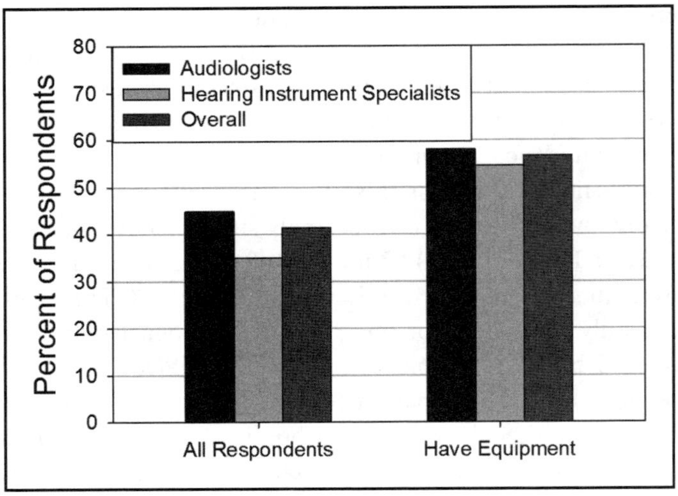

Figure 1–1. Survey results comparing "routine use of probe microphone measures" indicating across all respondents, about 41% use, and across practitioners who have the equipment, about 55% use. Adapted from Mueller and Picou, 2010.

One finding we find interesting is that in 1995, probe microphone use for audiologists, versus hearing instrument specialists (HISs), was 54 to 18%. Today, or at least in the 2010 survey, the use rate is essentially the same between these two groups, due to a considerable uptake by the HISs. Why is this? Although we have little data on the topic, we do have some opinions formed from discussions with individuals from both groups, as well as manufacturer's sales reps, who probably know the straight scoop the best. Here are our thoughts:

- There are fewer "mom and pop" HISs today than there were 20 years ago. Currently, HISs are younger and more tech savvy.
- Many HISs in private practice are no longer with a franchise company, but are now selling the same hearing aids as the audiology practice down the street. This places a greater emphasis on the quality of the fitting, using the right equipment, and a contemporary fitting protocol.
- More and more, the fitting is driven by consumers, as they become better educated regarding the right and wrong way to fit a hearing aid. In July 2009, *Consumer Reports* reported that in their sample, about two-thirds of hearing aids sold were fitted incorrectly. The article concluded: "The provider should do several tests to verify that they (hearing aids) are working optimally. Of that battery of tests, one stands out as a must-have: the real-ear test."
- Finally, in recent years the hearing aid distribution system has changed, with many chains and big-box stores dispensing hearing aids. These are common employment sites for HISs, and many, if not most of these stores, make an *effort* to follow Best Practice guidelines; sadly, perhaps more so than some audiology practices. Individuals

working at these sites are strongly encouraged to follow the established Best Practice protocols.

Much of the MarkeTrak VIII report focused on verification, including the administration of tests such as probe microphone measurements (e.g., Kochkin et al., 2010; Kochkin, 2011). The approach taken by MarkeTrak VIII was different from that used in the other surveys we have reported. Rather than asking audiologists and HISs if they conducted the testing, individuals purchasing hearing aids were queried if they had received testing using a probe tube inserted in the ear. Survey findings reported that 42% of the respondents stated that they received this testing, and there was not a significant difference in the frequency if the patient had been fitted by an audiologist or an HIS—findings which more or less agree with the Mueller and Picou (2010) survey.

Possible Ethics Violation?

Ever since it became obvious that audiologists were not adopting the use of probe microphone measures at the rate that everyone expected, many of us have publicly commented that not doing probe microphone assessment when hearing aids are fitted is clearly *poor clinical practice*. In a 2009 article in *Audiology Today* titled, "It's a Matter of Ethics," Catherine Palmer took it to a different level. She questioned if not doing probe microphone testing is a violation of the code of ethics of our major audiology professional organizations. She specifically stated, "If we talk about ethical practice, then we have to be comfortable saying that there are hearing health care providers (audiologists) who are not practicing ethically" (p. 32).

Most of us think of unethical practice related to the fitting of hearing aids as things such as free trips to Hawaii or giving kickbacks to referral sources. But the Code of Ethics for professional organizations also includes items related to how we perform clinical audiology. For example, Principle 2 of the AAA Code of Ethics states, "Members shall maintain high standards of professional competence in rendering services." Principle 4 states, "Members shall provide only services and products that are in the best interest of those served." Principle of Ethics II from the ASHA *Code of Ethics* states that "Individuals shall honor their responsibility to achieve and maintain the highest level of professional competence."

Consider this example: If you don't use probe microphone measures, how would you know if you had even made soft sounds audible—one of the most basic components of the hearing aid fitting? If you actually sold a pair of hearing aids and *didn't* make soft sounds audible (simply because the necessary software adjustments were not made), would this be a "high standard of professional competence?" Would it be "providing services that are in the best interests of those served?" Not really.

Palmer (2009) concludes her article with the following.

> I hope we can continue to discuss the reasons that hearing aid acceptance is not higher in the hearing-impaired population. The fact that a doctoral profession is arguing about whether or not to individually verify the gain and output of a hearing aid in a patient's ear that takes less than 5 minutes might just be a good place to start. If you are wondering if providing this level of verification will establish you as an expert and set you apart from other providers, keep

in mind that it does not require any particular expertise to attach cords to a HI-PRO Box, double click on NOAH, enter a patient name, click hearing thresholds on a graph, double click on a manufacturer icon, and click "first fit." This level of "expertise" does not require a doctoral degree. As a profession, it is time to be an expert. An expert knows exactly what levels of sound are being produced in an individual's ear canal and how those levels correspond to the listener's residual dynamic range of hearing. (*Audiology Today*, p. 34)

Reasons for Not Conducting Probe Microphone Measures

More important than the recommendations of best fitting practices and experts, is that the research evidence that we detail in the following discussion clearly demonstrates the importance of completing probe microphone measurements. Despite being the intuitive thing to do, the right thing to do, and therefore, we think the ethical thing to do, as surveys reveal, probe microphone testing is *not* conducted by most audiologists when they fit hearing aids. Over the years, there have been many reasons postulated regarding why this is true, as well as articles written on the topic (Mueller, 2005b). We review several of those reasons here.

Equipment Isn't Available

Why would one choose to set up a practice without the necessary equipment? Certainly, the overall cost of essential equipment must be considered, but used systems, in good working condition are available for a few thousand dollars, and the more basic new systems sell for only a little more. Lease-to-buy deals are available for around $100.00 per month. Given that many clinics and offices will have gross annual hearing aid sales of $300,000 to $500,000, a $5000 equipment purchase that leads to improved patient satisfaction and benefit does not seem very unreasonable. Would an audiologist decide to whistle pure tones, and open a clinical practice without an audiometer?

Not Enough Time

If you unbundle your products and services, what percentage of the total cost of a pair of hearing aids is for the hearing aids themselves, and what portion is for our services? Even when the price of hearing aids is bundled (e.g., average cost of $6000. for a pair of premier hearing aids), we know that a good share of the money paid by the patient is for our professional services. Isn't the patient paying for our time? How much time does $6000.00 buy? 5 hours? 10 hours? 20 hours?

These professional services include optimizing gain to provide as much hearing aid benefit as possible, while ensuring satisfaction and comfort. This is the very goal of many of the validated prescriptive gain and output procedures we are verifying through probe microphone testing. As professionals, we take as much time as necessary to get the job done right.

Not Valid with Today's Technology

Those of us fitting hearing aids for several years have heard a lot of "what you can't do." It started with you can't do probe microphone testing with wide dynamic range compression (WDRC) hearing aids. Then we heard, you can't do probe micro-

SOAPBOX: Let's Just Do It Right!

Several years back, we transitioned to a doctoral profession because we realized that being an audiologist involved a lot more than what could be learned in Master's program. Along with being a "Doctor" comes responsibility—it's "okay" to be the one who does things right. You're the only student who refuses to go to a placement because they don't use probe microphone verification for fitting hearing aids? Good for you. You're a practicing audiologist and you're the only one in the clinic doing probe microphone? Good for you. The place where you work doesn't have probe microphone equipment? Buy it yourself. Your employer tells you that there isn't time to do probe microphone testing for your hearing aid fittings? Find a new job!

There is considerable evidence to show that the use of hearing aids will improve individual's lives. There is also evidence to show that well-fitted hearing aids will have an even greater impact.

phone testing with programmable hearing aids, which then led to you can't do probe microphone testing with digital processing hearing aids (Mueller, 2001a). Even today we often hear a clinician say, "I was told by my rep that probe microphone testing really doesn't tell you much with their product." All this simply is not true. In fact, in many cases, the more sophisticated the processing, the more things that you can verify, and the more important it is to verify. With today's real-speech inputs, the probe microphone findings provide a very reasonable estimate of real-world audibility for speech. Sure, there are a few caveats to this, but they are easy to overcome. We will discuss those in Chapter 5. The bottom line is, if one of our primary goals is achieving the right amount of audibility for speech, it seems to make good sense to measure it in the real ear.

Poor Training?

Could it be that AuD students simply are not trained properly regarding the importance and use of probe microphone measures? This has been suggested by some. We find it unlikely that an accredited AuD program would *not* teach the verification procedures recommended in best practices guidelines. However, there is sometimes a disconnect between academic training and clinical practice and mentoring. Here is a comment on the topic from professor Mike Valente, certainly one of the strongest advocates of probe microphone testing that you will find in an AuD training program.

> According to the clinic coordinator at one graduate program, in 16 of 20 external clinical sites where she sends her students for clinical experience, probe microphone equipment is never used or used only in "special cases." Therefore, some students wonder if probe microphone verification really is necessary if seasoned audiologists with successful practices do not use it. Also, I believe a majority of students graduate understanding the need for probe microphone measures to implement a "best practice," but the facility in which they are then employed either does not

> have the equipment and/or has staff who do not promote its routine use. It is very difficult, if not impossible, for new graduates to arrive at their first job and change the method of practice. (Comments of Valente, taken from Mueller, 2005b.)

We agree with Mike's comments, as we have heard the same thing from others. You would think that doctoral students in audiology would only be allowed to do practicum at sites that follow Best Practices, but for some reason that doesn't always seem to be possible. The critical need to change the culture in the workplace is probably related to the reason we discuss next.

The Fitting Software Gets It Right

The biggest factor in the failure to use probe microphone verification is probably the general belief of many audiologists that the fitting software will somehow get things right. That is, if you click the default button in the fitting software, the cartoon on the fitting screen shows a match to target, the patient will most likely have the best fitting. If you click the NAL-NL2 button, the patient will most likely be fitted to NAL-NL2. Or, if you look at the simulated gain or output displayed by the fitting software, you actually see a true representation of the actual gain or SPL levels in the real ear. Unfortunately, research has shown that none of these assumptions are true, as we detail in the following sections.

Of course we would not expect the software fitting to be perfectly accurate for individual patients, as average correction values are used, and there are differences in individual ears. What we are talking about here, however, is something different: Variances that are much larger than the usual 3- to 4-dB differences in RECDs or CORFIGs. In general, the issues surround both the manufacturer's proprietary fitting (what actually happens in the ear when you activate the default fitting for a specific hearing loss) and the manufacturer's software implementation of a validated prescriptive method, such as the NAL-NL2. We will address each of these issues separately.

Proprietary Fittings Are Best?

As discussed in Chapter 2, all major manufacturers have a proprietary fitting. How this fitting was developed probably varies from manufacturer to manufacturer. To some extent, this fitting relates to specific processing of a given manufacture's product, but for the most part it is based on two types of data from research studies and/or patient or clinician complaints compiled by the manufacturer: (1) preferred sound quality including naturalness, and (2) initial acceptance data (e.g., reports from dispensers and/or return for credit rates). Sometimes, these proprietary fittings have been simply employed to compensate for past problems, or perceived problems. For example:

- Patients say our first fit sounds tinny, let's roll off the highs;
- Patients (or audiologists buying our instruments) say our first fit results in feedback, let's roll off the highs;
- Patients (or audiologists buying our instruments) say the first fit of Brand X sounds better than ours, let's make ours just like Brand X.

How this relates back to the non-use of probe microphone assessment is that it is very difficult to verify a proprietary fit in the real ear, starting with the term *proprietary.* If you want to verify to the NAL-NL2 or DSL v5, you simply select this in the software of your probe microphone system, and the prescriptive targets will appear on the screen. But if you want to verify to Starkey Fit, or Signia Fit, or Phonak Fit . . . there are no real-ear targets in your probe microphone system. Now, it could be that there are some simulated curves in the fitting software, and you could maybe print these out, and then maybe eyeball them while conducting probe microphone testing, but this is more trouble than most audiologists want to go through. And, even if you went through the trouble of trying this, your results would only be valid if the LTASS used to construct the proprietary gain and output curves was the same as the as the LTASS of the input signal with your probe microphone equipment when the real-ear measure is performed. This is probably unlikely, and ensuring that the same LTASS is used is sometimes difficult to even determine.

So, maybe the first question should be, "Are proprietary fittings a reasonable starting point for the fitting?" If so, then maybe you really don't need to do probe microphone testing. Experts have commented on the use of proprietary fittings for some time. Denis Byrne, for example, expressed his concerns in 1996:

> Scientifically, the concern is that amplification may become prescribed by a wide variety of proprietary formulae of which few, if any, are validated by published research. A possible philosophical problem is that control of the fitting process is taken away from the fitter, who is responsible for the care of the client. (p. 378)

The concerns of Byrne (1996) appear to be well founded. Here is a brief summary of research that has looked at how these strategies compare to validated approaches, adapted from Mueller (2006):

- Keidser, Brew, and Peck (2003), in a study examining the recommended algorithms of five different major manufacturers, showed that it is common for prescribed gain to differ by 10 dB or more from the NAL-NL1 targets in the high frequencies for average-level input signals.
- Bentler (2004) examined the default algorithm of the premier product from six leading hearing aid manufacturers using a real-speech input (long-term 65 dB SPL input). In general, all algorithms prescribed gain below the NAL-NL1 target levels. Of particular concern was that for key frequencies, such as 2000 Hz, the difference in prescribed gain was as much as 15 to 20 dB, with some algorithms only prescribing 5 dB of gain for the sample patient with a 50 dB hearing loss at that frequency.
- Bentler, Wu, and Jeon (2006) calculated the real-ear insertion gain (REIG) for four different open canal (OC) products based on the manufacturers' recommended fitting. The hearing aids were programmed for an individual with a high-frequency hearing loss (50 dB at 2000 Hz, 60 dB at 3000–6000 Hz). They observed about a 5 dB difference among manufacturers, but in general, the average "recommended" gain fell 10 to 15 dB below NAL-NL1 targets in the 2000 to 4000 range. Two of the four products provided no more than 7 dB of gain at 4000 Hz for this sample patient with a 60 dB hearing loss at that frequency.

These studies suggest that the default proprietary fittings fall seriously short on providing appropriate audibility. Even if you are not a believer in validated fitting methods such as the NAL prescription, Hearing Aids 101 and a little horse sense tells us that a patient needs more than 5 dB of gain when they have a 50 dB hearing loss. It's true, however, that the studies we cited are somewhat dated, but we have evidence that things haven't gotten any better.

In a unique and eye-opening study, Leavitt and Flexer (2012) reported how modern-day default fittings actually impact speech recognition in background noise. They compared the premier 2012 product of the six major manufacturers to a single-channel analog product from 2002. Subjects were fitted bilaterally and tested using the QuickSIN, presented at 57 dB SPL—slightly below average speech. The old analog hearing aids were programmed (and verified) to NAL-NL1 for each subject. Two different settings were used for the six pair of premier hearing aids: the hearing aids were tested while programmed to the manufacturer's default setting, and also when programmed to NAL-NL1. The old hearing aids did not have directional technology or digital noise reduction. The new hearing aids did, and these features were activated at the levels suggested in the default software. The mean results of QuickSIN speech recognition testing are shown in Figure 1–2.

As we describe later in Chapter 6, the QuickSIN is scored as signal-to-noise (SNR) loss, and therefore, the lower the bar extends downward in Figure 1–2, the worse the performance; the greater the deviation from individuals with normal hearing. Note that the average SNR-Loss for the old hearing aid was about 8.5 dB. What stands out, however, is the poor performance for all the modern-day hearing aids, when fitted to the manufacturer's proprietary fitting. Note that for HA-3, HA-4, and HA-5, the SNR-Loss is

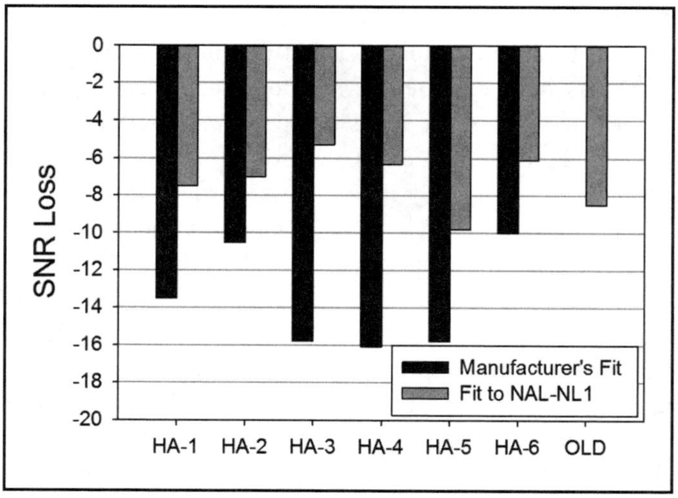

Figure 1–2. SNR-loss is shown across five premier hearing aids and one older style analog hearing aid as a function of the manufacturer's default setting and the NAL-NL-1 fitting. Values closer to 0dB indicate better performance. Adapted from Leavitt and Flexer, 2012.

greater than 15 dB, about a 7-dB drop from the mean performance obtained with the old analog hearing aids.

Let's put the Leavitt and Flexer (2012) findings into practical terms—we'll say that an audiologist has fit someone with a pair of new high-end hearing aids, programmed to the manufacturer's default settings. The patient was a previous user of old analog hearing aids programmed to the NAL-NL1, similar to what was used in the study. The audiologist's counseling would have to go something like this. "Bob, thanks again for the $5000, but I do have to tell you that when you go back to your favorite restaurant this weekend, you'll somehow have to convince management to reduce the background noise level by 7 dB if you want to understand as well as you were with your old hearing aids." Why would an audiologist ever do that to a patient?

Notice, referring back to Figure 1–2, that by simply programming the hearing aids to the NAL-NL1 prescriptive targets, average SNR-Loss improved significantly for all models; 9 to 10 dB for HA-3 and HA-4. When programmed to NAL-NL1, all products except HA-5 had performance better than the old hearing aids. Patients often walk in the door looking for the best and latest technology. These findings clearly show that's it is not just the technology. Simple technology programmed well will outperform fancy technology programmed poorly almost every day. And, when you don't do things the right way (e.g., allowing the patient to walk out the door with the hearing aids programmed incorrectly), the outcome may have long-term consequences for the patient—inability to understand in background noise often leads to reduced activity and social isolation, which can impact cognition, which can lead to other long-term effects.

In a recent study examining today's proprietary fittings, Sanders, Stoody, Weber, and Mueller (2015) conducted probe microphone measures for the premier hearing aids of the five leading manufacturers, using products and software current in 2015. The hearing aids were all programmed to the respective proprietary fitting, for a common gradually downward sloping hearing loss (e.g., 25 dB in the lows, dropping to 75 dB in the high frequencies), and real-ear output was obtained (16 ears) for inputs of 55, 65, and 75 SPL. The testing was conducted with the Audioscan® Verifit®, which calculates the SII, and these values also were used for comparison.

In Figure 1–3 we see the output for the five different products for the manufacturers' default fitting for the input levels of 55, 65, and 75 dB SPL (male shaped-speech signal). While these algorithms are not intended to match NAL-NL2 targets, we include these values as a reference.

In general, these proprietary fittings are relatively close to the NAL-NL2 for the 65 dB SPL input, at least for the mid-frequencies, but considerably below the NAL-NL2 for the 55 dB SPL input (especially for the high frequencies), and result in output considerably above the NAL-NL2 targets for the 75 dB inputs, particularly for the mid frequencies. There also appears to be considerable variation among manufacturers, and this varies by frequency. Note, for example, for the 55 dB SPL input that HA-4 falls about 10 dB below HA-3 in the mid frequencies with smaller differences for the high frequencies, while HA-3 falls nearly 10 dB below HA-5 at 3000 Hz. Another interesting finding is that if we view the changes in output going from the 55 dB SPL input signal to the 75 dB SPL input signal (a 20 dB change), we notice that the output also changes by nearly 20 dB for most instruments.

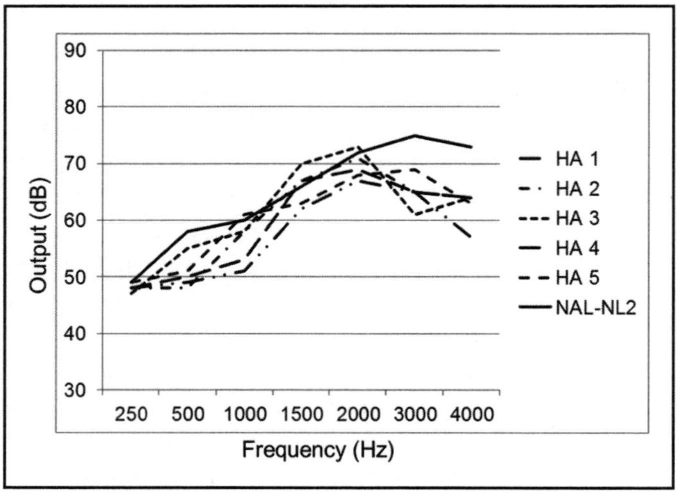

A

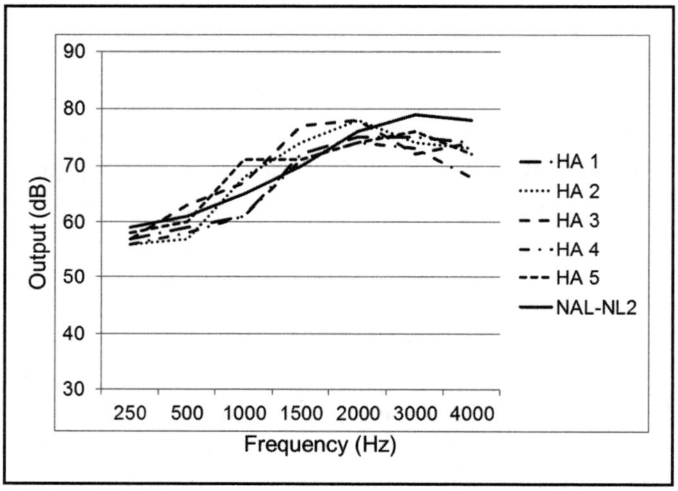

B

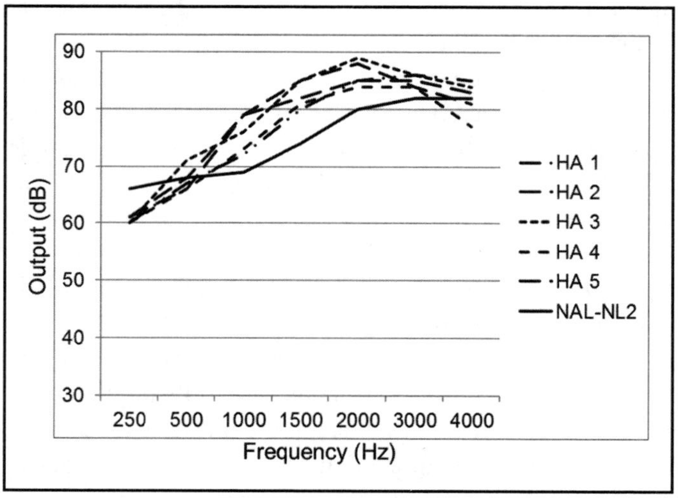

C

Figure 1–3. Shown here are the REARs (mean findings for 16 ears) for five premier hearing aids programmed to the manufacturer's default prescriptive method. The NAL-NL2 fittings targets also are included as a reference. Results are shown for a 55 dB SPL input (**A**), 65 dB SPL input (**B**), and a 75 dB SPL input (**C**). Adapted from Sanders et al., 2015.

The SII findings from Sanders et al. (2015) are shown in Figure 1–4. The SII values reflect a familiar theme—reduced audibility. It appears, however, that the differences among manufacturers, and the variance from the NAL-NL2, become smaller as the input signal increases (most probably because the proprietary methods are more linear than what would be prescribed by NL2). For example, for the 55 dB SPL input, SIIs among manufacturers vary from a low of 0.25 to 0.40, compared to a 0.47 values for a NL2 fitting. For average inputs, the different products vary from 0.46 to 0.57, compared to 0.65 for the NALNL2. For the 75 dB SPL input, the products were similar, and were only 0.1 to 0.5 below the NAL-NL2 SII. The authors did not measure speech recognition directly, and it is somewhat difficult to predict speech recognition from SII values; however, if we look at the 55 dB SPL input, we would expect that the lower SIIs from some instruments would results in 20% to 50% poorer speech recognition than if the patient had been fitted to the NAL-NL2 (e.g., based on the SII conversion chart of Killion and Mueller, 2010, shown in Figure 1–5).

Validated Fittings Are Best?

Of course, the most critical factor when comparing default fittings to validated methods is the patient outcome. The laboratory data of Leavitt and Flexer (2012) are quite compelling—improvements of the average SNR of 6 to 10 dB for most manufacturers. One would think that this would have a significant effect on benefit. But, if you happen to be a skeptical reader, at this point you still might be asking, "Is there any real evidence that sending the patient out the door with a verified prescriptive method instead of using manufacturer defaults leads to better outcomes?" Good question. We will look at this using research from two different areas. The first area relates to studies using trainable hearing aids. We would assume that if a patient were allowed to train their gain and output, and train their degree of compression, if the default fitting was really the best,

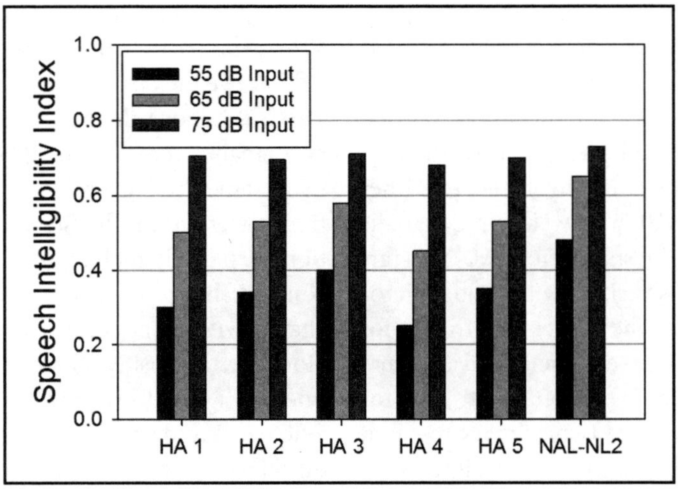

Figure 1–4. Derived Speech Intelligibility Index (SII) values (ANSI, 1997a) across five premiere hearing aids and compared to the NAL-NL2 prescriptive gain as a function of the input level. Adapted from Sanders et al., 2015.

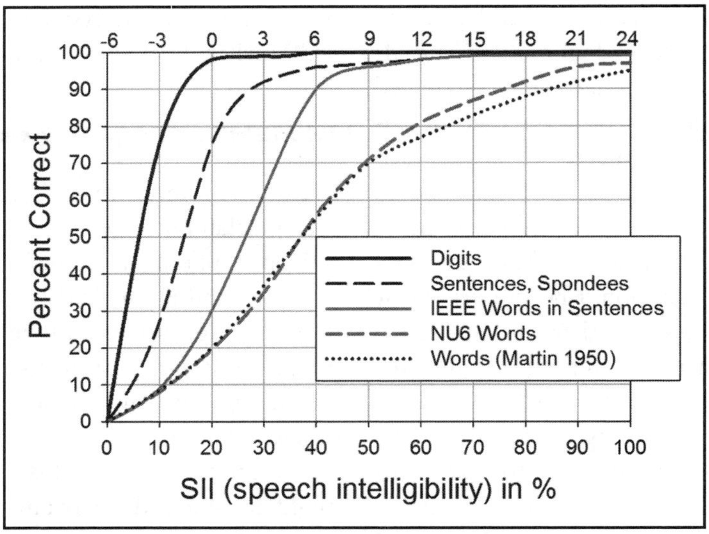

Figure 1–5. Predicted speech recognition performance as a function of SII for different types of speech materials. As contextual content increases, a lower SII will result in higher speech recognition performance. Adapted from Killion and Mueller, 2010.

they would train to something similar. The second area we'll examine is clinical studies in which the validated method has been compared to the default fitting.

Using Trainable Hearing Aids to Validate the NAL. Mueller, Hornsby, and Weber (2008) used a crossover design to study the first generation trainable product, which had an algorithm contained that allowed training for overall gain. Each of their 22 participants was initially fitted to either 6 dB above or 6 dB below NAL-NL1 targets (LTASS originally shaped to NAL-NL1 targets), which was verified with probe microphone measures. The participants trained for this fitting for two weeks, returned and were fitted to the other condition, and trained for two more weeks. The two primary research questions were as follows: (1) Will the subjects tend to train toward the NAL-NL1 prescription targets? (2) Will the starting point influence the end point for gain training? The investigators found large variability among participants—for example, one trained to 14 dB above the NAL target and another trained to 14 dB below the NAL target. Interestingly, however, when the two sets of data were combined (6 dB above and 6 dB below), *the mean and the median trained gain for the group were within a dB or so of the current NAL-NL2 prescription.* When the participants were initially fitted 6 dB above the NAL, they tended to train to 2 to 3 dB above the NAL. When the same participants were fitted 6 dB below the NAL, they trained to 5 dB below the NAL. These trends were not influenced by what condition the participant had first. There was also considerable variability in the magnitude of change within patients across the two trials. However, the positive slope of the regression line in Figure 1–6 indicates that patients who decreased gain less for the +6-dB condition were more likely to increase gain for the −6-dB condition.

- Take-Home Points: For the participants in this study, there appeared to be a wide range of acceptable gain, and

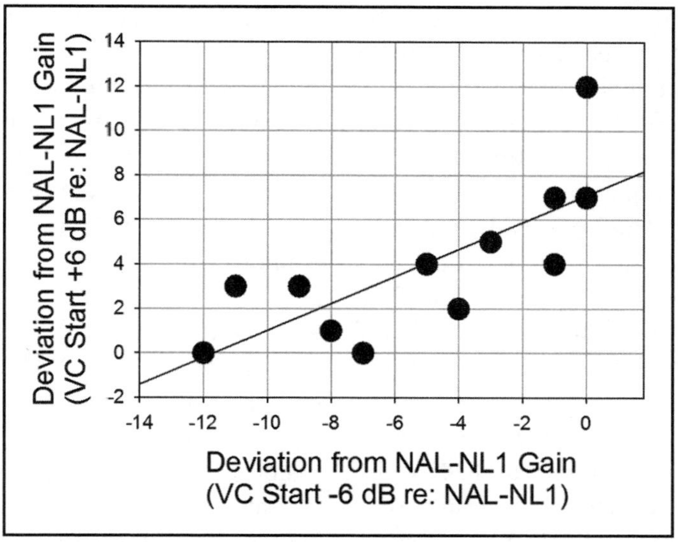

Figure 1–6. Deviation of trained gain from the starting VCW position for the +6-dB and –6-dB conditions. It is clear from the graph that when the participants were initially fitted 6 dB above the NAL (*abscissa*), they tended to train to 2 to 3 dB above the NAL. When the same participants were fitted 6 dB below the NAL (*ordinate*), they trained to 5 dB below the NAL. Adapted from Mueller et al., 2008.

the starting point for training can have a significant impact on the final trained gain. Remember that speech recognition benefit is highly dependent on audibility, and patients in this study trained down in gain much more than they trained up. Therefore, we view these results as indicating a strong need for initially fitting patients using validated prescriptive targets, even when they subsequently use a trainable hearing aid. Moreover, related to our discussion in this chapter, it is important to again say that the mean and the median trained gain for the group were within a dB or so of the current NAL-NL2 prescription.

Palmer (2012) studied trainable hearing aids with new hearing aid users, all initially fitted to the NAL-NL1. She questioned whether the starting time for training had an impact on the outcome. For the control group (n = 18), training was turned off at the initial fitting and then activated a month later at the second visit. The experimental group (n = 18) had training activated from the very beginning. Accordingly, the first group had only one month of total training, whereas the second group had two months of training. Prior to training, the aided Hearing in Noise Test (HINT) was administered to both groups, and there was no difference between groups on the pre-training HINT speech recognition. The findings following training revealed that gain for soft sounds was reduced slightly for both groups. The speech intelligibility index (SII) for soft-level sounds for the control group was reduced by about 2%, as calculated by the Audioscan Verifit. The SII for soft-level sounds for the experimental group that trained for two months was reduced about 4%. Unfortunately, we do not know if this was simply because the experimental group had an extra 30 days to train, or if the initial use of the NAL-NL1 fitting influenced the subsequent training for the control group. Post-training HINT performance was the same for both groups, and it was not significantly different from pre-training scores for either group. Following a real-world comparative trial of the trained setting versus the NAL-NL1, 65% of the participants favored the trained setting.

- Take-Home Points: When new users are initially programmed to the NAL prescription, on average, they do not train far from this gain setting. Using the gain prescribed by NAL-NL1 for a month may influence training. Group findings show that allowing patients to alter their gain and frequency response through training does not reduce speech recognition in background noise. Interestingly, about one-third of participants did not show a significant preference for their new "trained" gain setting. Of course, if their trained gain was similar to the NAL-NL1 (and it was for many), then when forced to choose one or the other, we'd expect a 50/50 split.

Keidser and Alamudi (2013) reported on 26 hearing impaired individuals (experienced hearing aid users) who were fitted with trainable hearing aids, initially programmed to NAL-NL2. Following three weeks of training, they examined the newly trained settings for both low and high frequencies, for six different listening situations (the training was situation-specific). The participants did tend to train down from the NAL-NL2, but only by a minimal amount. For example, for the speech in quiet condition at the high frequencies, the average value was a gain reduction of 1.5 dB (0.95 range = 0 to −4 dB), and for the speech in noise condition, there was an average gain reduction of only 2 dB (0.95 range = 0.5 to −4.5 dB). The trained gain for the low-frequency sounds for these listening conditions was even closer to the original NAL-NL2 settings (Figure 1–7, Panels A and B).

- Take-Home Points: When initially programmed to the NAL-NL2, individuals tend to train to values similar to the NAL-NL2. Training does not vary significantly for different listening situations, such as speech in quiet versus speech in background noise. Importantly, the authors repeated training and found about 60% of patients reliably trained to similar settings, although all trained settings were reasonably close to the NAL-NL2 prescribed values.

Mueller and Hornsby (2014) questioned whether experienced hearing aid users would train to the gain that they had previously used when fitted to the NAL-NL1, using new trainable instruments. They studied 20 experienced hearing aid users: six females and 14 males between the ages of 52 and 80 years (mean age 68.3 years). On average, these participants had been using hearing aids that were programmed about 10 dB below NAL-NL1 targets for soft sounds and 5 dB below for average speech inputs. The hearing aids used in this research had compression training, so it was possible to train the gain for soft sounds without impacting gain for loud inputs. As shown in Figure 1–8, these authors found that, after two weeks of training, the participants did not train to their previous use gain, but rather trained to gain similar to the NAL-NL1. For soft-level inputs, only four of the participants trained more than 5 dB away

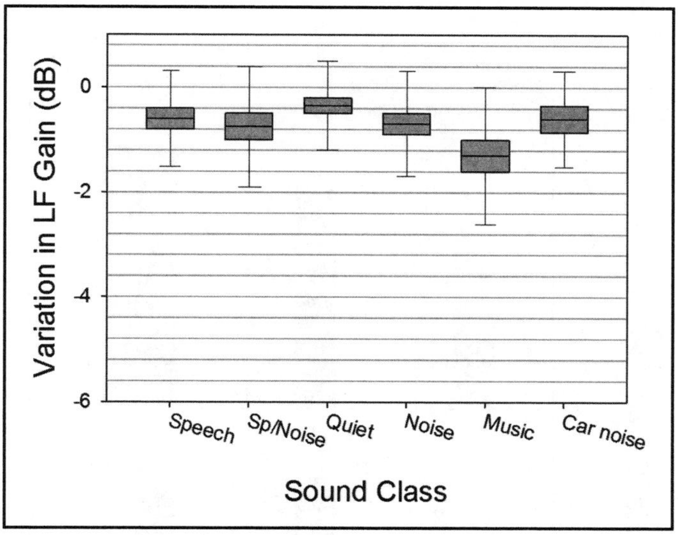

A

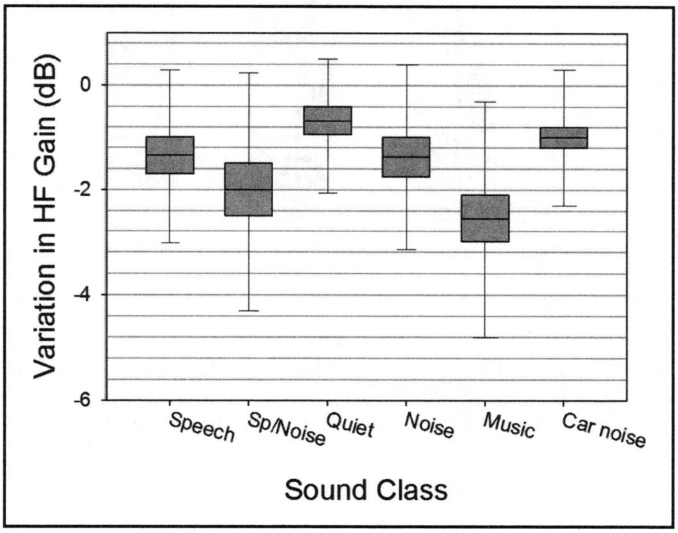

B

Figure 1–7. Average trained deviation from baseline for experienced, bilateral hearing aid users following a training period. Negative values indicate that the participants preferred less of the low-frequency (LF) or high-frequency (HF) gain than was prescribed. The boxes show +/−1 SE, and the bars show +/−.95 times the standard deviation. Adapted from Keidser and Alamudi, 2013.

from the programmed NAL-NL1, and the overall findings showed that 55% were using 10 dB or more gain for soft inputs following training than they had previously been using.

- Take-Home Points: Individuals who have been using gain substantially below NAL-NL1 targets and are then fitted to NAL-NL1 prescriptive targets,

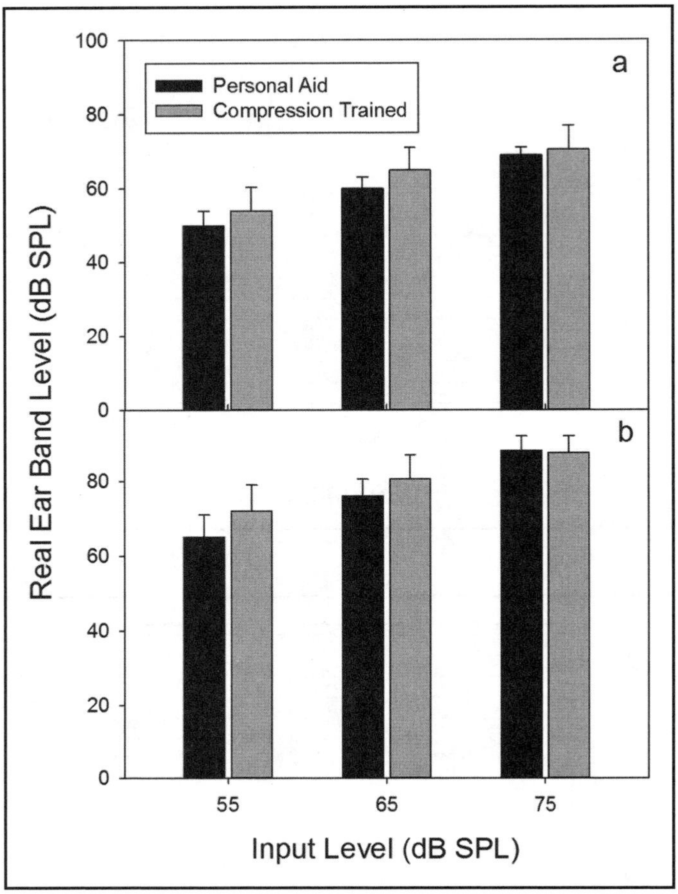

Figure 1–8. Average real-ear band level measured across 20 experienced hearing-aid users after two weeks of training. The top panel (*a*) is the average of the low-frequency band, and the lower panel (*b*) is the average of the high-frequency band. The different shaded bars show the average output for the participants' own hearing aids and the trained gain. Adapted from Mueller and Hornsby, 2014.

do not train to their previous use gain. Rather they train to a fitting very similar to the NAL.

Comparative Clinical Studies to Validate the NAL. Another way to validate the NAL prescriptive algorithm is to compare it to an alternative, such as a manufacturer's proprietary fitting. This was conducted indirectly by Cox, Johnson, and Alexander (2012). We say indirectly, as these authors did not specifically use the proprietary algorithm of a given manufacturer, but rather programmed the hearing aids to mimic the typical proprietary real-ear output as shown in Figure 1–3. Making this research even more intriguing, the authors also studied the NAL-NL2 vs. proprietary fitting with individuals with cochlear dead regions.

The study was a double-blinded, nonrandomized intervention design with 18 matched pairs of adult subjects. In each pair, one subject had high-frequency cochlear dead regions and the other subject did not. Each subject was fitted with two active programs: the NAL and the mimic of a typical proprietary fitting (gain roll-off in the high frequencies). Outcomes included aided speech recognition in quiet and noise measured in the laboratory, real-world ratings of speech understanding in daily life, and final preference for the NAL or LP program.

The results follow:

- In laboratory testing, speech recognition in quiet was significantly better when using the NAL program. This result was observed for subjects with dead regions and without.
- When listening in noise, speech recognition was significantly better when using the NAL program for subjects without dead regions. For subjects with dead regions, results were equivalent for the two programs.
- In daily life, the NAL program received significantly higher ratings for speech understanding, and this result was observed for subjects with and without dead regions.
- Regarding final preference for listening in daily life, roughly two-thirds of the participants preferred the NAL fitting. The reason most frequently given for preferring the default program was that the NAL fitting was too loud.

Overall, adult hearing aid wearers with mild to moderately severe hearing loss benefitted from the additional high-frequency gain provided by the NAL algorithm, whether or not they had dead regions.

- Take-Home Points: In laboratory testing, and real-world field studies, the NAL fitting out-performed the typical default. This was true even for individuals with high frequency dead regions, athough they did not expericne as much benefit. However, provision of NAL high-frequency gain never resulted in poorer performance in either group.

Abrams, Chisolm, McManus, and McArdle (2012), in a crossover design, compared manufacturer's first fit to a verified prescriptive NAL-NL1 fitting across 22 subjects. In this study, the authors began with the verification of a validated prescriptive target (NAL-NL1), and the manufacturers' default. Several manufacturers and models were used, so there was a sampling of different manufacturer default fittings. For both types of fittings, the researchers made minor gain modifications based on patient input. The "verified" fitting was still somewhat below the NAL-NL1 prescribed targets, however, it was significantly closer than what was obtained with the manufacturers' recommended fittings (as you would predict from our earlier discussion). The participants used the hearing aids with the two different fittings in the real world, and following each trial, completed the APHAB (see Chapter 6). After using both prescriptive methods, the participants selected their "preferred fitting."

The APHAB-mean group results showed significant self-perceived hearing aid benefit with the verified NAL-NL1 fitting for the speech in quiet, reverberation, and listening in background noise subscales. Of the 22 participants, 17 selected the verified NAL as their preferred fitting. For some of the participants, the verified NAL and the initial-fit were not significantly different after modification based on patient input. In total, the RMS error was significantly closer to the prescribed NAL-NL1 target for the modified NAL-NL1 fit than for the modified initial-fit approach for 13 participants.

Of those 13 listeners, 11 preferred the verified fit at the conclusion of the study. In other words, starting with the NAL-NL1 fit did not lead to a different fitting for everyone, but in those that it did, there was a clear preference over the manufacturer's first fit as a starting point AND there was a significant real-world outcome advantage for the entire group.

- Take-Home Points: The NAL fitting leads to better real-world outcomes (compared to the manufacturer's proprietary fitting) for speech recognition in quiet, background noise, and reverberation. The majority of participants also preferred this fitting.

A similar study to that of Abrams et al. (2012) was recently conducted by Valente, Oeding, Brockmeyer, Smith, and Kallogieri (2017). These researchers used a randomcontrolled design to compare the manufacturers' default fitting to the NAL-NL2. Comparisons were made using three different metrics: clinic performance for speech recognition, real-world self-assessment scales, and final user preference for one algorithm versus the other. In all three areas, the NAL-NL2 was the superior algorithm. When this fitting was employed, the results showed that there was significantly improved speech understanding for the clinical setting, and the participants rated this fitting significantly higher on the APHAB self-assessment scales compared to the proprietary fitting—by about 10% for both the background noise and reverberation sub-scales. At the completion of the field trial, 19 of the 24 participants preferred the NAL-NL2 fitting.

The APHAB results of Valente et al. (2017) are summarized in Figure 1–9. Of course, even individuals with normal hearing have some problems understanding

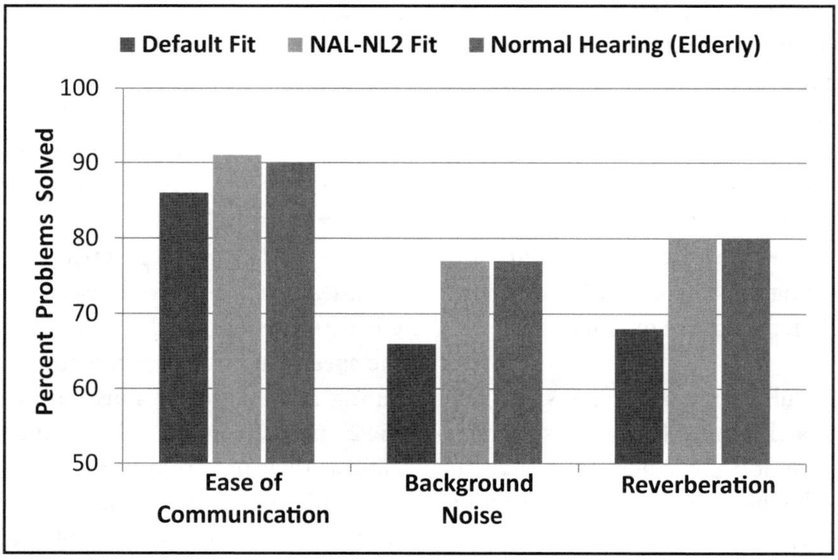

Figure 1–9. Median aided APHAB "problems solved" for an NAL-NL2 fitting compared to a manufacturer's proprietary fitting for Ease of Listening, Background Noise, and Reverberation. Also shown is 50th percentile APHAB problems solved for unaided elderly individuals reporting no hearing problems. Adapted from Valente et al., 2017. Normal hearing data from Cox, 1997.

speech in the real world, which is reflected in their APHAB scores. We have added the APHAB 50th percentile for elderly listeners with normal hearing (reporting no hearing problems) for comparison (Cox, 1997)—the mean age of the subjects in the Valente et al. (2017) research was 72 years, so these are reasonable comparative data. Note, that not only did the NAL-fit subjects have substantially better APHAB ratings than the default fittings; the real-world performance for this algorithm was rated equal to that of individuals with normal hearing (see Figure 1–9).

- Take-Home Points: When directly compared to the manufacturer's fitting, the NAL-NL2 algorithm results in superior performance in speech understanding in clinical testing and also for real-world self-assessment. The algorithm also was preferred by 79% of the participants.

TAKE FIVE: Some Worldly Questions Are Quite Easy to Answer!

What is the meaning of life? Does free will really exist? Is there life after death? Some questions are very difficult to answer! But on the other end of the continuum, we have, "Should I use the manufacturers' fitting algorithm rather than NAL-NL2 or DSL 5?" As we point out in this chapter, there is clear evidence that a better outcome will result when a validated prescriptive method is used. It's not a debatable topic. So why, why do the majority of audiologists persist is using their favorite manufacturer's default fitting? Does free will really exist?

NAL-NL2 on the Screen Is NAL-NL2 in the Ear (NOT)

Hopefully, the previous section convinced you that a validated prescriptive method is the best starting point. And, of course, by "prescriptive method" we are referring to the gain and output that is present in the ear canal. A final area that we believe is one of the leading reasons why audiologists do not conduct probe microphone measures is the misconception that selecting "NAL-NL2" or "DSL v5" in the fitting software will result in the output in the real ear that corresponds to these fitting targets. This is different from what we discussed in the previous section. In this case, the audiologist indeed does want to use a validated prescriptive method rather than the manufacturer's proprietary method, but incorrectly assumes this only requires a couple mouse clicks in the fitting software, and then believes that what is displayed on the software screen is correct.

There are at least two good reasons why real-ear verification is needed, even when a validated prescriptive method is selected in the fitting software. First, as we discuss in Chapter 2, when real-ear gain and output curves are software-simulated based on 2cc-coupler data, there are several factors that must be considered, such as the individual's RECD and REUG, and also microphone location and vent effects. So, even in the best case, we would only expect the fitting to be "correct" if: (1) all the correction factors were applied appropriately, (2) the patient has an average ear, (3) the hearing aid or earmold is at average depth in the ear canal, (4) the microphone is at the average location, and (5) the clinician's description of the tightness of the fit agrees with the manufacturer's definition. While some of these variables amount only to a few dB, when added up, the effect can be considerable and noticeable to the patient. If we look at the patient and fitting factors we just mentioned, given that most patients are not "average" we would expect to see real-ear differences from the prescribed targets, with the variances expected to be both above and below the desired levels.

While all this is important, this does not appear to be the major problem. A second issue that has been commonly observed, at least for the NAL prescription, relates to the manufacturer's calculation of prescriptive targets. Specifically, the average fitting does not actually reflect prescribed targets, but rather falls below them, especially for the higher frequencies. This suggests there are errors, or intentional alterations, other than patient variability when applying a manufacturer's version of a validated prescriptive method. Mueller (2014a) illustrated this with examples of real-ear measures from three different leading manufacturers. The hearing aids were programmed to the manufacturers' NAL-NL2 algorithm, but when compared to the NAL-NL2 targets in the real ear, output in the high frequencies fell below target by 10 dB or more for all three manufacturers—*despite that fact the on-screen display in the fitting software showed a perfect match to target.*

Past research has suggested that the mismatch to target reported by Mueller (2014a) has been common for many years. For example:

- Aazh and Moore (2007) tested four different products from major manufacturers, all programmed to the manufacturers' NAL-NL1. Probe microphone measurements on 42 ears revealed that 64% of cases failed to come within +/−10 dB of the target at one or more of the key frequencies, from 250 to 4000 Hz. After adjusting the frequency-gain response of the hearing aids, 83% of cases came within +/−10 dB of the target, and the fit rate was 100% for the hearing aids with four or more software handles. This shows that it was not that the aids were not capable of matching the prescriptive target, but rather, that the fitting software did not apply the correct gain. And, note that the window of acceptance used by these authors was 10 dB, which is pretty generous and larger than we would normally use clinically.
- In 2012, Aazh, Moore, and Prasher conducted a similar study, although this time they examined fittings for open-canal (OC) fittings. As before, the hearing aids were all programmed to "NAL-NL1" and then tested in the real ear (30 individuals, 51 ears). Fittings were considered "acceptable" if the real-ear gain was within +/− 10 dB of prescribed target; only 29%, however, met this rather lax criterion. After adjustment, 82% were fitted to within 10 dB, and for the remaining 18%, the primary factor was gain for 4000 Hz, where feedback was an issue (recall that these were OC fittings).

To put these latter findings in simple clinical terms: Without conducting probe microphone testing for your OC fittings, you would expect that when you click on "NAL" in the fitting software, only 29% of cases will be fitted close to NAL target. In contrast, by taking a few minutes to conduct probe microphone testing, and making appropriate adjustments, you would expect that 82% of your fittings will be close to NAL target (and this could be even higher if feedback can be resolved). That's more than a 50% improvement in fitting accuracy!

These data suggest that trusting the manufacturer's NAL algorithm to be the true NAL algorithm is risky practice. However, the Aazh and Moore (2007) findings are somewhat dated, the Aazh et al. (2012) research was only with one manufacturer, and the Mueller (2014a) data showed only isolated examples. Fortunately, however, we have relatively current findings that address this issue, and for the most part they reveal that the long-standing software/real-ear mismatch continues to be common. We are referring to the previously mentioned Sanders et al. (2015) research, which used hearing aids and software current for 2015. In this study, the authors selected the premier model hearing aid from the five leading companies, and programmed each instrument to the NAL-NL2 using the respective manufacturer's software. Probe microphone measures were then conducted (16 ears; 8 male and 8 female) and the hearing aid output was compared to the NAL-NL2 targets generated by the Audioscan Verifit (factors such as experience, bilateral fitting, and so forth were matched between the software and the probe microphone equipment). The hearing loss used for the comparison was a typical downward sloping configuration, 30 dB in the lows to 70 dB in the high frequencies. The input signal was the Verifit male speaker (carrot passage); inputs of 55, 65, and 75 dB SPL were used.

Figure 1–10 shows the deviation from NAL-NL2 targets for the average of the 16 ears. Panels A, B, and C are the inputs of 55 dB, 65 dB, and 75 dB SPL, respectively. It appears that only one of the five manufactures has used an algorithm that is reasonably close to the NAL-NL2 for all inputs (HA5). The greatest variation from target is for the 55 dB input signal—observe that at 3000 Hz, the average output for four of the five products are 10 dB or more below prescribed target. But even for the 65 dB input, the measured output falls 7 to 10 dB below target in the high frequencies for the majority of products.

The pattern of deviation from NAL-NL2 seems to be fairly consistent among manufacturers:

- Reduced gain for soft inputs
- Roll-off of high frequencies above 2000 Hz
- Boost in gain for mid-frequencies, to the extent that output exceeds NAL-NL2 targets for the 75 dB inputs
- A generally more linear fitting than prescribed by NAL-NL2

Interestingly, while the real-ear findings of four of the five manufacturers' NAL-NL2 algorithms differ significantly from the desired NAL-NL2 targets, they are quite similar to the respective manufacturer's proprietary fittings. If we examine the individual fittings, we see results similar to what Aazh et al. (2012) reported for a single manufacturer. Individual data for the 80 fittings (16 ears times five products) at the 55 dB SPL input revealed that, in 59 of the 80 cases (74%), the measured output varied from the NAL-NL2 target by 10 dB or more for at least one frequency (250–4000 Hz). If HA-5 (the product that resulted in a reasonably close fitting to NAL-NL2) is removed, of the remaining 64 fittings, 86% varied by 10 dB or more from the desired NAL-NL2 fitting targets. For these later 64 fittings, compliance with the NAL-NL2 was somewhat better for the 65 dB SPL input, but there still were 35 (55%) of the fittings where the ear-canal SPL deviated by 10 dB or more from the desired output.

In general, these data add to the body of literature showing that most manufacturers are using a NAL-NL1 or NAL-NL2 "fitting" that has been modified from the validated version. This is not an issue, of course, if probe microphone verification is conducted, and appropriate gain corrections are made.

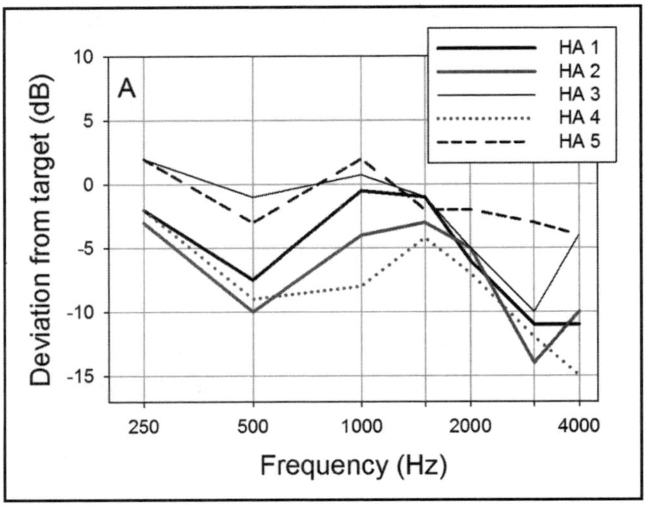

A

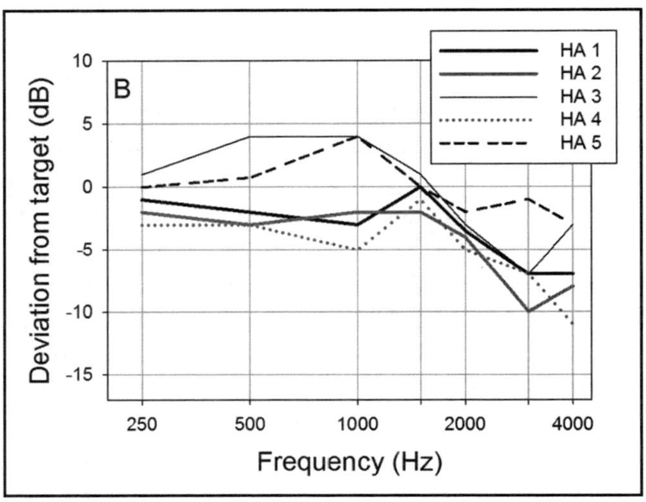

B

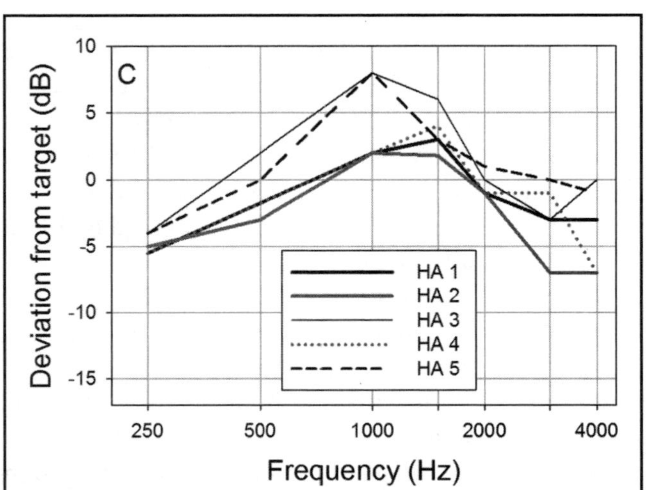

C

Figure 1–10. Actual deviation from prescribed NAL-NL2 gain is shown for the soft (**A**), average (**B**), and loud (**C**) inputs for each of the five premier hearing aids. Adapted from Sanders et al., 2015.

Accuracy of Software Display. A related issue to our discussion is the accuracy of the gain and output values displayed in the fitting software. Going back to our previous discussion, if you knew that the NAL-NL2 prescribed output for your patient for a 65-dB-SPL LTASS signal was 90 dB at 3000 Hz (reference ear canal SPL; you could obtain this target from your NAL-NL2 stand-alone software), and after clicking the "NAL-NL2" button of your favorite manufacturer's software, their fitting screen showed an output of 80 dB SPL at 3000 Hz, you would know that you needed to turn up gain by 10 dB. What if the software showed an output of 90 dB SPL? Then you would assume that all is well, right? But what if it showed 90 dB, but only 80 dB was being delivered in the real ear? Now we have a problem. A big problem. Unfortunately, this problem seems to exist.

Hawkins and Cook (2003), using five different manufacturers, reported that there was a poor match with the measured average REIG, compared to the REIG values shown on the fitting screen. Up to about 2000 Hz, the differences appeared to resemble what you might see for individual ear differences (e.g., +/−3 to 5 dB or so). For the higher frequencies, however, their research showed a distinct pattern of deviation; there was an average real-ear *reduction* of high-frequency gain of 5 to 10 dB, present for all manufacturers. That is, even if an audiologist selected a validated procedure, such as the NAL-NL1, and the computer display showed an excellent match to target, it was possible, if not probable, that the real-ear gain above 2000 Hz would fall well below this prescriptive target. Similar findings to Hawkins and Cook (2003) were obtained by Aarts and Caffee (2005). And, remember the Sanders et al article that we just discussed? Where real-ear measures were common missing target by 10 dB or more? These authors report that the four manufacturers who had large deviations from targets in the real ear (e.g., greater than 10 dB in the high frequencies), *all had fits to targets within 1 dB on the fitting screen.*

We mention that some of the research data we are citing on this topic is somewhat dated, but we can say anecdotally that we commonly hear clinicians say that when they fit the hearing aids to prescriptive target in the real ear, using the target displayed by the probe microphone equipment, the match on the software fitting screen is nowhere close. We do not find this surprising at all. Fortunately, if you verify using probe microphone measures, you do not care what the fitting screen shows, because you have data showing what is really happening in the ear canal. That's more or less the point we've been making the last several pages.

Verification and Patient Satisfaction

We have already reviewed well-controlled studies that have provided research evidence regarding the benefit of probe microphone testing (i.e., target verification), but we also have some long-term satisfaction data related to these measures, and hearing aid verification in general. As the name indicates, MarkeTrak VIII was the eighth in series of consumer satisfaction surveys. What makes MarkeTrak VIII unique, however, is that not only was patient satisfaction assessed, but also considerable information was collected regarding how the hearing aids were fitted. The relationship between the fitting process and subsequent satisfaction has led to several articles discussing these data (e.g., Kochkin, 2010, Kochkin et al., 2010, Kochkin 2011, Kochkin, 2014).

> ### *AUDIOID: Hearing Aids for Norma-Rae-ville?*
>
> In this section we talk about the findings from MarkeTrak VIII, and since that version, we have had MarkeTrak9, and someone is probably planning MarkeTrak10 about now. The whole MarkeTrak thing started way back in 1984. One of the most provocative elements of the 1984 MarkeTrak findings was the use of the so-called PRIZM segmentation of the potential hearing aid market. That is, giving labels to the different purchase groups. The resulting cluster analyzes used some jaunty descriptions to define the different groups: *Shotguns and Pickups*, *Norma Rae-ville*, and *Furs and Station Wagons*. Not sure you could get by with that today!

The Survey Process

The MarkeTrak VIII survey process has been explained in detail by Kochkin (2009), but a brief overview is as follows:

- A short screening survey was sent to 80,000 members of the National Family Organization households (balanced for age, income, location, etc.).
- This survey was completed by 46,843 individuals. Of this group, 14,623 stated that at least one family member had a hearing loss; 3,789 were owners of hearing aids.
- In 2009, a detailed seven-page survey was sent to the 3,789 hearing aid owners. There was a response rate of 84% (3,174).
- Narrowing this database to individuals who had hearing aids that were no older than 4 years resulted in 1,141 experienced users and 884 new users (total $n = 2{,}025$).
- The mean age (~71 years), gender (~55% male) and hearing aid age (~1.8 years) was similar for both groups. (Note: new users identified individuals using their first pair of hearing aids, not newly fitted users.)

As with most of the previous MarkeTrak surveys, satisfaction was assessed for several factors using a 7-point Likert scale. Using these data, overall success was measured using a statistical composite of the following factors:

- Hearing aid use
- Benefit and satisfaction
  - Satisfaction with hearing aids to "improve hearing"
  - Perception of problem resolution for 10 different listening situations (only ones that applied to them)
  - Satisfaction for different listening situations
- Patient purchase recommendations (e.g., recommend hearing aids for friends)

Important for our discussion here, the respondents also reported on tests/services they received during the fitting process with a "yes" or" no" response. If they were "not sure," that also was provided as an optional response. Each of the items listed below was described in a manner that would be meaningful to the lay individual:

- Hearing tested in sound booth
- Loudness discomfort measurement
- Probe microphone measurement used for verification
- Measurement of objective benefit (e.g., pre-post measurement of speech understanding)

- Measurement of subjective benefit
- Outcome measure of patient benefit/satisfaction
- Auditory training software/therapy
- Enrollment in aural rehabilitation group
- Received self-help book/literature/video
- Referred to self-help group (e.g., HLAA)

As is probably obvious from the lists just presented, data analysis of these survey results could easily be used to examine if there was a relationship between the verification and validation testing conducted, and patient success with hearing aids. Also, using other data from the survey, Kochkin was able the examine relationships between the testing conducted and repeat visits and patient loyalty. We will review each of these research questions.

Test Protocol and Patient Satisfaction

The findings of greatest interest to individuals fitting hearing aids from the MarkeTrak VIII survey was the relationship of patient satisfaction to the test protocol used in the fitting process. Does Best Practice pay off? To derive a total measure of success, a factor analysis was conducted on the outcome measures, resulting in a single index that was standardized to a mean of 5 and standard deviation of 2. In comparing above-average and below-average hearing aid user success, individuals were compared in two different categories: those who were at least one standard deviation below the mean ($n = 331$) on success and those who were at least one standard deviation above the mean on success ($n = 407$). This analysis revealed that hearing aid users with above-average success were most likely to have received objective benefit measurements (+26%), subjective benefit measurements (+25%), loudness discomfort testing (+24%), probe microphone verification (+20%), and a patient satisfaction measurement (+17%).

These data are summarized in Figure 1–11. Overall, some of the tests were administered more than others; the average of "above average" and "below average" values is roughly the number of people who

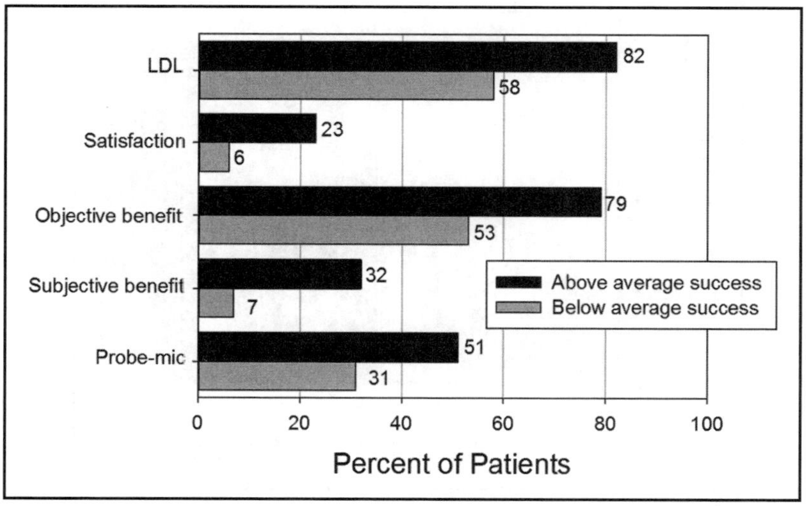

Figure 1–11. Example of the percent of patients with above average and below average success who were administered tests of LDL, satisfaction, objective benefit (e.g., speech recognition tests), subjective benefit (e.g., self-reported success), and probe microphone measures. Adapted from Kochkin, 2014.

received a given test (the n's are slightly different, but close enough). For example, the overall test rate for probe microphone measures was around 40%. (Interestingly, this is similar to what has been found when dispensers report their procedures.) Of course, those of us who favor Best Practice procedures might predict (or hope) that the difference between these groups would be even larger, but that's why we use data, rather than expert opinion, whenever possible. The trend favoring Best Practice, however, certainly is present. We, of course, do not know if the increased satisfaction is a result of the test procedure itself (e.g., the MPO was changed when loudness testing was conducted) or simply that increased testing means that the patient spends more time with the audiologist, which probably gives the audiologist more time for counseling, gives the patient more confidence in the overall fitting process, and a greater respect for the audiologist's professional credentials.

A different way to view these findings is shown in Figure 1–12. These data reflect the answer to the question: Does pre-fitting testing, verification and validation steps performed during the hearing aid fitting process have an additive or multiplicative impact on real-world success? The patients were ranked on the number of items (range 0–12), or protocol steps, received during the hearing aid fitting process. The average total success scores were then derived by the number of protocol steps performed (see Figure 1–12). As is clearly shown, as additional steps were added—such as probe microphone measures—overall satisfaction rose steeply, from below 2.0 (hearing test only) to nearly 6.0. (Note: Steps 8 and above reflect post-fitting rehabilitation and counseling.)

If we consider that following Best Practice (Steps 1 to 7 in Figure 1–12) leads to improved satisfaction and success with hearing aids, then it's also important to consider other data from this research. The findings also revealed that 94% of the group in the top 15% of satisfaction would recommend their dispenser to others, whereas

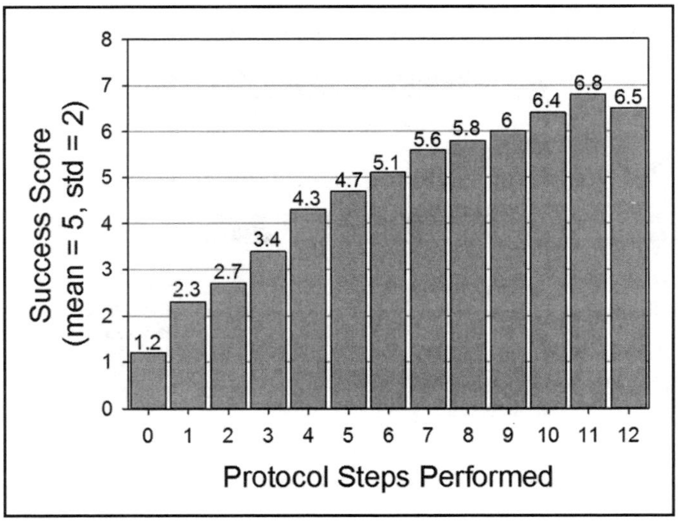

Figure 1–12. Success Score as a function of number of protocol steps performed during the hearing aid fitting. Adapted from Kochkin et al., 2010.

> **POINTS TO PONDER: What Influenced Satisfaction Outcome?**
>
> In the data we show in Figures 1–11 and 1–12, there certainly appears to be a strong relationship between the test protocol and success with hearing aids. What else could have influenced these findings? Kochkin et al. (2010) examined several possible variables. They report that age of the patient, gender, user (new vs. experienced), size of city (rural to metropolitan), price of hearing aid, style of hearing aid, and degree of hearing loss explained less than 1% of variance. In this study, 69% of hearing aids were fit by audiologists and 31% by hearing instrument specialists. Did this impact the results? The professional training/occupation of the hearing aid fitter explained less than one-half of 1% of the protocol used or hearing aid user real-world success. Yes, you just read that correctly: The professional training/occupation of the hearing aid fitter explained less than one-half of 1% of the protocol used or hearing aid user real-world success. Why no difference? We think this is directly related to evidenced-based practice procedures. While audiologists are typically trained to use best practice procedures such as probe microphone measures, we already told you that most of them do not. As you saw in Figure 1–1, data examining use of probe microphone verification suggest very similar percentages for audiologists and hearing instrument specialists. Being trained for best practices does not really help us if we don't apply them in our clinical practice.

only 39% of the group with the bottom 15% of satisfaction would consider doing this (Figure 1–13). More on patient loyalty later.

Return Patient Visits

Unscheduled repeat visits during the fitting process can be considered an indirect measure of patient success. Kochkin (2011), using the MarkeTrak data, examined how the test protocol might influence repeat visits. To do this, he divided the patients into four groups (Figure 1–14), separating those that had both verification (probe microphone measures) and validation from those that had one or the other. Note that 22% had neither.

The trend is what we would expect, with the big jump in visits present for those patients who did not receive any verification or validation measures (average of 2.4 visits vs. 3.6 visits). Kochkin also provides the following data from this analysis:

- For patients with above average success, 76% were fitted in one or two visits compared to 40% of patients who experienced below average success.
- For patients with below average success, 47% required 4 to 6 visits to fit their hearing aids compared to only 7% of patients who experienced above average success.

Kochkin (2011) goes on to report that in 2010, nearly 2.7 million hearing aids were fitted in the United States, representing over 1.5 million patients (e.g., estimating bilateral fitting rate of 75%). Assuming the same distribution of best practices as noted by patients in Figure 1–14, and the

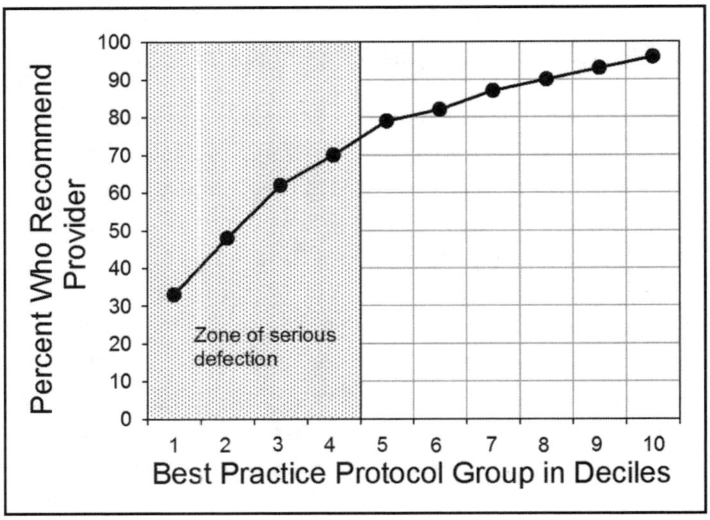

Figure 1–13. The relationship between the protocol used during the hearing aid fitting, and the probability that the patient would later recommend that provider (Adapted from Kochkin, 2011).

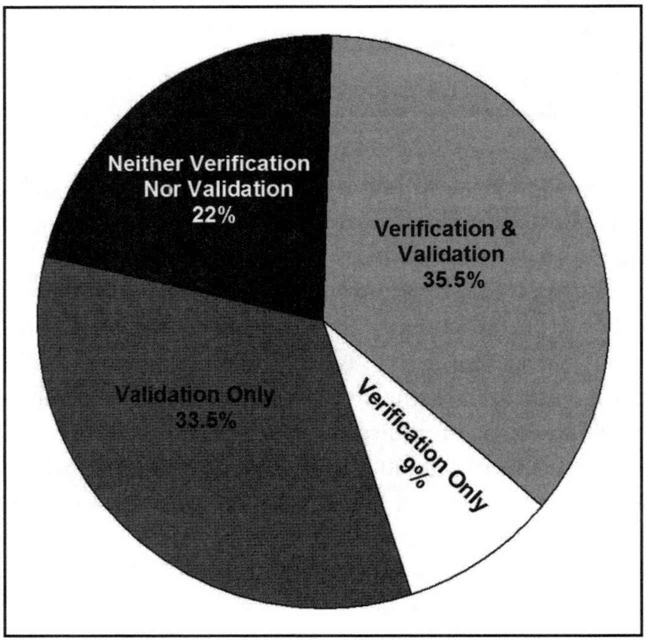

Figure 1–14. From Kochkin, 2011, the percent of survey respondents that had verification only (9%), validation only (33.5%), verification and validation (35.5%), and neither (22%).

estimate of reduced patient visits, Kochkin suggests that the systematic utilization of both probe microphone measures and validation procedures while fitting hearing aids will reduce unnecessary patient visits by a total of 521,779. He goes on to point out that this additional service consumes a lot of the audiologist's time (~400,000 hours/year) that could be better spent counseling others or fitting new patients with hearing aids. Moreover, and perhaps most importantly, he adds that these extra and unnecessary visits can be a huge inconvenience to the older patients, who often need a ride to the clinic, and often have multiple disabilities that can include challenges in mobility, danger from falls, and other potential problems. We agree.

Patient Loyalty

Most of us fitting hearing aids are pretty confident that most patients leave our office with their new hearing aids and with pretty positive thoughts about us and the fitting process. Based on this positive experience we probably also assume that these happy patients will steer their friends and relatives who need hearing aids our way. Further, they will certainly be back to see us when they need replacement hearing aids. But how loyal are our patients? And how does our test protocol impact patient loyalty.

Patient loyalty and its relationship to the overall fitting process was yet another interesting area that could be examined by mining the MarkeTrak VIII data. Going back to 1986, in the classic book by W. Edwards Deming, *Out of the Crisis*, we've often heard that a happy customer (patient) who comes back is worth 10 new prospects. As the story goes, happy customers spread their good news to eight other potential customers, but unhappy customers spread their bad news to 16 potential customers. This was before the days of Facebook and Twitter so you can imagine the current multiple of these numbers! We also know that the cost of acquiring a new customer is five times higher than keeping a customer satisfied. There has not been a lot of research in this area related to hearing aid sales, but to a large extent, a customer is a customer, whether its repeat business for an airline, a coffee shop, or an audiologist's office.

In the MarkeTrak survey that we explained earlier, hearing aid users were asked to rate their dispenser (either audiologist or hearing instrument specialist) on seven factors using a 7-point Likert scale: "Very dissatisfied," "Dissatisfied," "Somewhat dissatisfied," "Neutral" (equally satisfied and dissatisfied), "Somewhat satisfied," "Satisfied," and "Very satisfied." They also then completed Likert scale ratings for the dispenser/audiologist on the following factors: (a) professionalism, (b) knowledge level, (c) explained care of the hearing aid, (d) explained hearing aid expectations, (e) quality of service during the hearing aid fitting, (f) quality of service post-fitting, and (g) level of empathy. For data analysis, an average of these last seven attributes was obtained to reflect a single dimension.

It is, of course, important to see how patient loyalty relates to the verification and validation procedures. Recall from our earlier discussion, an overall index of best practices was standardized to a Z-score with a mean of 5 and standard deviation of 2. For this analysis, scores were converted to percentile rankings and then grouped into 10 levels of best practices (BP) in deciles, where BP1 = minimal hearing aid fitting protocol = 10%, BP5 = average (50%) protocol, and BP10 = comprehensive (100%) protocol. Kochkin reported that those with the highest level of best practices (BP10) have a 96% loyalty rating. Loyalty ratings rapidly decline to 34% for those using minimalist fitting protocols. In general, as shown in Figure 1–15, there was an average loyalty rating of 57% for audiologists who do not conduct verification or validation, and an average loyalty rating of 84% for those audiologists who do.

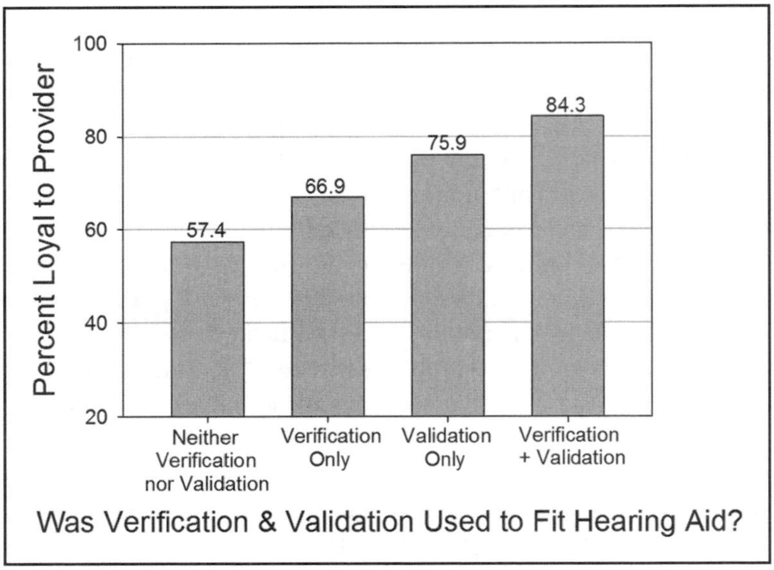

Figure 1–15. Relationship between patient loyalty and groupings as per best practice. Adapted from Kochkin, 2011.

TAKE FIVE: Practical Thinking Regarding Loyalty Ratings and Hearing Aid Sales

Figure 1–15 shows that doing things the right way can move our loyalty ratings from 57 to 84%. Let's take these average patient loyalty findings and compare two different practices, Practice A and Practice B. Practice A conducts probe microphone measures and self-assessment validation, Practice B does not. To provide more background data, both practices have been in business for 10 years, and every year they each sell hearing aids to about 100 patients.

Approximately 80% of their fittings are bilateral, which then results in 180 hearing aids/year. After 10 years of practice, many of their patients should be returning to replace their hearing aids. But, about 20% have either died or moved away, or are not in a position to obtain new hearing aids, so we'll consider the potential annual return rate for both practices is 80% or 80 patients.

We would predict the Practice B return rate to be 57%. To do the math: 57% of 80 (potential) × 1.8 (bilateral fittings) = 81 hearing aids sold to return patients. Now how about Practice A, where they work a little harder? Their patient return rate should be 84%. Again, to do the math: 84% of 80 (potential) × 1.8 (bilateral fittings) = 120 hearing aids—a 39 hearing aid difference, which we would predict to be present every year. So not only is best practice ethical practice, it is also good (and profitable) practice.

Professionalism and Perceptions

In the preceding section, we discussed how following best practice can have a long-term impact regarding patient loyalty. Certainly, a big part of this is that when conducting testing such as probe microphone measures, the patient views you as more professional. How many times have you heard a long-time hearing aid user say, "Wow, I've never had that test before," only for you to tell them that probe microphone measures have been around since the mid-1980s!

In the MarkeTrak VIII findings, probe microphone measures were just one aspect of the verification process, and in some cases, were mixed with validation measures. We do have recent data, however, which provides insight regarding the effect that specifically conducting probe microphone measures has on patient perceptions. Amlani, Pumford, and Gessling (2016) studied three groups of 20 adult listeners (n = 60) with mild to moderately severe sensorineural hearing loss. These included experienced users, owners of hearing aids who did not use them frequently, and non-adopters of amplification who experienced hearing difficulties and were interested in a trial period. One-half of each group were fit by simply selecting the manufacturer's default NAL-NL2 setting (no probe microphone verification), the other half received probe microphone verification with appropriate adjustments to meet target for three input levels. Both subgroups were allowed to rate the fitting for speech inputs, and during and after the fitting process, each subject was counseled on the procedures being performed by the same experienced clinician. At the conclusion of the protocol, each listener's perception toward the service received was quantified using two measures: (1) willingness-to-pay (WTP), price anchored at $250, for professional services, and (2) a modified version of the Perceived Value Measurement (PVM) designed to assess a respondent's attitude toward professional services assessed in five dimensions: perceived quality, perceived value, behavioral intent, emotion, and price (rating on a 7-point scale—"1" equals very satisfied).

The authors report that all three groups showed a significant increase in WTP, with overall values going from $170 for the "quick fitting" approach versus $340 when probe microphone measurements were included. A similar significant finding was obtained for the PVM, which revealed that the protocol including probe microphone measures improved patient satisfaction while reducing anxiety (i.e., emotional distress) for all three groups. For example, for the experienced-user group, satisfaction improved from 4.1 to 2.2 when probe microphone testing was included.

In this chapter, we have primarily focused on the importance of probe microphone verification for the purposes of improving audibility, speech understanding, and overall patient benefit. As the above data revealed, it is worth remembering that by conducting these measures, we also are improving the perceived value and patient satisfaction in the overall fitting process. As hearing aid distribution channels continue to multiply and become more diverse, it is critical that the hearing aid fitting services proved by audiologists are indeed different from what can be obtained from the neighborhood pharmacy or big box store.

In Closing

Mueller (2015) reported that recent data indicate that when we look at the number of audiologists who simply use the manufacturer's proprietary fitting, and then add a second group of audiologists who select NAL-NL2 (or NL1) in the fitting software, but do *not* verify, we are left with the disturbing low number of about 15 to 20% of hearing aids that actually are being fitted (verified) based on a validated prescriptive method. Yet, we know that the patient's success with amplification will be greater when fitted to a validated prescriptive method, or at the least, when aided audibility is appropriate. There is no other way to reliably verify that this has occurred except through the use of probe microphone measures. Failure to do so is poor clinical practice, and often results in poorer audibility, benefit, and satisfaction of our patients. We agree it may even be a violation of the ethics of our professional organizations. Hopefully we have convinced you that these measures are critical for fitting hearing aids. Now let's move on to the nuts and bolts of how to select a gold standard, and how this testing is conducted.

2 Developing a Gold Standard

If you don't know where you are going, you might wind up someplace else.
—Lawrence "Yogi" Berra

One of baseball's legends, Lawrence Peter "Yogi" Berra, died in 2015 at the age of 90. Yogi was an all-star catcher with the great New York Yankee teams of the 1950s and early 1960s, and certainly, one of the top catchers of all time. Yogi was a huge fan-favorite, and also a favorite target for New York reporters. He soon became known for his malapropisms and paradoxical quotes. The popularity and use of these quotes has spread outside of baseball, and today they are referred to as Yogi-isms (or Yogisms). They have certainly spread to the profession of audiology, as in 2016, Mueller and colleagues revealed how many of Yogi's quotes could be applied to how we select and fit hearing aids. And the same can be said for the quote above—it is critical that we know where we are going when we select the gain and output for a given patient. And yes, as Yogi said, if you don't, you might end up someplace else. And that might not be a very good place for your patients. Fortunately, we know where we are going, because we have well-researched prescriptive fitting methods to guide us. That's what we'll be discussing in this chapter.

As recent as 30 years ago, we were often faced with fitting a patient with an analog hearing aid that had, at best, one screw-driver potentiometer that allowed us to vary gain in the 500 Hz region by 5 to 10 dB. There was only one channel, no input or output compression, and very little control of the frequency response. Much has changed. It is clear that with today's highly adjustable digital products, with multiple channels of gain and compression, we have the capability to select most any frequency response and output characteristics desired for a given patient. Now that we have the capability to craft almost any frequency response and input/output function characteristics that we desire, how do we know what is best?

Most would agree that a *good* hearing aid fitting must be a combination of optimizing audibility and speech recognition, matching preferred loudness levels for different input levels, avoiding loudness discomfort, and providing good sound quality. For a reluctant new hearing aid user, we might also want to consider using an algorithm that would be rated *acceptable* during initial use. These goals have led to the development of several prescriptive gain/output methods over the years, including the original methods that were developed more than 80 years ago, to the resurgence of newer prescriptive methods aimed at fitting amplitude compression that have been proposed in the past 20 years or so.

Let's consider your Monday morning patient. She has a relatively flat bilateral

60 dB HL sensorineural hearing loss. Not surprisingly, she is having significant problems understanding speech, even in quiet, and is anxious to purchase hearing aids from you. You are ready to program channel-specific gain for her for average-level speech inputs. How much gain is enough? How much is too much. Your knowledge of average-level speech tells you that 10 dB of gain isn't enough, and 50 dB of gain certainly seems like too much, but you still have a 40 dB range to choose from. We need to narrow the range and try to define an optimal starting point given the specific hearing loss, and that is exactly the purpose of prescriptive fitting approaches. In general, prescriptive methods are based on the assumption that using the patient's pure-tone thresholds, and perhaps some suprathreshold measures, hearing aid gain, and/or output can be *prescribed* that will result in the best fitting for the average patient for the desired attributes (e.g., intelligibility, sound quality, listening comfort, etc.). With modern hearing aids, the intent is also to accomplish these goals for a wide range of sound input levels and listening environments. There are a number of variables to consider, and no one procedure is going to get it perfect for all patients all the time. But we need a starting point, and research studies have shown that the chances for success will be maximized when we use validated procedures.

The moment that one attempts something as simple as selecting the maximum gain, or what instrument to fit to a given patient, at least some rudimentary form of a prescriptive method is being used. This is true even if the fitter themselves doesn't actually know it! Denis Byrne (1982) said it best,

> The only choices are whether we admit to using a theoretical procedure, or even realize that we are doing so, and whether we are prepared to say what procedure we are using. . . . The only problem with confessing to using a theoretical procedure is that it inevitably exposes our inadequacies. (p. 176)

Denis Byrne was a noted Australian audiologist who died in April of 2000. He didn't invent hearing aid prescriptions, but through his work we are able to use these methods based on a sound rationale and self-critical research. If we had to name a "father of prescriptive hearing aid fittings," he certainly would be the man. If you are new to fitting hearing aids, Byrne's statement above might not make much sense. Consider that if you didn't know that the aided output at 4000 Hz should be 90 dB SPL (ear canal sound pressure level) for a 55 dB speech signal input, it probably wouldn't bother you at all when the ear canal output for this signal was only 80 dB. Or maybe you wouldn't even measure it!

In 2015, Mueller wrote a paper on the disturbingly low use of prescriptive fitting methods among audiologists, which he subtitled "What would Denis say?" In his paper, Mueller mentioned that some audiologists believe that "clinical experience" trumps a prescriptive method—we've often heard, "I don't use the NAL-NL2, I have a better way to fit hearing aids." In November of 2001, Harvey Dillon gave the Denis Byrne Memorial Lecture at the annual meeting of the American Speech and Hearing Association (Dillon, 2001). Here is what Harvey had to say about Denis's thoughts on clinical experience:

> From time to time, Denis encountered critics of his work who claimed they selected and adjusted hearing aids using their considerable "clinical experience." Furthermore, they claimed, such methods were more effective than anything based on a formula could ever be, as they took many more aspects of the

patient into account than did any prescriptive approach. While Denis readily agreed that there was more to a patient than an audiogram, he was scathing of "experience" as a scientific approach to audiology. His attitude can be summarized in the following three paraphrases:

- If you can't write down the rules you use, you probably don't understand what you do.
- If it's not written down, no one else can do it, and no one can test whether it's better or worse than some alternative approach.
- If you can't evaluate your procedure you can't improve it.

With those thoughts in mind, let's talk more specifically about prescriptive fitting approaches.

A Little History

Today, most audiologists take it for granted that when they are fitting hearing aids, a computerized algorithm will do some number crunching and desired gain and output values will appear, and in most cases, with a single mouse click, the hearing aid will automatically be programmed to these desired values. But it wasn't always like this, and we're not just referring to the automation aspect. The underlying philosophical issues regarding how hearing aids should be fitted have also evolved over the years.

In the 1930s and 1940s, the term *selective amplification* was often used, which meant that the frequency response of the hearing aid would be tailored from the audiogram, similarly to what we now call *prescriptive fitting.* As is the case today, approaches varied then, although often the general notion was to restore normal hearing, and in fact, one method suggested was to mirror the audiogram (gain = amount of hearing loss). Several early pioneers of this time, however, did point out the importance of considering the range of comfort, equal loudness curves, and uncomfortable loudness level (Watson & Tolan, 1949). The Harvard Report (Davis et al., 1946), however, concluded that patient-specific information might not be that critical, as they concluded that even for people with different audiometric configurations, the best performance

TAKE FIVE: You Have to Start Somewhere!

We often hear people question the value of prescriptive fitting methods, suggesting that they have a better way to fit hearing aids. Maybe that's true, but as we've said a couple times already in this chapter—you have to start some place. Audiologist Earl Johnson made that point nicely in one of his articles (Johnson, 2012). His example was that of an experienced clinician who was skillful enough to narrow down the possible choices to a 20 dB range/frequency for a given patient, simply based on the patient's audiogram. The clinician was fitting a 16-channel hearing aid. Johnson's calculations reveal that even when the choices have been narrowed to 20 dB, there are still 1,430 possible frequency responses to choose from (see the article for the formula he used). And that was just for one input level! So as we said, you have to start someplace, so why not use a validated fitting method?

AUDIOID: What Was on THEIR Play List?

In addition to developing one of the first hearing aid fitting protocols, Raymond Carhart is one of the individuals credited with coining the word "audiology" in the mid-1940s. And you might wonder how the musician John Kirby fits in? In the late 1930s, the New York-based John Kirby Sextet was known as "The Biggest Little Band in the Land." The group also went by the name John Kirby and His Onyx Club Boys. Most of his music was recorded between 1938 and 1941, and one of his original songs that you might be interested in was something called "Audiology." Could it be that Raymond Carhart or Hallowell Davis listened to a little John Kirby before naming this new professional a few years later?

was with a frequency response that was relatively flat, or gradually upward sloping (+6 dB/octave). In general, during this period, audiometric data were used for hearing aid selection, although no specific prescriptive method emerged other than the general recommendations of the Harvard Report.

In the mid-1940s, Army Rehabilitation Centers were established, and one of their missions was to fit hearing aids and conduct aural rehabilitation for returning World War II veterans. One such center was at Deshon Army Hospital in Butler, Pennsylvania, and the director of the Acoustics Section was Captain Raymond Carhart, now often referred to as "the father of audiology." During this time, Carhart developed an extensive 12-step test protocol for selecting appropriate amplification (Carhart, 1946). In one respect, this procedure could be considered *prescriptive*, in that the selection process included an extensive preselection procedure, which at that time included only hearing aids that were subjectively rated as superior. The selection was narrowed down to three or four hearing aids, which were then comparatively tested using different speech tests over several weeks. Ultimately, the patient would receive the hearing aid that provided the best performance on aided speech recognition tests. We say hearing *aid*, in the singular, as at that time everyone was fitted monaurally.

In the 1950s, 1960s, and through the mid-1970s, audiologists shortened the 3 to 4-week comparative procedure of Carhart to one hour, or maybe two hours in university settings. In addition, rather than conduct a battery of speech tests, often no more than a 25-word list of live-voice monosyllables-in-quiet was delivered. It was still common to test three different hearing aids, and the hearing aid that resulted in the *best* percentage correct score was usually recommended (even though it often was only 2 to 4% superior to another—so not actually statistically different at all). Audiologists using these procedures tended to report that they were using the Carhart fitting method. Surveys taken during this time indicated that this fitting approach was used by 80 to 85% of audiologists (Burney, 1972).

The move toward the current routine use of prescriptive fitting methods for hearing aid selection began in the mid-to-late 1970s. There were several converging reasons why audiologists began to abandon their repeated speech testing and began to measure aided gain in order to determine if it met some predetermined desired value.

Factors, which probably impacted this transformation, included:

- At national meetings, opinion leaders were presenting new data revealing the poor reliability and validity of using monosyllabic word lists to select the *best* hearing aid.
- Audiologists were going into private practice, and it was now ethical for them to sell hearing aids. This increased the interest level in finding an efficient and effective method to select the appropriate hearing aid. The traditional two-hour university fitting method did not lend itself to a busy private practice.
- Custom hearing aids were becoming popular. Unlike their behind-the-ear (BTE) counterparts, there was not a stock of hearing aids to use for comparative testing.
- New prescriptive methods were emerging, and audiologists like Kenneth Berger were presenting workshops on prescriptive fittings, and the use of functional gain testing for verification.

Prescriptive formulas continued to proliferate after the 1980s. This was due, in part, to the emergence of the first multichannel programmable hearing aids in the late 1980s, and the introduction of the first commercially viable digital hearing aids in the United States in the mid-1990s. Prior to this time, only rough changes in hearing aid frequency response were possible via analog potentiometers (trim pots), or through the plumbing modifications. In addition, there was a surge of software and tools to ensure the fittings were "accurate." For example, probe microphone systems allowed for easier visualization of the hearing aid gain "targets" and the actual gain and output present in the patient's ears. More than any era before, using prescriptive hearing aid fitting methods was actually defensible because frequency specific hearing aid gain and output could be precisely adjusted and verified.

A Few of the Older Prescriptive Methods

By the mid-1980s, it was common for probe microphone equipment to include prescriptive fitting methods as part of the operating software. You might still see some of these methods from the 1980s and 1990s on equipment today. In this section, we'll go down memory lane for a little while, reviewing a few of the more popular methods over the years.

Lybarger Half-Gain Rule (1944, 1953, 1963)

Samuel Lybarger first proposed that gain should be "equal to one-half of the hearing loss." This is now referred to as the half-gain rule indicating that the gain at each frequency should be equal to one-half of the hearing threshold at that frequency. These values were defined as user gain, not full-on gain. To establish full-on gain, 10 to 15 dB of reserve needed to be added to each result from the formula. Additional gain was also added to compensate for conductive or mixed losses. It should be mentioned that this formula had no specific rationale or data to examine its effectiveness. However, because Lybarger worked for a major hearing aid company (RadioEar), one might assume that the formula was based on experience with patients and was consistent with placing average speech inputs near expected MCL. Methods introduced in later years continued to use Lybarger's one-half-gain rule.

AUDOID: From Talcum Powder to Hair Spray

Sam Lybarger is known for his one-half-gain fitting rule, but on the lighter side, he also was known for his definition of a hearing aid. His parent company, RadioEar, had his definition printed on a small poster, and was distributed nationally, often seen hanging in the offices of audiologists and dispensers. His one-sentence, 84-word definition went like this:

> A hearing aid is an ultra-small electroacoustic device that is always too large, that has to faithfully amplify speech a million times without bringing in any noise, that has to work without failure—in a flood of perspiration or a cloud of talcum powder, that one usually puts off buying for 10 years after he needs it because he doesn't want anyone to know he is hard-of-hearing, but which he can't do without for 30 minutes when it needs to be serviced.

This definition was written over 60 years ago. If we substitute the words hair spray for talcum powder, you may have thought it was written yesterday. Some things do not change much.

Berger (1976 and 1984)

This prescriptive method was the first to consider prescription of both frequency specific gain and the hearing aids maximum power output (MPO). Additionally, this prescription included gain modifications for unilateral or bilateral fittings as well as for conductive hearing loss components. This method required only measurement of pure tone thresholds, and all suprathreshold data were interpolated, as Berger believed that MCL measurements were too variable (and we agree on this point). For some frequencies, the Berger method called for more than one-half gain, as the formula called for dividing the audiometric threshold by 1.5 (2000 Hz) and 1.7 (3000 Hz). The Berger method enjoyed moderate success, partly because of numerous workshops conducted by Berger promoting this fitting approach.

Prescription of Gain and Output—POGO (1983)

This prescriptive approach for selection of gain and OSPL90 was developed by Gerry McCandless and Poul Erik Lyregaard. The POGO was very similar to the Lybarger half-gain rule, except it also provided real-ear insertion gain (REIG) targets. Audiologists were eager to adopt the POGO method as a fitting guide for prescriptive gain, as even the math-challenged were able to divide by 2 without the use of calculator (dividing by 1.6 for the Berger method presented some concern). And, we think people just liked saying the word POGO! Interestingly, the portion of the method used for calculating maximum output was largely ignored. For most, the prescription method actually was "POG," not "POGO."

In 1988, modifications were made to the original POGO formula to extend it to lis-

TIPS AND TRICKS: Uncomfortable Loudness—Alphabet Soup?

As you're reading about these prescriptive methods, you will notice that we talked about the uncomfortable loudness level (UCL) and the loudness discomfort level (LDL). And, of course, there is also the Threshold of Discomfort (TD). Confusing? If we want to know the point that loud sounds are uncomfortable (which is what many prescriptive methods call for), we would be talking about the UCL, LDL or TD—Loudness anchor #7 on the Cox Contour Chart (Cox, 1995; see Chapter 6). One could argue, of course, that we would never want the output to be uncomfortable, and therefore, the value we should be calculating in our prescriptive methods is the Upper Level of Comfort (ULC; used by the DSL) or the Highest Comfortable Level (HCL: used by Robyn Cox in the MSU procedure; Cox, 1985, 1988) This would be loudness anchor #6 on the Cox Contour Chart. For adults with hearing loss, with a typical residual dynamic range, the difference between #6 and #7 is usually around 5 dB.

teners with severe hearing loss (i.e., when hearing loss was greater than 65 dB HL). The POGO II prescribed the same gain as POGO for losses equal to or less than 65 dB HL, however, for greater losses, gain was increased by 1 dB for every 2-dB increase in hearing loss (Schwartz, Lyregaard, & Lundh, 1988).

Libby (1986)

This prescription was very similar to the POGO procedure except, based on his own experiences using probe microphone measures fitting hearing aids, E. Robert "Cy" Libby concluded that people with mild or moderate hearing losses prefer gain that is equal to one-third (rather than one-half) of their hearing loss, and there was less gain reduction in the low frequencies (250 and 500 Hz). Furthermore, he concluded that the proportion of hearing loss used for calculation of gain should increase with increasing degrees of hearing loss. Specifically, for moderate-to-severe hearing loss, one-half of the hearing loss was used to establish gain, whereas two-thirds of the hearing loss was used for severe hearing loss. In the early days of probe microphone measures, the Libby 1/3 method was popular among clinicians, simply because it was quite easy to obtain 1/3 gain—1/2 gain (POGO) often led to feedback.

Visual Input/Output Locater Algorithm (VIOLA)

In 1992, a group of 12 audiologists formed the Independent Hearing Aid Fitting Forum (IHAFF), with the primary goal of developing a prescriptive method for fitting the new nonlinear hearing aids being introduced. The method that evolved from this group, sometimes referred to as the IHAFF method, is the VIOLA. Robyn Cox, a member of the IHAFF, was largely responsible for developing this method (Cox, Goff, Martin, & McLoud, 1994; Cox, Taylor, Gray, & Brainerd, 1994, 1994; Cox, 1995).

TAKE FIVE: Did They Really Prefer One-Third-Gain?

As we discussed, the "Libby one-third method" was based on observations made by Libby, an optometrist in Philadelphia who sold audiologic equipment and dispensed hearing aids. Libby was one of the first in the United States to distribute the Rastronics probe microphone system (ca. 1984), and was an early adopter of routinely conducting probe microphone measures when fitting hearing aids. He observed, having tested hundreds of individuals, that even though he was attempting to fit his patients to the POGO prescription (~one-half-gain), when they returned for follow-up, many patients tended to use and prefer something closer to one-third-gain (based on their use-gain VC adjustments). Consider, however, that these were linear instruments, with relatively high OSPL90s (common at the time), and in most cases, there was no maximum power output (MPO) control on the hearing aid. We suspect that for many of these individuals, one-half-gain caused loud sounds to be too loud and/or distorted, and they turned down gain to closer to one-third of their hearing loss, because that was what was required to keep loud sounds below their LDLs. Consider that a hearing loss of 50 dB HL would result in a POGO gain prescription of 25 dB, which might be just fine for average inputs, but would most often be too much gain for inputs of 75 to 80 dB SPL, as these individuals typically have LDLs similar to people with normal hearing. Today, of course, we have adjustable compression and output settings, so that the patients preferred listening level for one input level, is not influenced by inputs of other intensity levels.

The VIOLA strategy attempted to restore "normal" loudness growth of speech by restoring the relationship between the loudness perception of soft, comfortable, and loud warble tone stimuli and the corresponding levels of unfiltered, wideband speech, observed in normal-hearing listeners. The VIOLA method provided 2cc targets, not REIG or REAR targets. This limited its use, as many audiologists were not prepared to run coupler measures just for this purpose. It was also discovered early on, that most audiologists did not want to take the time to conduct the seven-point loudness contour. The software did provide the option, however, to simply enter the thresholds and the LDLs for each frequency, and the intermediate values would be predicted. While the VIOLA was never widely accepted as a fitting method, the software provided by Cox and colleagues was extremely valuable in helping audiologists understand WDRC, as input/output functions could be observed by inserting a wide range of gain values, output levels, compression kneepoints, and ratios.

FIG6

The most popular WDRC circuit of early 1990s was the K-Amp, developed by Mead Killion. Not surprisingly, therefore, Killion and his staff were interested in developing a fitting method that could be used with this compression strategy. As an alternative to methods that measured individual loudness growth, Killion (1994) proposed that normal loudness impression for a *preferred dynamic range* could be restored based on average loudness growth data. The FIG6 strategy (Killion, 1994) utilized previously collected cross-modality loudness matching data categorized by average threshold (Hellman & Meiselman, 1990, 1993). Hearing aid gain was then calculated at octave frequencies based on differences between average, normal, and impaired loudness growth, given a particular hearing loss. This gain calculation was made at three different inputs assumed to reflect the preferred listening range of speech inputs (40, 65, 90 dB SPL). The 40 dB SPL input gain calculation was based on audibility considerations rather than loudness. Specifically, Killion suggested that gain sufficient to bring aided sound-field thresholds to 20 dB hearing level was necessary in order to ensure the audibility of the lowest intensity elements of speech.

The National Acoustic Laboratories (NAL) Family of Prescriptive Methods

The first version of NAL was published by Byrne and Tonisson (1976). In the United States, the procedure was not commonly referred to as the *NAL procedure*, but rather identified by the authors as *the Byrne and Tonisson method*. Because this prescriptive approach was competing with the much simpler methods developed in the United States (e.g., Berger, POGO, Libby) it received little attention.

Approximately 10 years after the introduction of the first NAL method, a revised prescription was published (NAL-R; Byrne & Dillon, 1986). The authors of the original NAL continued to advocate for equal loudness across frequencies; however, they corrected the original formula after deciding their original method for arriving at equal loudness was incorrect, particularly for sloping hearing loss. The authors reported that the NAL-R prescribed frequency response was seldom inferior to, and usually better than, any of several variations having more, or less, low and/or high-frequency amplification, and on the average, use-gain was approximately equal to prescribed gain. In 1990, Bryne, Parkinson, and Newall further revised the NAL-R procedure to address gain prescription for severe-to-profound hearing losses.

The next modification of the NAL algorithm was a fitting method for nonlinear hearing aids, the NAL-NL1, which became available for clinical use around 1998. As stated by Dillon (1999), the aim of the NAL-NL1 was to provide the gain-frequency response that maximizes speech intelligibility while keeping overall loudness at a level no greater than that perceived by a normal-hearing person listening to the same sound. This is then a nonlinear method, as the gain-frequency response that achieves this varies with input level. The principle of the NAL-NL1 includes the idea of normalizing loudness; however, this notion applies to the total or overall loudness, not the relative loudness at each frequency.

Dillon (1999; 2001) described the development of the NAL-NL1, which we summarize here:

- One theoretical model used was a modification of the speech intelligibility index (SII) method, with allowance for desensitization (see related Tips and Tricks) and for listening at high input levels.
- A second model was a method for calculating loudness, allowing for the effects of a sensorineural hearing loss.

- Using a high-speed computer, the loudness and intelligibility programs were linked using data that were generated using a method known as a "constrained numerical optimizer." That is, a best fit for the two models was determined for 50 to 90 dB SPL inputs (see related Clinical Concept).
- So that the findings of this analysis could be easily used clinically, for any audiogram and speech level, in order to predict gain for all frequencies, a formula was constructed based on the following:
  - Hearing threshold at that frequency
  - Three-frequency average hearing threshold (500 Hz, 1000 Hz, and 2000 Hz)
  - Slope of the audiogram from 500 to 2000 Hz
  - Overall level of the speech input signal
- Dillon adds that the gain at any frequency ended up depending on the hearing loss at several frequencies, rather than only the frequency in question, just as with its NAL-RP predecessor. For a speech input level of 65 to 70 dB SPL, the NAL-NL1 prescribes a gain-frequency response similar to that prescribed by NAL-RP.

The NAL-NL1 was available as stand-alone software, where clinicians could enter in audiometric data and then view the gain and channel-specific compression parameters. This procedure also was quickly adapted by both hearing aid and probe microphone equipment manufacturers. Although the NAL-NL1 was somewhat of a latecomer to the nonlinear prescriptive party, it quickly became the method of choice for both clinicians and researchers. One factor that led to its popularity was that the software calculated targets in just about any form one might want. Gain could be expressed as REIG, REAG, 2cc-coupler gain, or ear-simulator gain, with test signals being pure tones or broadband speech-shaped noises (different targets for the different test signals). The availability of REAG targets encouraged verification using ear canal SPL values, rather than REIG, making the NAL verification process similar to what previously had been used only for the DSL.

CLINICAL CONCEPT: Loudness Normalization Versus Loudness Equalization

A reasonable question when selecting a prescriptive fitting approach is whether your goal is to *normalize* or *equalize* loudness, and, yes, there is a difference, and different approaches will result in different gain prescriptions (much of the time).

Loudness normalization intends to restore, usually for certain frequency bands, the loudness perception of the listener with hearing impairment to the same loudness perceived by a listener with normal hearing. Loudness normalization can also mean that soft, medium, and loud speech as heard by a normal hearer are appropriately amplified to the categorical rating descriptor of *soft, average,* and *loud* by an individual with hearing impairment. In other words, soft sounds are soft and loud sounds are loud. Because the specific loudness patterns differ in individuals with the same hearing loss, trying to precisely normalize loudness would require consideration of individual loudness growth patterns. Further, in order to control the loudness of all segments of sound precisely, gain changes in hearing aids would need to be very rapid. Fortunately, evidence does not support the assumption that precise loudness normalization leads to better outcomes. More generally accurate, frequency specific loudness normalization provides much more gain in the low frequencies and much higher compression ratios than provided by current, validated prescriptive methods such as DSL v5 and NAL-NL2. Consequently, whereas the general concept of loudness normalization makes intuitive sense, evidence suggests precise loudness normalization is probably not an appropriate hearing aid fitting goal. There also was a critical flaw inherent to strict loudness normalization procedures. They did not account for the fact that all speech frequencies are not equally important and we have only so much loudness to work with before patients find amplified sounds too loud. Wisely allocating loudness to optimize audibility for the most important frequency ranges of speech as an alternative to strict loudness normalization now seems somewhat intuitive. Consequently, it is not surprising that the majority of the loudness normalization fitting methods of the 1990s have since been abandoned.

In contrast to loudness normalization, *loudness equalization* aims to equalize the perception of loudness over a range of frequencies instead of having lower frequencies dominate loudness as is the case for listeners with normal hearing. For example, the frequency range of 500 to 4000 Hz can be amplified such that the loudness perception of 500 Hz and 4000 Hz as well as the various narrow bands in between are equivalent in the unit of sones. This process was explicit in the earlier years of linear NAL prescriptions and carries forward in the current iterations as well. The assumption made by the authors of the NAL procedure was that loudness equalization would better distribute loudness to the speech frequencies that were most important for speech understanding when compared to loudness normalization.

The Desired Sensation Level (DSL) Family

We mentioned earlier that the work from the NAL has helped guide us in the programming and fitting of hearing aids for decades. Much of the same can be said for the work from the University of Western Ontario. Richard Seewald and his colleagues published the original Desired Sensation Level (DSL) method in 1985, although the conceptual work on this fitting method actually started when Seewald began his studies with Mark Ross in 1976. The first algorithms were being studied around 1982. As stated by Seewald, Moodie, Scollie, and Bagatto (2005):

> The DSL method was originally developed to provide clinicians with a systematic, science-based approach to pediatric hearing instrument fitting that ensures audibility of amplified speech by accounting for factors that are uniquely

AUDIOID: The DSL Beginnings

The DSL fitting method came out of Richard Seewald's work as a clinician in Halifax in the 1970s—his concerns and frustrations associated with fitting children with hearing loss. Richard decided to study under Mark Ross at the University of Connecticut, and they collaborated in the late 1970s on the first version of the DSL. Seewald states, "We had developed a really interesting protocol, but the down side was that it took about 45 minutes to do the calculations by hand to determine the desired amplification characteristics for each child." Shortly thereafter, Richard moved to the University of Western Ontario, and took on the task of speeding up the calculation processes. As the story goes, the first computerized version of DSL was developed in his living room, by hooking up his 16K Sinclair computer to the family black-and-white Motorola TV. And, as they say . . . the rest is history.

> associated with the provision of amplification to infants and young children who have hearing loss. (p. 145)

The basic philosophy driving the development of the algorithm focused on optimizing speech recognition for children with hearing loss, knowing that speech must be amplified to a certain sensation level (SL) to maximize intelligibility. Further, they argued that, based on the work of Erber and Witt, the SL for maximum speech intelligibility in children needed to be quite high. The findings from these studies were then used to define target SLs for amplified speech for children with hearing loss (Seewald, Ross, & Spiro, 1985) as a function of degree of hearing loss. According to the developers, a longstanding goal of this prescriptive method is to amplify speech to the DSLs across as broad a frequency range as possible to support auditory learning via audibility of speech cues. Another goal of the DSL method has been to provide targets that limit the maximum output, while still providing appropriate headroom and comfort for loud sounds.

The original versions of this procedure required some time to calculate on paper and pencil worksheets—but things soon changed. An updated version of the DSL method was developed to address the fitting of WDRC instruments. In 1995, Cornelisse and colleagues designed the *input/output formula* (DSL [i/o]) by using Steven's power law to map a wide range of input levels to target hearing aid output levels across various frequencies. The DSL [i/o] method version 4.1 prescribed targets for gain, output limiting, and compression ratios. The average speech SLs were approximately equivalent to those recommended by earlier versions of the DSL (Cornelisse et al., 1995); however, the listener's residual dynamic range (from frequency specific threshold to predicted LDL) was used to assign compression parameters. This was labeled a *loudness normalization* procedure at the time, although restoration of the normal dynamic range may be a more accurate description of the goal of the calculations for compression parameters.

A key feature of the original DSL method was to display the characteristics of the hearing aid output together with the child's auditory characteristics in an *SPL-O-Gram* format. The SPL-O-Gram uses a real-ear SPL reference scale across frequencies to permit direct comparison of the output levels of the hearing aid for known input levels with the listener's thresholds and LDLs. Clearly this had considerable influence on hearing aid fitting as this approach has been adopted, at least as an option, in nearly all current probe microphone equipment.

TAKE FIVE: They Even Had the Audiogram Upside Down!

Consider that when the first DSL method was introduced, audiologists were living in a pretty simple gain-based world for fitting hearing aids. The patient has a 50 dB loss at 2000 Hz? Okay—he needs 25 dB of gain. Compared to this simplistic way of selecting amplification characteristics, the early calculation of the DSL targets by hand was a bit overwhelming for some. Worksheets, workbooks, and workshops were provided to facilitate the use of this method. Adding to the confusion was that the common audiogram was now upside down, and called an SPL-O-Gram. This had been advocated by Norm Erber and others years earlier, but was still foreign to most. As time went on, however, dedicated pediatric audiologists realized that there was a payoff for the extra math, as they began fitting their hearing aids differently. The computerized version, however, introduced a few years later, was still warmly welcomed. Today, of course, looking at a patient's audiogram and an average speech signal referenced to ear canal SPL, and then attempting to obtain appropriate audibility with amplification is commonplace.

TIPS AND TRICKS: *Considering* Desensitization *in Prescribing Gain*

It has been shown that as hearing thresholds increase above 60 dB, particularly in downward sloping hearing losses, the usefulness of high-frequency speech information is reduced significantly. That is, there is a range of effective audibility, and beyond that point, increased audibility does not provide the benefit that might be predicted. In some individuals, increased audibility may even cause a reduction in speech understanding. This has been referred to as hearing loss *desensitization* (see Pavlov, Studebaker, & Sherbecoe,, 1986; Ching, Dillon, & Byrne, 1998; Ching, Dillon, Katsch, & Byrne, 2001). Accordingly, methods such as the SII may overestimate intelligibility when the hearing loss is severe to profound. Some prescriptive methods, in particular those of the NAL, have taken desensitization into account when prescribing gain. This factor often causes concern among audiologists when fitting a downward sloping hearing loss, as they see real-ear target NAL-NL2 values in the high frequencies that appear to provide insufficient audibility. The issue is that increasing audibility where it will be of questionable use will increase overall loudness, which may prompt the patient to turn down gain, losing audibility for other frequencies where it is of much greater value.

Today's Prescriptive Approaches

Our history lesson is over. We are now to the point of talking about the prescriptive methods that we currently use. The good news is that there are only two survivors! Both have been modified in the fairly recent past, are available from all, or nearly all manufacturers, and have been incorporated into all probe microphone equipment. We are talking about the NAL-NL2 (a revision of the NAL-NL1) and the DSL v5.0 (a revision of the DSL4.1 [i/o]). The DSL v5.0 has been out the longest, so we will talk about that first.

DSL v5.0

In 2005, the DSL Multistage Input/Output v5.0a—or simply the DSL v5.0—was first released. The authors reported that the fitting targets were now more flexible than they had been in past versions. There was no longer a single DSL target but rather a family of targets that vary based on the type of fitting. Another obvious outcome of this change was the introduction of targets that differ as a function of age. These changes were based on data demonstrating clear differences in the preferred listening levels for adults and children. Although the habilitative audibility goals are the same as previous versions of the DSL Method, DSL v5.0a provides compatibility with frequency specific ABR threshold estimates (nHL), updated RECD normative data for infants and children, infant-friendly RECD measurement techniques, targets for quiet and noisy environments, adjustments for conductive losses and bilateral fittings, and accounts for multichannel compression characteristics of modern hearing aids. Detailed descriptions of these modifications and additions can be found in Scollie et al. (2005) and Bagatto et al. (2005).

Scollie (2007) provides a comprehensive review of the different areas where DSL v5.0 varies from the previous DSL 4.1 [i/o], based on the Scollie et al., 2005 publication. A revision of DSL v5.0 (v5.0b) added conversions from nHL to eHL to further enhance implementation of ABR estimates of threshold, as well as providing new corrections for mixed hearing loss and conductive components. A summary of the changes, from Scollie (2007) is provided here and in Table 2–1:

- Age and Etiology: A fairly significant modification to DSL v4.1 is the change in fitting targets based on the patient's age and etiology of the hearing loss. The DSL v5.0 was adjusted to recommend a higher listening level for pediatric patients (presumably with congenital hearing losses) than for adult patients (presumably with acquired hearing losses). Clinically, this is selected by the clinician rather than automatically based on birthdate, so that either target type can be chosen. For example, for adults who have congenital hearing losses or who prefer a setting that provides maximal audibility of speech, the higher listening levels would be chosen. As reviewed in Scollie et al. (2005), the size of this difference appears to be greater than 5 dB and likely less than 10 dB, where children both require and prefer greater gain than do adults. The DSL v5.0 accommodates this difference by reducing the gain recommended for adults by 7 dB for a 50 dB HL audiogram and a 60 dB SPL speech

Table 2–1. Summary of Changes in DSL v5.0

Change Description	*Change Amount and Direction*
Adult/acquired versus pediatric/congenital target	A 7 dB reduction for moderate losses, 3 dB for severe losses
Interpolation	Greater number of target values across frequencies when working with partial audiograms
Compression threshold	Less gain and output for low-level inputs due to prescribed compression threshold. Inputs of 70 dB and above are not affected.
Output limiting	Narrowband output limiting targets are largely unaffected. Output limiting for speech may cause target reductions of 5 to 10 dB if hearing loss is severe or test level is high.
Quiet versus noisy environment	Compression threshold raised by 10 dB and gain reduced at low-importance speech frequencies by about 5 dB
Bilateral fittings	This is optional. When implemented, targets for speech are reduced by 3 dB. Output limiting targets are not affected.
Conductive or mixed hearing loss	Increases gain by up to 9 dB for mild losses, 5 dB for severe losses, depending on magnitude of air-bone gap.

Source: From Scollie, 2007.

input. As hearing levels increase, the method uses a gradually decreasing adult-child difference in order to maintain audibility of the speech signal for both populations. For hearing losses greater than about 80 dB HL, the age-related difference in target is very small. A general guideline is that the DSL v5.0 targets are most similar to DSL v4.1 targets with the age variable set to "child" and with the bilateral correction disabled.

- Treatment of Missing Data: With pediatric fittings, it is common that thresholds are not available for all frequencies of interest. DSL v5.0 includes an interpolation routine to derive a full spectrum of targets for any audiogram from two or more thresholds. This interpolation may not be shown in the fitting screens of all systems, but will be implemented whenever a manufacturer chooses to provide interpolation.
- Compression Characteristics: Version 5.0 of DSL uses a new input/output algorithm that is based on DSL v4.1. It was modified so that the target input/output functions can be clustered according to the channels of the hearing aid, so that compression targets per channel are computed. It also allows for the appropriate calculation for hearing aids with expansion. Scollie (2007) notes that the matching of channel structures between the prescription and the hearing aid will be done within hearing aid fitting software and is not something the audiologist must do. Also, probe microphone systems using speech as a test signal can derive DSL v5.0

targets without adjustments for channel structure because the effects of channel structure are minimized by testing with speech. Compression thresholds (CTs) are also revised in DSL v5.0; a channel-specific CT prescription recommends a low compression threshold for milder hearing losses. The prescribed CT is about 50 dB SPL for moderate hearing losses, and is gradually raised as hearing loss increases, to about 70 dB SPL for severe to profound losses. The prescribed CT may be overridden by the clinician or by fitting software.

- Limits to High-Level Speech: Scollie et al. (2005) report that experimental evidence with today's hearing aids with multichannel processing show that high-level speech exhibits at least 9 dB of crest factor. That is, the speech peaks fall about 9 dB above the LTASS. In DSL v5.0, the targets for aided speech are limited so that speech peaks do not exceed the listener's upper limit of comfort (ULC—as a reminder, #6 on the Cox Contour Test). This can have the effect of limiting the LTASS target values through a target variable called the Broadband Output Limiting Thresholds, or BOLT. This makes targets appear somewhat lower than they were in DSL v4.1 for the same audiogram. BOLT-limited targets are most likely to occur for higher input levels and/or severe hearing losses, and can be identified by a target LTASS that parallels the ULC contour, and is exactly 13 dB below the ULC.
- Listening Environments: The DSL targets for speech are computed assuming that spoken communication is taking place in a quiet environment, and therefore aims to provide full, or nearly full, audibility of speech. Scollie (2007) notes that in noisy environments, this degree of audibility may decrease comfort without improving intelligibility. The DSL v5.0 provides targets for a noise program that combine less gain at speech frequencies of lower importance with a raised CT.
- Bilateral Fittings: The DSL v5.0 includes an optional bilateral correction that reduces speech targets by 3 dB. Sloping losses receive a small adjustment that provides more mid-frequency and less high-frequency gain.

There also are a few other features of the DSL fitting method, which we will discuss later when we compare this method to the NAL-NL2. As we mentioned, the DSL v5.0 software has been implemented by nearly all major manufacturers and is a verification option in most probe microphone equipment. There is not stand-alone software, however, to purchase for clinical use.

NAL-NL2

In 2011, the current version of the NAL prescriptive formula was released. It is referred to as the NAL-NL2. The rationale behind this newest version of NAL is consistent with previous versions focusing on optimizing speech intelligibility and loudness comfort. The aim is to maximize intelligibility by increased gain in the frequency response, while modifying the gain so that the loudness is not greater than that perceived by normal-hearing listeners. The newest NAL makes use of a neural network to calculate the gain based on the audiogram. The authors state that they now have available more extensive data on how much information people with hearing loss can extract from speech once it has been made audible, which has enabled the development of an improved method for predicting speech intelligibility.

Following the release of NAL-NL1, there was some concern from both the audiologists using the method, and the patients being fitting with hearing aids programmed to the method, that the NAL-NL1 called for a little too much gain. Specifically, the NAL research group reported the findings from several studies, involving 187 adult hearing aid users who had their hearing aids fitted and fine-tuned to preferred gain. This research revealed that the NAL-NL1 prescription was "just right" for 49%, "too soft" for only 5%, and for 46% of the sample, the NAL-NL1 gain was "too loud" (Keidser & Dillon, 2006). Dispensers using the NAL-NL1 had similar opinions, especially when fitting new users. One change, therefore, that was applied in the NAL-NL2 was an overall reduction in loudness.

There are specific modifications that have been made to the earlier formulas based on data gathered from previous NAL prescriptions users. Some general findings that resulted in prescriptive changes for NAL-NL2, based on research from the NAL laboratories and the experience gained from using NAL-NL1, include:

1. Males prefer slightly more gain than females.
2. Individuals who are experienced hearing aid users and have a moderate/severe loss prefer more gain than new users with a similar hearing loss (Figure 2–1).
3. Hearing aid users prefer slightly higher compression ratios than what was prescribed using NAL-NL1 (Figure 2–2).
4. There should be less gain for bilateral fittings (especially at high input levels) than unilateral fittings to account for loudness summation (Figure 2–3).
5. Children prefer more gain than adults, particularly at low input levels. While the measured differences in preferred level were smaller than those reported by the DSL group, this finding led to different prescriptions for adults and

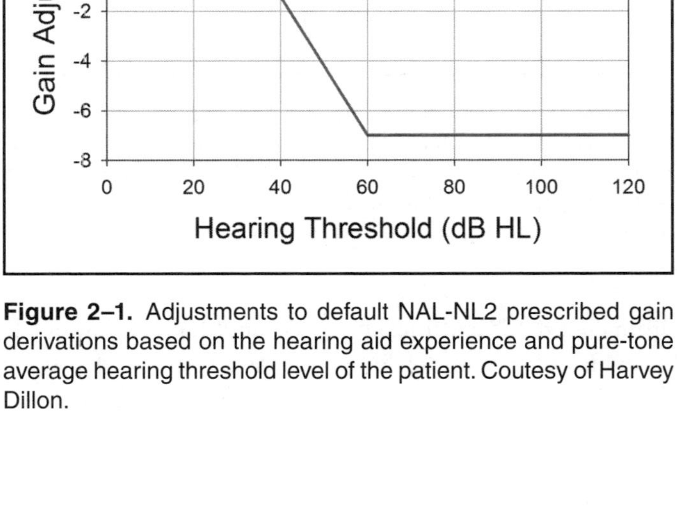

Figure 2–1. Adjustments to default NAL-NL2 prescribed gain derivations based on the hearing aid experience and pure-tone average hearing threshold level of the patient. Coutesy of Harvey Dillon.

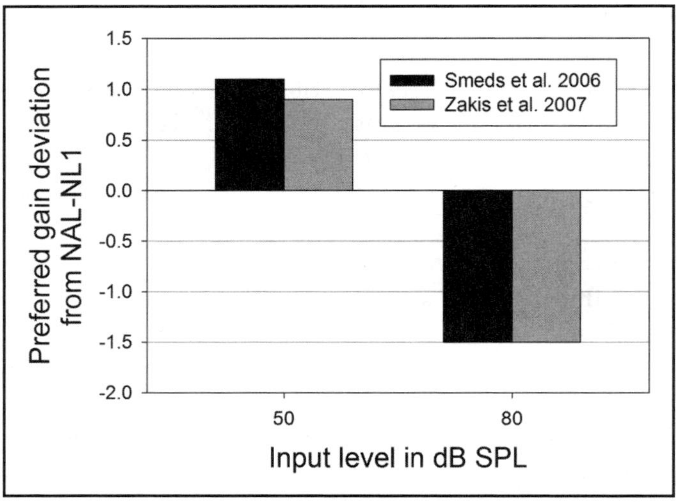

Figure 2–2. Evidence to support higher compression ratios than prescribed by NAL-NL1. Subject preferred more gain for soft sounds and less gain for loud sounds, a feat accomplished by increasing the compression ratio. Courtesy of Harvey Dillon.

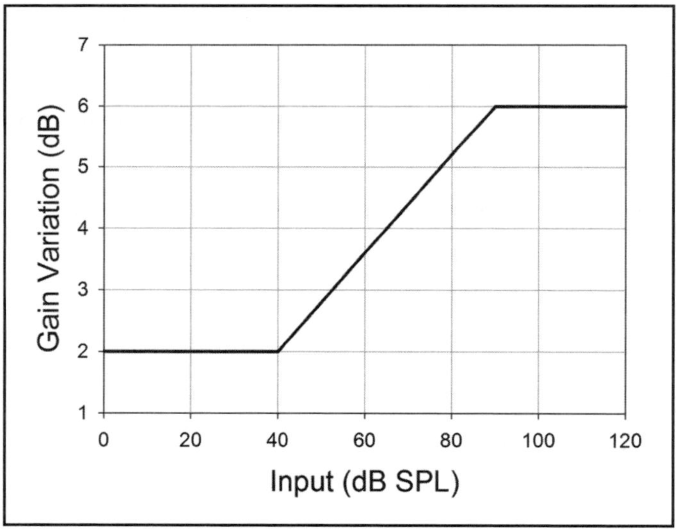

Figure 2–3. Adjustments to default NAL-NL2 prescribed gain derivations based on the binaural fitting of hearing aids. The correction for binaural summation is 2 dB at low input levels and up to 6 dB at high input levels for symmetric losses (but less for asymmetric losses). Courtesy of Harvey Dillon.

children within NAL-NL2. Specifically, NAL-NL2 provides more gain for low inputs for children, but less gain at high input levels for adults than NAL-NL1. As a result, higher compression ratios are prescribed for children than adults.

There are also currently two versions of NAL-NL2 focused on tonal and non-tonal languages. This is important because low frequencies are more important in tonal languages; therefore, the version targeting tonal language is designed to give slightly more gain at low frequencies. The NAL-NL2 has been implemented by most manufactures of hearing aids and probe microphone equipment, and is also available as stand-alone software from the NAL Shop. (http://www.nal.gov.au/online-shop.shtml)

Comparing the Two Current Approaches

As we've previously stated, it is considered best practice to start a hearing aid fitting with a validated prescriptive approach for estimating optimal gain and output. We believe that either of the current NAL or DSL prescriptions is a good starting point, at least for our adult patients. If we consider adults only, just how different are the prescriptions from NAL-NL2 and DSL v.5.0? We compare them based on several different criteria:

Experience:

- DSL v5.0 does not incorporate a correction for gain based on new or experienced hearing aid user status (Scollie et al., 2005)
- NAL-NL2 incorporates adjustments that not only differ as a function of hearing loss but include an increase for experienced users and a decrease for new users (see Figure 2–1). It is important to note that in new users this correction could not be accounted for during the initial hearing aid fitting and verification; instead, it would need to be implemented over time by either the fitting clinician or automatically through the hearing aid.

Gender:

- DSL v5.0 does not include an adjustment for gender whereas NAL-NL2 includes a 1 dB increase in gain for male wearers and a 1 dB decrease in gain for female wearers.
- The NAL-NL2 adjustment was based on an analysis, irrespective of degree of hearing loss and experience with amplification, that females preferred 2 dB, on average, less gain than males (Keidser & Dillon, 2006, 2012).

Bilateral fittings:

- DSL v5.0 targets for speech are reduced by 3 dB across input levels for bilateral fittings re: unilateral fittings (Scollie et al., 2005).
- NAL-NL2 has a bilateral gain correction that increases with input level. The correction for binaural summation is 2 dB at low input levels and up to 6 dB at high input levels for symmetric losses, and less for asymmetric losses (see Figure 2–3).

Listening in noise:

- DSL v5.0 targets for speech are reduced by 3 to 5 dB for low-importance frequencies for listening in noise. It is important to note that actually applying this difference would require the hearing aid to change gain depending on whether noise was present or not. For clinical fitting and verification, the probe microphone manufacturer must either allow the fitter to choose between these two prescriptions, or default to a

single choice (typically the listening in noise prescription).
- The NAL-NL2 does not have corrections for listening in noise.

Correction for A/B gap:

- The NAL-NL2 first applies prescribed gain for the sensorineural component of the hearing loss, and then adds 75% of the air-bone gap to this value.
- DSL v5.0 raises the predicted ULC by 25% of the average air-bone gap, which raises the upper limit of the target input/output curve, resulting in small corrections for gain for most audiograms. For a maximal air-bone gap, the correction adds 5 to 9 dB of gain and output to the aided speech targets, depending on the hearing level.

Loudness discomfort measures:

- NAL-NL2 does not alter its prescription of gain and output at any input level based on patient-specific LDLs or uncomfortable listening levels (ULLs). In fact, an entry for patient-specific loudness discomfort measures is not an option (although some hearing aid manufacturers include this option in their version of the NAL-NL2).
- DSL v5.0 will accept patient-specific loudness discomfort measures; subsequently, it will alter its

CLINICAL CONCEPT: Should Experienced Users Be Prescribed More Gain?

There is a general thought among clinicians that experienced users should be prescribed more gain than new users. This certainly makes sense, as one would think that there would be some sort of adaptation to gain over time. Shortly after programmable instruments were introduced, manufacturers entered a box in the software to indicate if the user was new or experienced, and increased gain (usually around 3 dB) was added for he experienced user. But is there research to support that this is true? The NAL group believes there is. Keidser, O'Brien, McLelland, and Yeend (2008) reported on adaptation to hearing aid gain prescriptions based on the NAL-NL1 fitting algorithm. The researchers studied 50 new and 26 experienced hearing aid wearers. Gain preferences and comfortable loudness measures were obtained at 1, 4, and 13 months post-fitting for new wearers, and at 1 month post-fitting for experienced wearers. New wearers preferred progressively less gain (as hearing loss increased). The researchers concluded that for new users with a 4FA HTL of 25 dB HL, gain reduction from NAL-NL1 was approximately −2 dB, whereas for those with a 4FA HTL of 55 dB HL, gain reduction preference was −9 dB. A literature review by Convery, Keidser, and Dillon (2005) found little evidence to support a gain adjustment for new users of hearing aids, at least no more than 2 dB, which was not deemed to be statistically significant. Until recently, prescriptive fitting methods did not even consider a correction for experience, and the DSL v5.0 still does not. At what point does a new user become experienced? We don't know.

> prescription of gain and output for not only high input levels that approximate the loudness discomfort measure, but also the desired output for average and soft input levels as well.

Another difference is that NAL-NL2 includes a slight adjustment for less gain with an increasing number of channels (a channel summation effect). To illustrate how the differences we've discussed can impact prescribed gain, we show examples of what a clinician can expect for the current prescriptions, NAL-NL2 and DSL v5.0 in Figures 2–4 and 2–5. The examples, for three different input levels, are for a gradual downward-sloping and a flat hearing loss, respectively. It is clear that the difference in prescribed output depends on input level, and as expected, differs for children and adults.

Comparison of Outcomes?

We are not aware of clinical studies where a group of subjects have been fitted with both the DSL v5.0 and NAL-NL2 in some kind of real-world trial. There was a comprehensive comparison conducted by Johnson and Dillon (2011) that didn't involve real people, but did involve a lot of math. They reported the differences observed in prescribed insertion gain for seven different audiometric types (five sensorineural), and conducted an analysis of predicted specific loudness, overall loudness, bandwidth of

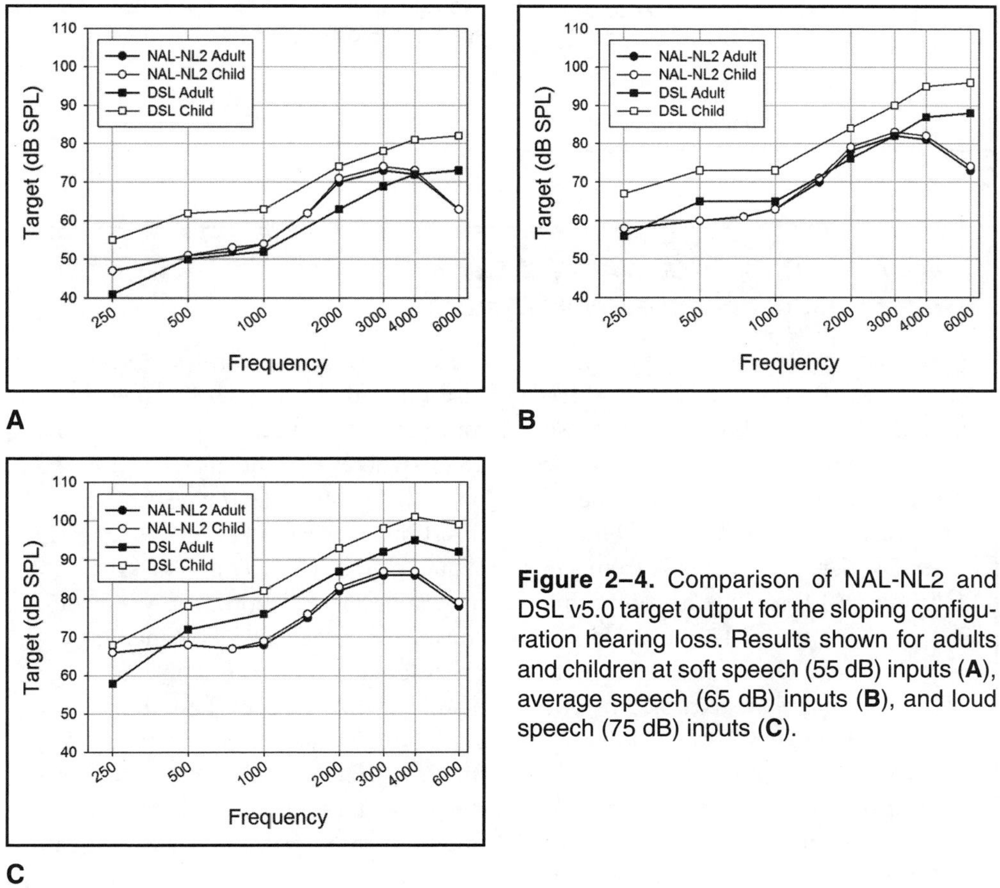

Figure 2–4. Comparison of NAL-NL2 and DSL v5.0 target output for the sloping configuration hearing loss. Results shown for adults and children at soft speech (55 dB) inputs (**A**), average speech (65 dB) inputs (**B**), and loud speech (75 dB) inputs (**C**).

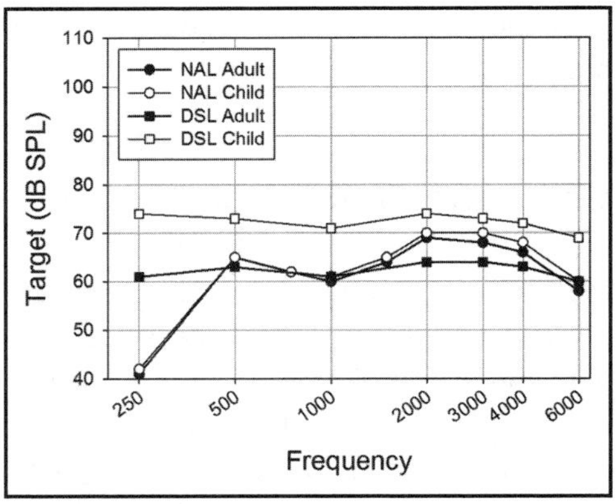

A

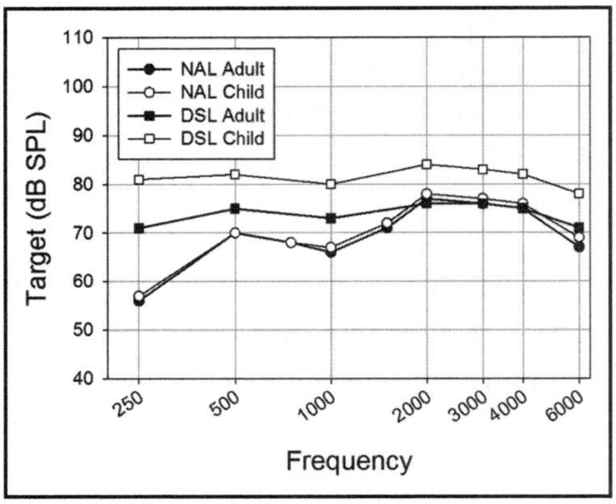

B

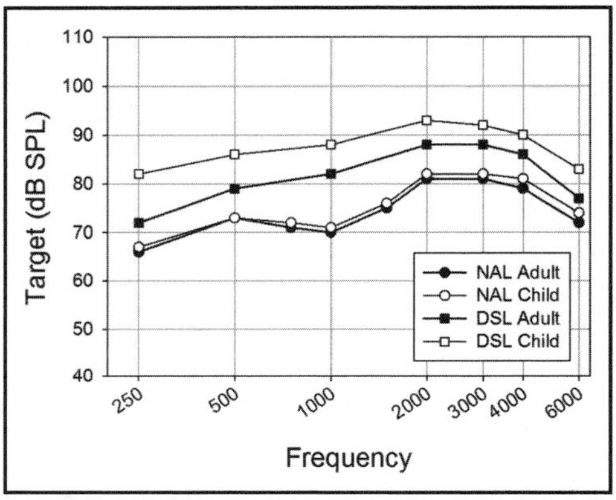

C

Figure 2–5. Comparison of NAL-NL2 and DSL v5.0 target output for the flat configuration hearing loss. Results shown for adults and children at soft speech (55 dB) inputs (**A**), average speech (65 dB) inputs (**B**), and loud speech (75 dB) inputs (**C**).

TIPS AND TRICKS: Do NAL-NL2 Corrections for Gender and Experience Really Matter?

As we have mentioned, the NL2 added some corrections that hadn't been used with the NL1 procedure. Two of these are for gender and experience. For the most part, the corrections are small, and one might ask if they really matter. They do. Here is an example from Johnson (2012) to illustrate this point. We start with two different patients with the same hearing loss, 20 to 30 dB HL in the low frequencies sloping down to 70 dB HL at 2000 Hz and above. One is a woman obtaining her first set of hearing aids, and the other an experienced male user, obtaining a new set of hearing aids. Even though they have the same hearing loss, the prescribed insertion gain at 2000 Hz for the female for a 65 dB SPL speech input would be 16 dB, whereas for the male it would be 21 dB. At 4000 Hz, the respective insertion gains would be 23 and 29 dB. Would gain differences of 5 to 6 dB make a difference? Probably, when you consider we are typically balancing provision of as much audibility as possible, while ensuring sounds are not too loud. This also points out why it is important to enter this information into the probe microphone equipment in order that appropriate fitting targets can be displayed.

cochlear excitation and effective audibility, as well as speech intelligibility using the international long-term average speech spectrum (ILTASS) at an average conversational input level. In general, they found that the NAL-NL2 and DSL v5.0 provided comparable overall loudness (~8 sones). The two prescriptive methods also provided comparable predicted speech intelligibility in quiet and in background noise.

There were some interesting differences, however, in the gain prescribed as a function of the audiometric configuration. Shown in Figure 2–6 are the five different sensorineural hearing losses used in the study, and Figure 2–7 shows the differences in the gain provided by the two methods. Values above the zero-line mean that more gain was prescribed by the DSL 5.0. Values below the zero-line mean that more gain was prescribed by the NAL-NL2.

At first glance of Figure 2–7, it appears that there are large differences between these two methods. Closer examination of the frequency scale, however, will reveal that the largest differences, at the low and high extremes, are at frequencies that we are not concerned with for the typical hearing aid fitting (or ranges where many hearing aids are unable to provide enough amplification to match targets). In fact, if we limit our observation to 500 to 4000 Hz, and use a +/− 5 dB criterion, we see that the two methods are within these boundaries for nearly all frequencies for all audiogram types. For two of the audiograms (A–1 and A–3, which are flat and gently sloping) the two methods are essentially identical. Where they differ the most are for either rising configurations, or very steeply sloping audiograms.

The bottom line is that we have two well-researched prescriptive methods to guide us in our hearing aid fittings. Their similarities seem to be greater than their differences. When differences do exist, the best method will probably depend on patient characteristics that would be difficult to predict prior to the fitting. We are quite certain, however, that using either of these methods places you far ahead of clinical

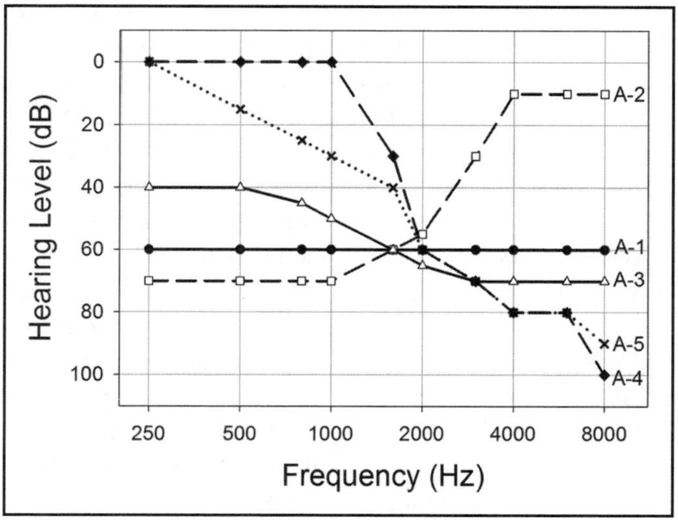

Figure 2–6. Five configurations of hearing loss used by Johnson and Dillon (2011) to determine differences in prescribed gain by NAL-NL2 and DSL v5.0 shown in Figure 2–7. Adapted from Johnson, 2012.

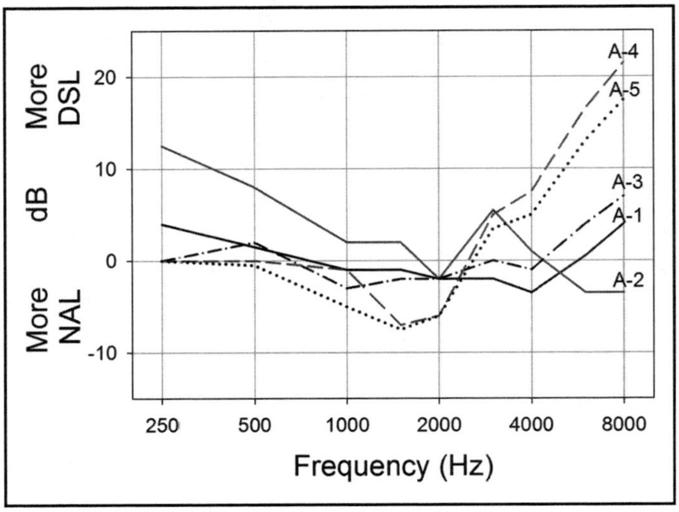

Figure 2–7. Differences in prescribed gain by NAL-NL2 and DSL v5.0 across the five configurations of hearing loss. Values above the zero-line mean that more gain was prescribed by the DSL 5.0. Values below the zero-line mean that more gain was prescribed by the NAL-NL2. Adapted from Johnson, 2012.

experience or other approaches derived by hearing aid manufacturers that have not been validated.

We mentioned a Denis Byrne quote in Chapter 1, but it's worth repeating. About 20 years ago in a 1996 *JAAA* article, Denis Byrne expressed concern that in the future, a scenario could exist that rather than using validated prescriptive methods, hearing aids would be fitted using manufacturer-specific proprietary formulae for calculating amplification requirements. He stated:

> The scenario described raises concerns, both scientific and philosophical. Scientifically, the concern is that amplification may become prescribed by a wide variety of proprietary formulae of which few, if any, are validated by published research. A possible philosophical problem is that control of the fitting process is taken away from the fitter, who is responsible for the care of the client. (p. 378)

Those Pesky Correction Factors

Our discussion of prescriptive methods isn't really complete unless we mention the correction factors that are involved. The fitting of hearing aids is frequently dependent upon calculations that convert measures obtained in a 2cc-coupler to gain in the real ear, or absolute ear canal SPL, or in other cases, convert hearing thresholds in dB HL to 2cc-coupler or ear canal SPL. This is true whether you use a validated prescriptive method (in which case the calculations are part of the method itself), a manufacturer's proprietary fitting algorithm (in which case the manufacturer has made these corrections), or if you simply view simulated gain on the fitting screen and "ballpark" a good fit (again, the manufacturer used correction factors to develop this display). These correction factors also are part of the verification procedures, as they are used by the manufacturers of probe microphone equipment to display thresholds, LDLs, and fitting targets.

Many audiologists fitting hearing aids prefer not to think about correction factors, but it really isn't a big deal, and actually can be somewhat fun once you get the hang of it. We often use mathematical conversions in our daily lives, especially when we travel, for example, converting temperatures from Fahrenheit to Celsius, or vice versa. Conveniently and appropriately, the same temperature conversion factors are used when the Sivantos Audiologische Technik people from Germany visit the SPAMfest in Minnesota, as when the Starkey Laboratories people of Minnesota take in the Oktoberfest in Munich. That is, 80°F is equal to 26.7°C regardless of where you live in the world. Unfortunately, this is not true for coupler-to-real-ear conversions. Different prescriptive methods use different correction factors, different hearing aid manufacturers use different correction factors, and different manufacturers of probe microphone equipment use even different correction factors. There is even some confusion as to whether some factors should be expressed with a "–" or a "+", which then determines if they should be added or subtracted (consider that adding "5 dB" versus subtracting "5 dB" results in a 10 dB mistake—a significant programming or display error). This lack of exactness is sometimes frustrating for audiologists when different data sets are compared during a hearing aid fitting (e.g., real-ear fitting targets on the probe microphone fitting screen versus the targets displayed in the manufacturer's fitting software). This also tends to be very frustrating to students who like preciseness, and can't quite understand why someone hasn't figured out the correct numbers to use. Indeed, the two most popular prescriptive methods today, the DSL v5 and the NAL-NL2, use somewhat different values for different correction factors. There are basically

AUDIOID: A "Semordnilap?"

One hearing aid-related term mentioned in this chapter is the CORFIG, although we won't be talking much about it. The CORFIG is a term used for COupler Response for Flat Insertion Gain, and was first used by Mead Killion and Ed Monser in a 1980 book chapter. In the second edition of that same book, published in 1993, Mead and Larry Revit wrote the chapter titled: "CORFIG and GIFROC: Real ear to coupler and back." In case it's not obvious, GIFROC is CORFIG backward, which makes the word CORFIG a Semordnilap (which of course is palindromes spelled backward; we're not making this up!). Killion and Revit realized that when making hearing aid gain calculations, there was some confusion as to whether you should add or subtract a CORFIG, so to, hopefully, simplify things, they added the GIFROC term, to remind us that when going from the real ear to the 2-cc coupler, you add the CORFIG, and when going from the coupler to the real ear, you would add the GIFROC (these are the same numbers). These are still important terms and numbers to remember for manufacturers and software developers, but really not part of the daily chatter of most practicing audiologists (whew).

four different corrections that are commonly applied related to hearing aid fitting and probe microphone measures:

- Coupler Response for Flat Insertion Gain (CORFIG): The difference between hearing aid *gain* in the coupler versus *gain* in the real ear.
- Real Ear Coupler Difference (RECD): The difference between hearing aid *output* in the coupler versus *output* in the real ear.
- Reference Equivalent Threshold in SPL (RETSPL): The difference between HL (audiometric dial setting) versus output in a 2-cc coupler.
- Real Ear Dial Difference (REDD): The difference between HL (audiometric dial setting) versus output in the real ear.

Putting It All to Practice

Now that you've heard all about today's fitting methods, we'll provide you a sample of how you would put this into practice with your probe microphone equipment. It's quite easy—just a few straightforward steps:

- Enter your measured hearing thresholds and LDLs into the probe microphone system. With some modern systems this can be conducted automatically, carried in from Noah.
- Using the systems prescription menu, select the desired fitting approach. For this example we'll select the NAL-NL2. As shown in Figure 2–8, for this probe microphone system we have several choices. We personally do not see the need for the older methods as they have been replaced. There are some audiologists, however, who still prefer the older methods, and we suspect that that is why they are still included by most probe microphone manufacturers.
- Following the selection of the specific method, it is then important to identify patient-specific factors that will influence the fitting. For the NAL-NL2, this would be such things as gender,

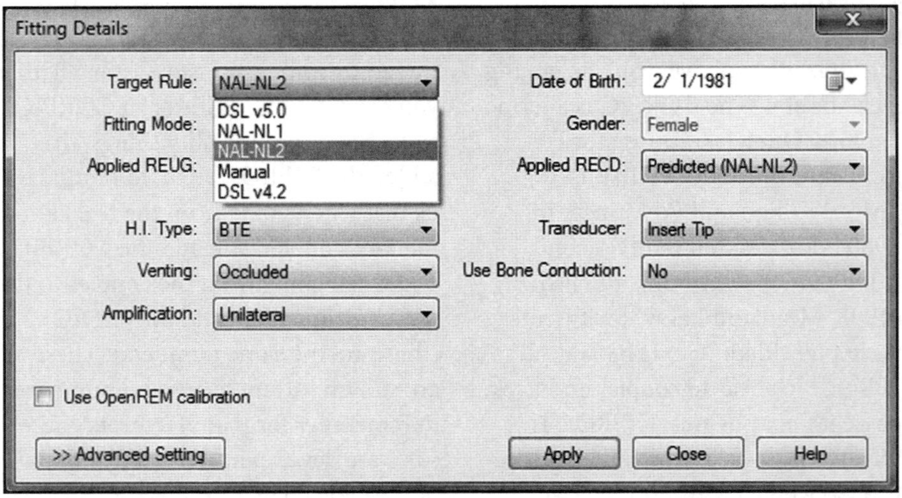

Figure 2–8. Example of prescriptive fitting methods available from a drop-down menu of a probe microphone system.

experience, and unilateral versus bilateral fitting (Figure 2–9).

- Once these are selected, you now will have a display on the fitting screen showing the desired targets, typically for three input levels (Figure 2–10).

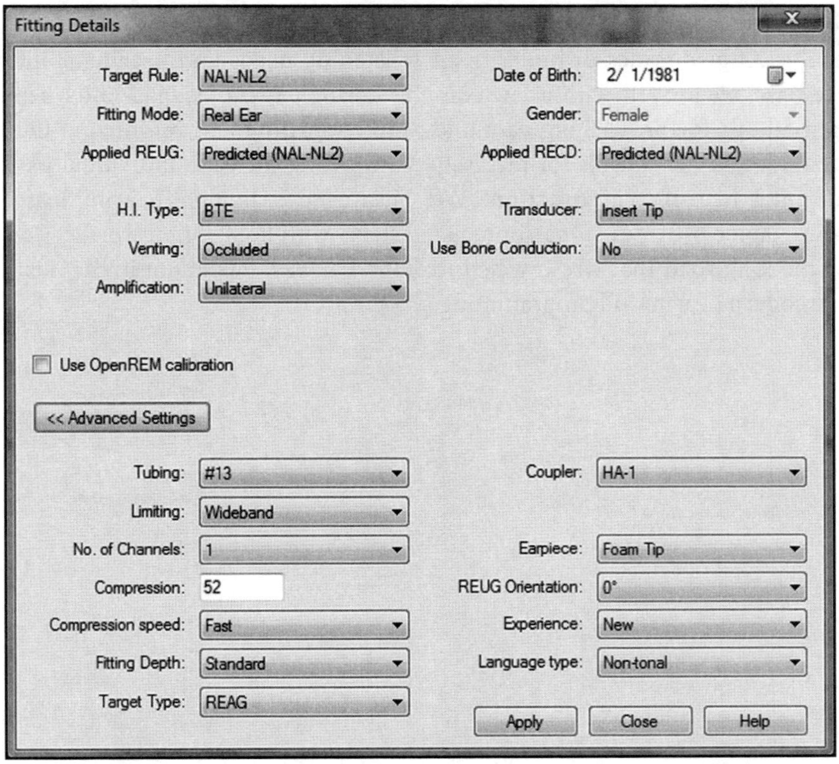

Figure 2–9. Example of patient-specific factors available from a drop-down menu of a probe microphone system.

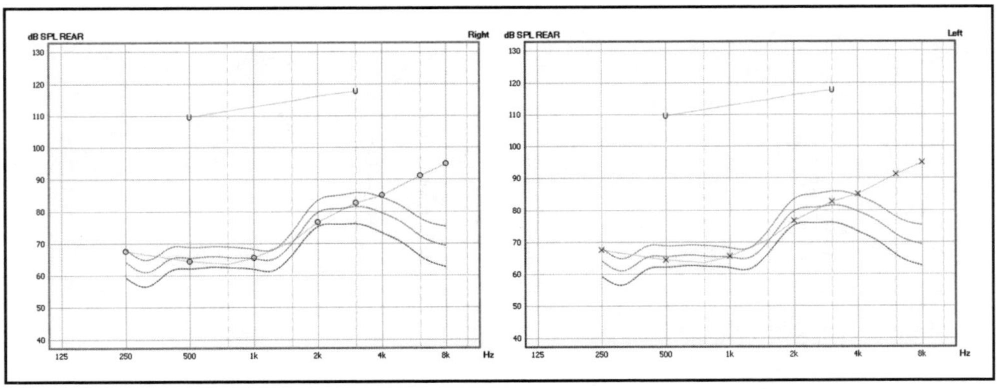

Figure 2–10. Example of screen display showing fitting targets for soft, average, and loud, after patient thresholds, prescriptive method, and patient factors have been entered and selected.

In Closing

We have come a long way from placing various hearing aids on a patient and attempting to choose the best based on word recognition results. After decades of building an evidence base, we are left with a few converging methods for prescribing gain and output, and a myriad of tools for precisely programming hearing aid function. We hope this chapter provides some appreciation for the long road that was traveled to arrive at modern hearing aid programming, and the underlying research evidence that has guided this process. Of course, these are just the basic tools. The true art (and *applied* science) of modern hearing aid fittings is applying what we learned during the hearing aid selection process about the patients listening needs and hearing abilities, considering patient feedback after being fitted, and adjusting and optimizing the hearing aid fitting for each individual patient, not just each individual hearing loss—this all starts with appropriate verification, which is what we'll talk about in the next chapter.

3 Getting Started

Excellence is achieved by mastery of the fundamentals.
—Vince Lombardi

Even if you're not a sports fan, you might have heard of Vince Lombardi, one of the greatest football coaches of all time, most famously with the Green Bay Packers. One of his strengths was assuring that his players were proficient in the fundamentals (blocking, tackling, etc.), as he knew that would carry them through the tough games. While audiologists typically don't participate in tough games, we do sometimes have tough hearing aid fittings, and knowing the fundamentals of our probe microphones measures is critical. The incorrect placement of the patient or the probe tube, or the use of the wrong input signal easily can have a significant effect on the success of the fitting. In this chapter, we review all these basic procedures and techniques, and by the end, you should be ready for the "big game!"

Probe Microphone Equipment

Probe microphone testing was conducted in the laboratory as early as the 1940s (e.g., the classic work of Wiener and Ross, reported in 1946); however, it was not until the late 1970s that a "dispenser-friendly" system was available for testing hearing aids in the real ear. In this case, the term "dispenser friendly," is used somewhat loosely. The late 1970s equipment that we are referring to was first described in a paper that was presented by Earl Harford, Ph.D. in September of 1979 at the International Ear Clinics' Symposium in Minneapolis, Minnesota. At this meeting, Earl reported on his clinical experiences of testing hearing aids in the real ear using a miniature (by 1979 standards) Knowles microphone. The microphone was coupled to an interfacing impedance matching system (developed by David Preves, Ph.D., who at the time worked at Starkey Laboratories), which could be used with existing hearing aid analyzer systems (see Harford, 1980, for review of this early work). Unlike today's *probe-tube* microphone systems, this early method of clinical real-ear measurement involved putting the entire microphone (about 4 mm by 5 mm by 2 mm) in the ear canal down by the eardrum of the patient. If you think cerumen is a problem with probe microphone measurements today, you should have seen the condition of this microphone after a day's work!

While this early instrumentation was a bit cumbersome, we quickly learned the advantages that probe microphone measures provided in the fitting of hearing aids. We frequently ran into calibration and equalization problems, not to mention a yelp or two from the patient, but the resulting information was worth the trouble. In the fall of 1980, at the ASHA convention in Detroit, Michigan, the first paper at a national meeting on this topic was presented by the Walter Reed group of Dan Schwartz, Brian Walden, Gus Mueller, and Rauna Surr.

In the early 1980s, the first computerized *probe-tube* microphone system, the Rastronics CCI-10 (developed in Denmark by Steen Rasmussen), entered the U.S. market (Nielsen & Rasmussen, 1984). This system had a silicone tube attached to the microphone (the transmission of sound through this tube was part of the calibration process), which eliminated the need to place the microphone itself in the ear canal. By early 1985, three or four different manufacturers had introduced this new type of computerized probe microphone equipment, and this hearing aid verification procedure became part of the standard protocol for many audiology clinics.

Due to changes in signal processing in hearing aids, it would be difficult to do even an "okay" job of verifying modern hearing aid gain and output using probe microphone equipment from the 1980s. This primarily is due to the fact that the majority of modern hearing aids use signal processing that provides differing amounts of gain for speech than for non-speech stimuli, as was used in early test equipment (swept-tones was the standard). Fortunately, there have been considerable improvements over the years in probe microphone equipment so that these systems have generally kept pace with changes in hearing aid technology. These improvements include new test signals, signal analysis, special tests for specific hearing aid features and types of processing and portability. Today's equipment certainly has different "looks," ranging from full size and portable clinical units (Figure 3–1, for example), some of which are integrated into a complete audiologic test system (e.g., audiometry, immittance, OAEs, etc.). On the other hand, there are *very* portable systems where the equipment includes a probe microphone assembly and a breakout box

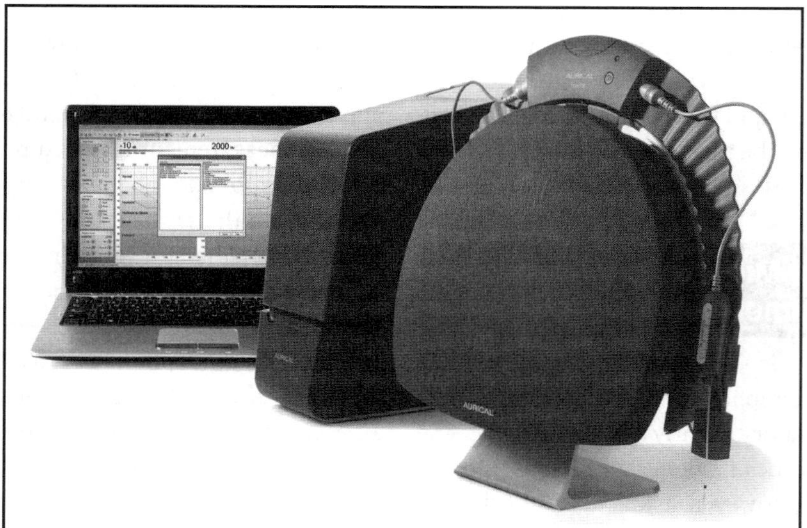

Figure 3–1. An example of complete probe microphone system. Photo courtesy of Otometrics (2017).

that is only slightly more than 3 inches long and plugs into the USB port of your laptop computer. Regardless of the size or the complexity, all of these units have some basic components, and can do the same basic measurements, which have not changed too much since the first Rastronics unit was released in 1982.

Test Signals

While not equipment per se, we will start our discussion with the test signals that are available for the different systems. Some of these are common among all or most manufacturers, others are unique to a particular system. Test signals can be categorized into three types:

- Signals that are intended to be used to verify validated prescriptive gain targets for speech inputs;
- Signals that are intended to test the operation or provide quality control for specific features, including maximum power output (MPO) and
- Signals that are intended to be used for demonstration or counseling purposes.

It should be noted that there is considerable overlap of these categories and some signals can be useful in multiple ways. Consequently, we may mention specific signals more than once as we discuss each of these three categories in turn. As shown in Figure 3–2, all of these signals are easy to access from a drop-down menu in the system software. Additionally, the equipment can be configured so that different test signals are automatically selected when a given test is chosen—the International Speech Test Signal (ISTS) could be automatically selected for target verification, whereas swept pure-tone signals would be selected for the REAR85.

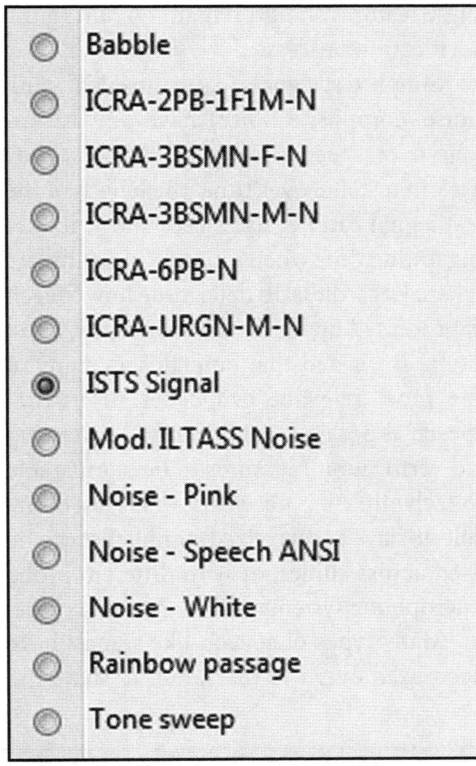

Figure 3–2. Example partial listing of test signals available from a test system, all easily accessed via a drop-down menu.

Prescriptive Target Verification

As we discussed previously, the most important goal of most validated prescriptive fitting methods is to provide optimal levels of speech. It is therefore imperative that signals used for verification of prescriptive targets are categorized as speech by the specific hearing aid processing being evaluated. Otherwise, the concurrent processing of DNR or feedback cancellation, for example, may indicate gain and output values that are not realized in a speech-laden environment. Moreover, because it is often desirable to test the instruments in their *use settings*, these features should remain *on* during the verification process.

Simple test signals (e.g., sinusoidal, pink noise, composite noise) have one advantage over speech, however. Because they are often stable over time, the length of the test signal can be made very short, reducing testing time when multiple measures are taken. Regardless, to determine how speech is processed by modern hearing aids, a test signal is needed that emulates as many of the most relevant properties of natural speech as possible. Additionally, for hearing aid verification measures to be comparable to each other, it is necessary, or at least desirable, to have standardized stimuli that can be used across clinics, or with different probe microphone systems within the same clinic.

Many types of speech-like signals have been used over the years, but all share the common feature of being *speech weighted.* That is, the signal is shaped (filtered) to match that of some LTASS. Some of the most simple signals used are speech-weighted steady-state noise or a rough approximate, such as Pink or Brown noise (Pink and Brown noise decrease in level at a rate of 3 dB and 6 dB per octave, respectively, when compared to white noise). Slightly more complex than these simple signals is a combination of pure tones, such as the composite noise provided by Frye Electronics in the early days, to simulate the speech spectrum. This stimulus was a speech-weighted composite of multiple (79) pure-tone signals, which are continuously presented in unison. As we will discuss, however, this stimulus did not have other characteristics of actual speech, and has been replaced by most probe equipment manufacturers by the real thing.

CLINICAL CONCEPT: The Effect of Vocal Effort on the Long-Term Average Speech Signal (LTASS)

The characteristic pattern for average vocal effort reveals a peak around 500 Hz and a spectral slope (drop in level across frequency) of about 9 dB/ octave. However, this shape is affected by vocal effort. Most studies have suggested that the spectral slope is slightly steeper for soft and average vocal effort and becomes flatter as speech level increases. The frequency range of the spectral peak is also higher for shouted speech than lower vocal effort levels. If you record shouted speech and play it at the same level as soft speech, one of the most striking (and perhaps surprising) features is that the shouted speech has a higher apparent pitch. While some probe microphone manufacturers apply the same spectral shape regardless of testing levels, others apply the level appropriate shaping based on published LTASSs. Based on reanalysis of published data, some probe microphone manufacturers have removed the distinction between *soft* and *average* vocal effort and only apply a different spectrum for *loud* and/or *shouted* vocal effort levels (for examples of specific levels, see Table 3–1). If you are curious regarding the signals of the probe microphone system that you are using, you could simply place probe module on the ear (anyone's ear will do), place the probe tip at the opening of the reference microphone (as you do for calibration), and then record the speech signal for different input levels.

Table 3–1. The LTASS level at octave frequencies for various vocal efforts as measured using spectral, 1/3 octave, and octave measurement bandwidths

		Vocal Effort				
Frequency	***Bandwidth***	***Soft***	***Normal***	***Raised***	***Loud***	***Shouted***
	S. Level	—	34.75	38.98	41.55	42.50
250	1/3 octave	48.00	52.38	56.61	59.18	60.13
	Octave	—	57.25	61.48	64.05	65.00
	S. Level	—	34.27	40.15	44.85	49.24
500	1/3 octave	50.00	54.88	60.76	65.46	69.85
	Octave	—	59.77	65.65	70.35	74.74
	S. Level	—	25.01	33.86	42.16	51.31
1000	1/3 octave	42.00	48.65	57.50	65.80	74.95
	Octave	—	53.52	62.37	70.67	79.82
	S. Level	—	17.32	25.32	34.39	44.32
2000	1/3 octave	40.00	43.96	51.96	61.03	70.96
	Octave	—	48.84	56.84	65.91	75.84
	S. Level	—	11.55	20.15	28.21	38.13
3000	1/3 octave	33.00	40.18	48.78	56.84	66.76
	Octave	—	—	—	—	—
	S. Level	—	9.33	16.78	25.41	34.41
4000	1/3 octave	32.50	38.96	46.41	55.04	64.04
	Octave	—	43.86	51.31	59.94	68.94

Source: Adapted from ANSI S3.46, 1997.

AUDIOID: Why Did Joe Take the Shoe Bench Out?

When we think of research regarding average speech, we simply can't ignore the sentence: "Joe took father's shoe bench out; she was waiting at my lawn." This is considered the shortest balanced passage, and was used for decades for acoustic research. Its use at Bell Labs goes back to at least the 1920s, although there is no record of who invented it. The most notable scientist from this group was Harvey Fletcher, who was employed there from 1916 to 1948. While the work of Dr. Fletcher in speech acoustics is widely known, it is not as commonly known that in 1907, while a student at BYU, he was involved in the design of the "Y" on the mountainside overlooking Provo, Utah (today referred to a "Y Mountain"). He was one of three university students who climbed the mountain to site the 322 by 120-foot landmark.

By the mid-to-late 1990s, it became clear to manufacturers of probe microphone equipment that more realistic test signals were needed because of early types of digital noise reduction processing in hearing aids. This processing commonly operates by providing less gain for signals that have amplitude modulations that are either faster or slower than those associated with speech signals.

Some of the earliest modified signals included those termed DigiSpeech, Dynamic Roving Tone, Digital Speech in Noise, and Modulated Speech Noise. In general, these signals were developed by applying the overall amplitude modulations that mimic speech to speech-weighted noise, randomly interrupting composite noises, or speech weighted noises (e.g., pulsing the signal off and on a few times a second at rates similar to speech modulations), or presenting short pulses of pure tones that *hop* in a semi-random fashion over the frequency range of speech. When examined as a group, the levels of these pure tones are speech weighted.

While some of these signals are still in use, increasingly modern hearing aids are better than ever at differentiating speech from non-speech signals. Consequently, some very sophisticated digital noise reduction schemes will classify at least some of these earlier test signals as noise (e.g., Scollie & Seewald, 2002). Another problem arises with test signals that have tonal components. In some cases, the hearing aid identifies tonal portions of the test signal as feedback, which the feedback suppression algorithm then attempts to cancel. In general, modern hearing aids typically apply compression and include adaptive characteristics that are applied based on signal analysis and classification. Consequently, they process speech much differently than nonspeech signals like sine waves and unmodulated noise.

In a further step to be even more speech like, ICRA signals (pronounced *eye-crah* in the U.S., *eek-rah* in Europe) were developed (Dreschler, Verschuure, Ludvigsen, & Westermann, 2001). The ICRA is an acronym for International Collegium of Rehabilitative Audiology, an international group of hearing aid researchers, and the signals were prepared by a mostly European working group dubbed Hearing Aid Clinical Test Environment Standardization (HACTES). The signals were developed by beginning with real-speech signals. Then a process of filtering into three bands, reversing some segments (called *Schroeder* processing), recombination of the bands, and smoothing of the spectrum was applied. This process resulted in noise signals that have the same modulation properties as the original speech in each of the three bands, but are completely unintelligible and have flat spectra. Spectral shaping was then applied to this modulated noise to reflect the appropriate level and shape of a variety of materials. In total, nine different ICRA signals are available, reflecting single or multiple talkers of both genders for different vocal effort levels (normal, raised, loud). A number of probe microphone manufacturers include ICRA signals, but whereas ICRA signals share many characteristics with speech, they are not without criticism or problems. Most importantly, they lack speech-like co-modulation characteristics (e.g., fundamental frequency) and are often classified by hearing aid algorithms as *noise* not *speech*. Hence, they are not commonly used by clinicians for hearing aid verification.

Of course, the most speech-like signal is speech itself. Recordings of a single talker (or one talker at a time) shaped to the desired LTASS are now used in some probe microphone systems. While recordings of real-speech signals have exceptional face validity, speech within any frequency range fluctuates greatly in level and the spectrum changes as a function of phonemic content, co-articulation and a variety of other fac-

> ### *TIPS AND TRICKS: Obtaining the ICRA Noises?*
>
> The ICRA noises can be obtained on Compact Disc from W. Dreschler, AMC University Hospital, Amsterdam, Holland. There is a nominal fee intended solely to cover the costs of shipping. No copyright is claimed and the CD can freely be copied. The noise files can also be downloaded from several websites, such as http://www.ICRA.nu, or by entering the term "ICRA noise" into your favorite search engine.

tors presents some challenges. To obtain a stable repeatable output measure across the wide range of gain processing available in response to the desired input spectrum is not entirely trivial and sometimes requires compromises such as making measurements over wider frequency ranges and the use of test signals that are longer in duration than the steady-state signals used in testing. That is, it is common for speech test stimuli to be several (10 to 60) seconds long in order to obtain a stable and repeatable measure. It is assumed that at least a 10-second sample of speech is needed to provide a reliable LTASS measure—some manufacturers allow you to determine the length of the speech sample using software adjustment which then becomes the default duration for each test condition. As we discuss later in this chapter, longer signals may be necessary for some types of gain processing, such as compression processing with very long time constants. The average levels, as well as the output dynamic range, for a single vocal effort (e.g., speech banana) of the speech signal over the entire duration of the signal can be calculated and displayed as shown in Figure 3–3.

Depending on the test equipment, speech signals may be available for male and female talkers as well as a child speech sample. These single talker samples may be shaped to multiple standard LTASSs to reflect conditions such as different vocal effort levels (casual, loud, shouted) or may remained unshaped (commonly no shaping is applied to child talkers). A specific LTASS shaping, however, must be applied for accurate verification of validated hearing aid fitting procedures if that shape was also used in generating prescriptive output targets. Most systems will guide you regarding the preferred input signal for target verification. For some shapes, there may not be fitting targets available.

One criticism of real-speech signals, even those that are shaped, is that they represent one specific language and gender. We think this is probably fine for the purposes of verification as most validated prescriptive gain procedures derive their targets for a specific LTASS shape, one gender at a time, and derived from a single language. The work of Byrne et al. (1994) revealed that the differences among gender and different languages are not as great as we might think.

In the interest of comparing hearing aid behavior in a more generalizable way, the International Speech Test Signal (ISTS) was developed (Holube, Fredelake, Vlaming, & Kollmeier, 2010). The goal of its development was to create a reproducible, standard test stimulus that included as many of the relevant properties of speech as possible, including average speech spectrum, modulation spectrum, variation of the fundamental frequency together with appropriate harmonics, and the co-modulation in different frequency bands.

The ISTS was created by segmenting (into 500-ms units) and then splicing back together the recordings of female speakers reading the internationally known passage, "The North Wind and the Sun," in six different languages (American English, Arabic,

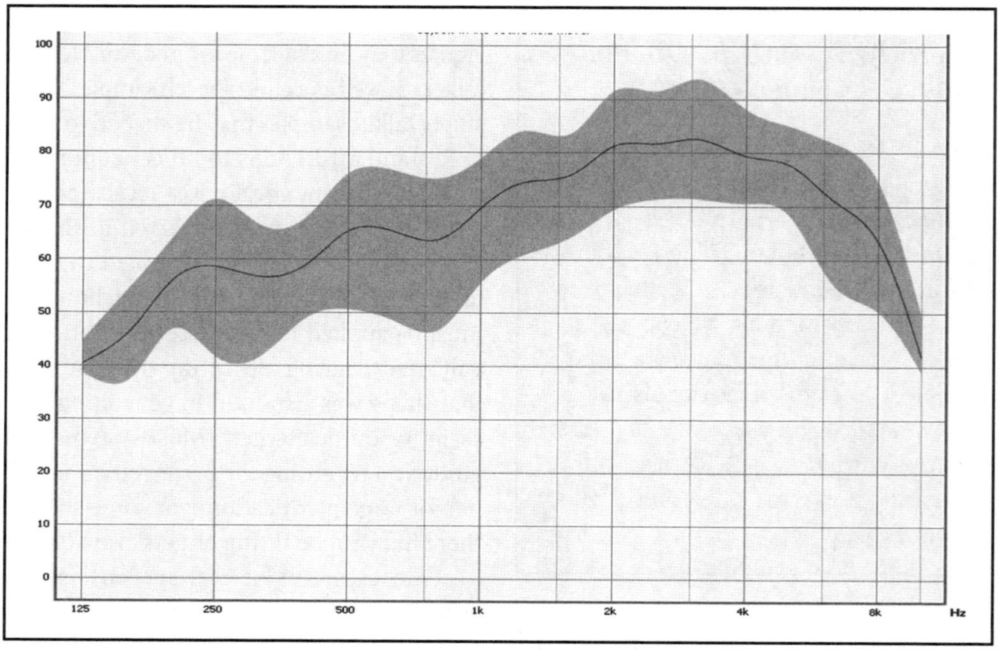

Figure 3–3. Display of the real-ear amplified output for the ISTS, including the 30th to 99th percentiles (i.e., the "speech banana).

> ### *TIPS AND TRICKS: The LTASS and Prescriptive Fitting Approaches*
>
> Although similar, several different speech spectra are used in clinical audiology and the fitting of hearing aids. It is of note that the two primary fitting algorithms, the National Acoustic Laboratories Nonlinear version 2 (NAL-NL2), and the Desired Sensation Level version 5.0a (DSL v5.0a) assume different speech spectra, as discussed in Chapter 2.
>
> - NAL-NL2: The development of the NAL-NL1 and NL2 algorithms has been based on the assumed input signal represented by the one-third-octave levels of the international long-term average speech spectrum (ILTASS) published by Byrne et al. in 1994.
> - DSL v5.0a: The evolution of the DSL fitting scheme has focused on placement of one-third octave speech levels at a desired sensation level for a given hearing loss. The actual values for that speech are an average of male/female/child recordings of speech obtained 30 cm in front of the talker and recordings taken at ear level of the child. The LTASS used is based on that recommended by Cox and Moore (1988).

Chinese, French, German, and Spanish). Because of splicing and segmentation, the ISTS is largely unintelligible. The final reassembled signal was then filtered to match the average female LTASS as described by Byrne et al. (1994). The resulting ISTS has been lauded for its speech-like characteristics including a realistic 20 to 30 dB

CLINICAL CONCEPT: Modifying Signals for Testing FM Systems

We mention that speech signals are often shaped for use with probe microphone measures. This could be related to male versus female versus child, or for vocal effort. With some probe microphone systems, the signals are additionally shaped to be used in the fitting of FM systems (FM only). The 84 dB SPL level and appropriate spectrum may be applied for a chest microphone location or a 93 dB SPL level and appropriate spectrum for a boom microphone location.

POINTS TO PONDER: What Needs to Be Considered to Develop a Good Speech Test Signal?

Given that the ISTS is becoming the most widely used input signal for probe microphone systems, you might be interested in the overall goals that were stated by the developers. They articulated 15 requirements based on available test signals and knowledge of natural speech. Of these, the eleven requirements deemed most clinically relevant are listed here:

1. The ISTS should resemble normal speech but should be nonintelligible.
2. The ISTS should be based on six major languages, representing a wide range of phonological structures and fundamental frequency variations.
3. The ISTS should be based on female speech and should deviate from the ILTASS for females by no more than 1 dB.
4. The ISTS should have a bandwidth of 100 to 16,000 Hz and an overall RMS level of 65 dB.
5. The dynamic range should be speech-like and comparable to published values for speech (Byrne et al., 1994; Cox, Matesich, & Moore 1988).
6. The ISTS should contain voiced and voiceless components. Voiced components should have a fundamental frequency characteristic of female speech.
7. The ISTS should have short-term spectral variations similar to speech (e.g., formant transitions).
8. The ISTS should have modulation characteristics similar to speech (Plomp, 1984).
9. The ISTS should contain short pauses similar to natural-running speech.
10. The ISTS stimulus should have a 60-second duration, from which other durations can be derived.
11. The stimulus should allow for accurate and reproducible measurements regardless of signal duration.

dynamic range, as well as having relatively natural combinations of voiced and voiceless speech segments.

There is at least one clinical disadvantage to this stimulus: the ISTS is somewhat longer than other speech samples with the original signal at 60 seconds long. If the entire sample is used, this can make probe microphone verification more cumbersome when multiple adjustments are made followed by repeated verification. However, shorter 10- and 15-second versions are commonly being used by clinicians to move through the process more efficiently. Generally, we find that to be adequate, as long as the impact of the signal processor can be accurately measured with the shorter durations. However, when fitting a hearing aid with long time constants (for example, with slow attack and release times, or slow acting noise suppression), a 10- or 15-second stimulus may not be sufficient to capture the characteristics of the hearing aid output when fully engaged, although we usually only are talking about differences of 1 to 2 dB or so.

In Figure 3–4, we show the LTASS of the ISTS compared with other common spectra used in hearing aid fittings. It is clear that there is little difference (2 to 3 dB) in level in the 250 to 4000 Hz range across samples.

The ISTS is copyrighted and belongs to the European Hearing Instrument Manufacturers Association (EHIMA). However, it is free and available for download at: http://www.ehima.com for use in the field of hearing aid testing. For use in other fields, permission must be obtained from EHIMA. It is available on most all probe microphone equipment.

Dynamic Range of Speech. The dynamic range for a single vocal effort—often referred to as the speech "banana"—is traditionally displayed by the distribution of one-third-octave band levels calculated for short time periods (120 to 128 ms). The level in each band that is exceeded only by 1% of the total number of samples is commonly referred to as the 99th percentile and is representative of the speech maxima. For long samples of speech, this level is about 12 dB above the

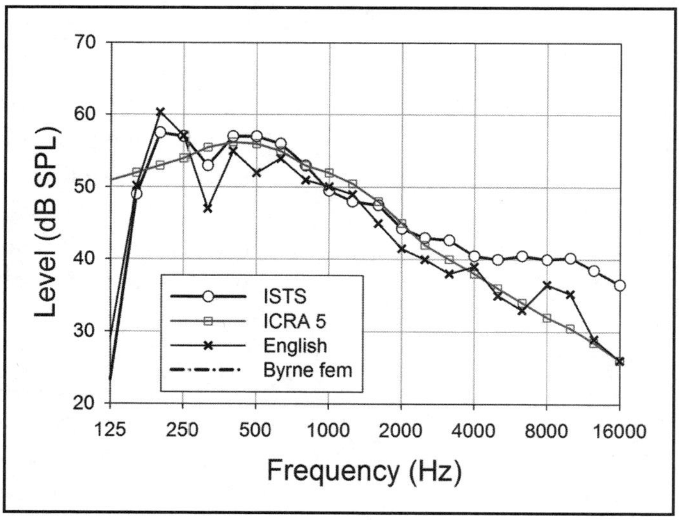

Figure 3–4. Long-term average spectrum of the ISTS (*circles*), the ICRA-5 signal (*squares*), the American-English speaker (*crosses*), and the international spectrum for female speech taken from Byrne et al. (1994) (*dashed line*), not visible because of its coincidence with the ISTS. Adapted from Holube et al., 2010

LTASS. The level that is exceeded by 70% of the total number of samples is commonly referred to as the 30th percentile and is representative of the speech minima. For long samples of speech, this level is about 18 dB below the LTASS.

Several probe microphone manufacturers not only display the approximate average (50th or 65th percentile) output or gain levels for single talker speech, ISTS and/or ICRA test signals, but also give some indication of this range (typically the percentile dependent real-ear output or gain levels for the 99th and 30th percentiles). This dynamic range information (sometimes referred to as *percentile analysis*) can be very useful in two ways: (1) reminding us of the effect of the compression on the banana and (2) reminding us that even in cases when the speech information present at *average levels* fall at or slightly below a listener's thresholds, considerable speech information may still be accessible to the listener. Refer back to Figure 3–3. In this example, the ISTS was presented at 65-dB SPL input, with the hearing aid set to the patient's preferred listening level (after initial verification to NAL-NL2 targets). The top curve of this range is the level exceeded 1% of the time (speech peaks), the lower curve is the level exceeded 70% of the time (speech valleys). The middle curve (dark line) is the average (LTASS).

The percentile analysis developed for the ISTS is similar. As described by Holube (2015), the 30th percentile represents the soft parts of speech, the 65th percentile is similar to average speech and the 99th percentile describes the peaks of speech. Note that both of these analyses use the 30th percentile, not the 1st percentile, as the latter one would be much more dependent on background noise in the measurement condition (and relatively impossible to measure given the noise floor in most test environments). The difference between the 99th and the 30th percentile, then, describes the dynamic range or *banana* of the particular speech signal. Holube (2015) provides examples of this ISTS analysis, shown in Figure 3–5, panels A and B. Shown in these examples are the LTASS and the percentile analysis for the ISTS for the output of the same hearing aid set to two different input compression settings. Notice how the range of the amplified signal (30th to 99th percentile) is different and even the LTASS changes somewhat. The left panel is a fast-acting compressor that reduces the speech range more than the slow-acting compressor in the right panel. This relates directly to our discussion of fitting to prescriptive target, which we'll be getting to in Chapter 4. If the patient has a small dynamic range, and your goal is to "squash the banana" with input compression, your match to target for a range of input levels likely will be better using a fast release time.

Percentile analysis is an excellent method to observe how the processing of the hearing aid impacts the speech signal. The differences in output for slow- versus fast-acting amplitude compression, for example, can easily be observed. Unfortunately, some audiologists think of this as more or less a "fitting method"—that is, a replacement for using the NAL-NL2 or DSL 5.0 validated prescriptive targets. It isn't. In stark contrast to what has been found during the validation of current popular prescriptive methods, some clinicians mistakenly believe that the goal of the fitting is to make all of the speech as audible as possible (e.g., the 30th percentile should be at or above the patient's threshold). Where this is usually an issue is in the higher frequencies, as most hearing losses we are fitting are downward sloping. This is certainly *NOT* an approach that we would recommend, and here are two reasons why (see Mueller, 2017):

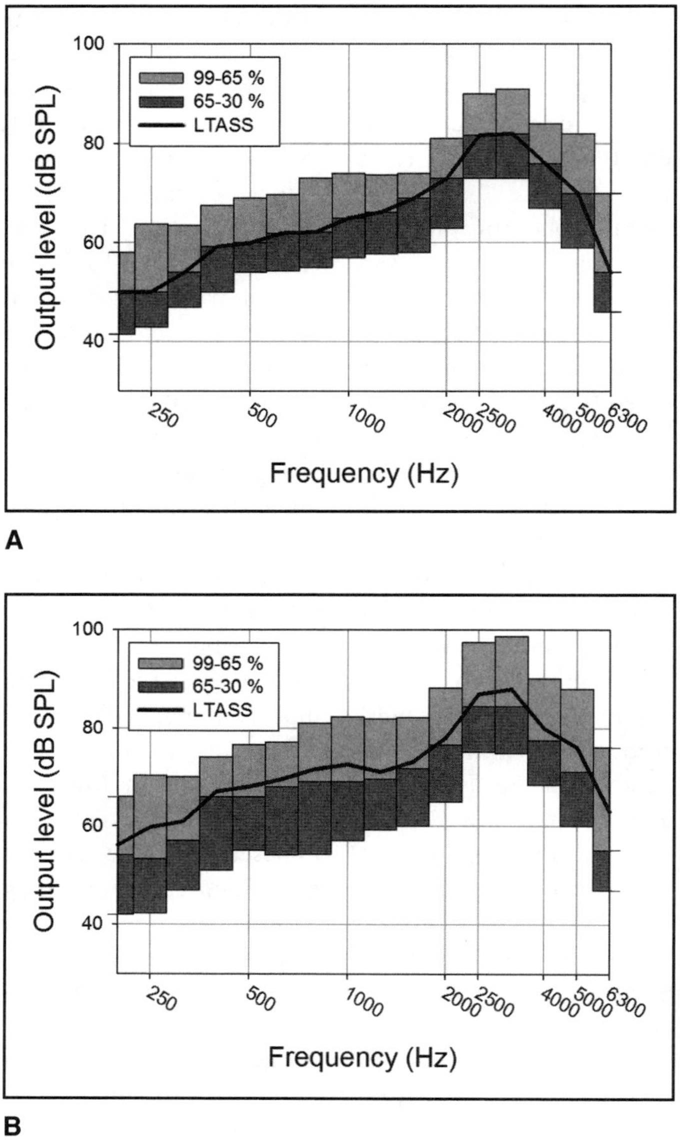

Figure 3–5. Percentile analysis of the output of two different hearing aids, with short (**A**) and long (**B**) release times. The overall gain of the instrument was not altered, only the time constants. Adapted from Holube, 2015.

- Each hearing aid user has a "preferred loudness" level. When we are shaping the frequency response, we have to decide where we obtain the best "bang-for-our-buck" regarding loudness. If we add considerable high frequencies, we likely will exceed the loudness limit, and the patient will turn down gain. However, it is not possible for them to just turn down gain for the highs, so this will result in less audibility for all the lower frequencies too. For most hearing losses, we would not want to sacrifice audibility at 2000 Hz for audibility at 4000 Hz.

- For all hearing losses, and in particular downward sloping cochlear hearing losses, there is a point of "effective audibility" (see Ching, Dillon, Katsch, & Byrne, 2001, for review). Audibility beyond that point no longer has a significant impact on speech recognition, and, in fact, can make speech understanding worse.

Test Signals for Evaluation of Specific Features

Several special test signals are included in probe microphone systems to test special hearing aid features. While the speech-like signals described in the previous section can be useful for testing certain hearing aid features such as the functioning of a hearing aid's feedback suppression system (e.g., additional gain before feedback or maximum gain/output before feedback), or quality control testing of the directional microphone system (e.g., front-to-back or front-to-side ratio), other special test signals often are needed to test features when the behavior for speech inputs is not of interest.

Evaluation of a hearing aid's MPO is one example of testing that often is completed with other types of signals. Specifically, warble tones, a pure-tone sweep, or bursts of pure tones are commonly used for evaluation of the MPO. These tonal signals are usually presented at either 85 or 90 dB SPL, referred to as the real-ear aided response (REAR) for these levels (REAR85 or REAR90). The maximum output of the hearing aid will be higher using a tonal input than with a broadband signal. This 15 to 20 dB higher output when a pure tone is used rather than a complex signal provides a good "worst case scenario," which is the very reason why it is used (see Chapter 5 for more details).

Since digital noise reduction processing is aimed at reducing the level of non-speech signals, it provides another example of when signals that *are* speech-like do not work very well. Many other signals, however, are available for evaluation of noise reduction processing ranging from steady-state-noise (e.g., pink, white, brown), to composite noise, to recordings of specific environmental noises (vacuum cleaners, air conditioners, airplanes), to recordings of music signals (Figure 3–6 provides a partial listing of some test signals, available from a pull-down menu from one manufacturer). Typically, these signals are available over a range of levels so the level specific behavior of the noise reduction processing can be accurately evaluated (e.g., the strength of the noise reduction often varies as a function of the intensity of the input signal).

Probe microphone manufacturers also sometimes attempt to distinguish themselves by introducing signal types for evaluation of specific features or outcomes that are not widely adopted or are novel to a specific manufacturer. At least one probe

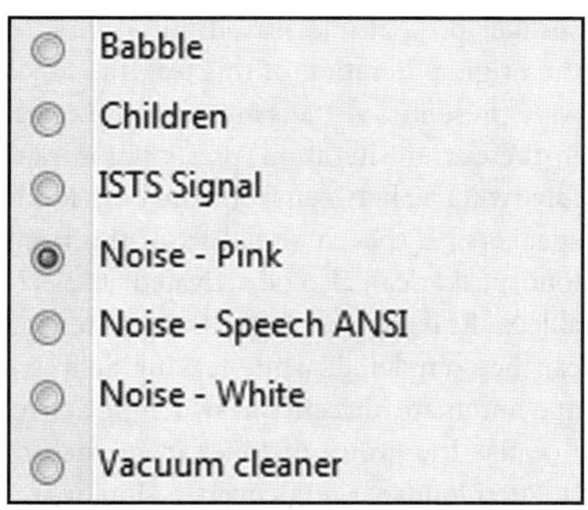

Figure 3–6. Example of different noise signals that are available for DNR testing, all easily accessed via a drop-down menu.

microphone system has narrow-band noise signals that can be used for aided loudness verification, both aided and unaided. While loudness contour measures were advocated for hearing aid fittings in the 1990s when fitting methods related to loudness normalization were popular, these methods are seldom used anymore (we think with good reason). That said, aided loudness verification continues to be useful for ensuring a patient's threshold of discomfort is not exceeded, and for the occasional patient who exhibits a very unusual loudness growth pattern necessitating changes to a standard fitting. For example, we have seen a few patients, who despite having a residual dynamic range of 50 dB, exhibited a most comfortable loudness level that was only 10 dB or so below their LDL. It is very convenient to conduct this aided MPO verification with the patient sitting at the probe microphone equipment, as calibrated signals are redily available.

One other type of testing that has been introduced is a special directional technology verification test, which presents interleaved pure tones from two loudspeakers. This test can be completed in the test box or using probe microphone equipment. In either case a "front" or a "back" loudspeaker present interleaved pure tones. In the original iteration of this test, the tones were presented at the same time; however, in the current iteration, presentation rapidly switched between front and back loudspeakers. A speech signal from the front loudspeaker can also be activated at selectable SNRs during testing so that this testing can be completed, while leaving adaptive and automatic directional switching active. Because the group of tones from each of the two loudspeakers covers a similar frequency range, but are not of exactly the same frequencies, it is possible to display the real-ear response for each loudspeaker position separately. Shown in Figure 3–7 is a screen display of the directional measurement. The top curve represents the output from the test signal from the front, while the lower curve represents the output from the test signal from the back. In this case, we would say the directional microphone is working well!

Another special type of signal that we will discuss is aimed at assessing frequency-lowering technologies. As we'll discuss in Chapter 5, traditional speech mapping with a signal such as the ISTS will reveal that frequency lowering has been activated (reduction in high- frequency output), but is unable to show the location or amplitude of the lowered signal, as it is blended in with the overall output at the frequency region. In an attempt to solve this problem, one probe microphone manufacturer begins with a real-speech signal that has been shaped with the appropriate LTASS for verification of validated prescriptive targets. This signal is then filtered to reduce the level of the one-third-octave bands above 1 kHz by 30 dB with the exception of a single high-frequency one-third-octave band. Three different signals are included with a high-frequency band centered at either 4000 Hz, 5000 Hz, or 6300 Hz. These three signals may be used to determine the amount of frequency shift provided by frequency lowering technology, as well as the average sensation level of the lowered components of the speech signal after averaging over the length of the sentence. Importantly, this is not truly representative of audibility of the speech peaks at these frequencies. While these signals have been in common use for the past few years, there are several limitations, as pointed out in University of Western Ontario (UWO) Protocol for the Provision of Amplification (2014). They cite the following issues:

- The one-third-octave-band is narrower than the frication band of naturally

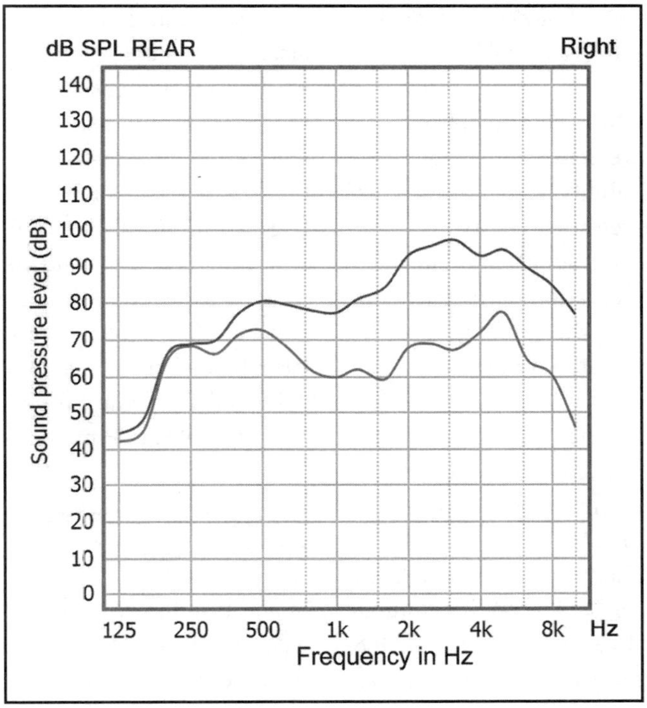

Figure 3–7. Real-ear findings obtained for a directional hearing aid. The top curve is the REAR for the signal from the front, and the bottom curve is the REAR for the signal from the back.

produced speech sounds (e.g., /s/ or /ʃ/). This may lead to a conservative estimate of audibility.

- The one-third-octave-band is presented at the level of the LTASS at the test frequency. This presentation level is slightly lower than the level of /s/ or /ʃ/ would be in speech that is similar to the ISTS passage.
- This test signals available only allow for evaluation to 6300 Hz, while a female /s/ is typically higher in frequency.

More recently, probe microphone manufactures have introduced recorded Ling sounds and excised phoneme sounds for evaluation of frequency lowering technologies. These signals can be quite helpful for evaluation of changes in speech audibility for specific sounds and overlaps and other distortions that can result when applying frequency-lowering technologies too aggressively. The /s/ and /sh/ test signals have been developed by the researchers at UWO, and have been adopted by some of the probe microphone manufacturers. The researchers state that in order to obtain calibrated /s/ and /sh/ signals with fricatives, they extracted these phonemes from the ISTS, measuring each fricative's average spectrum. Synthetic fricatives were then generated that match the observed spectra.

They report that these fricatives fall close to the peaks of speech, and represent average female production of the fricatives. It's important to point out that excised ISTS sound samples are different from the Ling /s/ and /sh/ signals—the latter were developed for threshold testing with children, not for adjustment of frequency lowering. The

UWO group cites the following advantages of using the escised ISTS signals:

- The signal has been calibrated to a consistent level and frequency to improve replicability of measures. This improves test-retest reliability.
- Calibrated speech signals offer an accurate representation of the frication band. This allows the audiologist to estimate hearing aid output of the fricative.
- Measurement of the frication band of /s/ and /ʃ/ allows the audiologist to assess the spectral separation (i.e., how far apart do /s/ and /ʃ/ lie in the frequency domain), which is correlated with the listeners' ability to discriminate between these two sounds. In Figure 3–8, we see an example of the /s/ and /sh/ as extracted from the ISTS.

The measurement of the occlusion effect also involves somewhat unique signals, as we describe in more detail in Chapter 5. The most commonly used is the person's own voice—the vocalization of a vowel such as the /ee/, held constant at a determined SPL (e.g., 75 to 80 dB SPL) for a few seconds. Alternatively, the occlusion effect can be roughly assessed by using pure tones (e.g., 250 and 500 Hz) generated by a bone oscillator placed on the patient's head, either delivered from the probe system itself, or by a portable audiometer.

Signals for Demonstration or Counseling Purposes

In addition to verification of validated prescriptive methods, it is sometimes of interest to demonstrate the amount of audibility a listener may have for specific signal types.

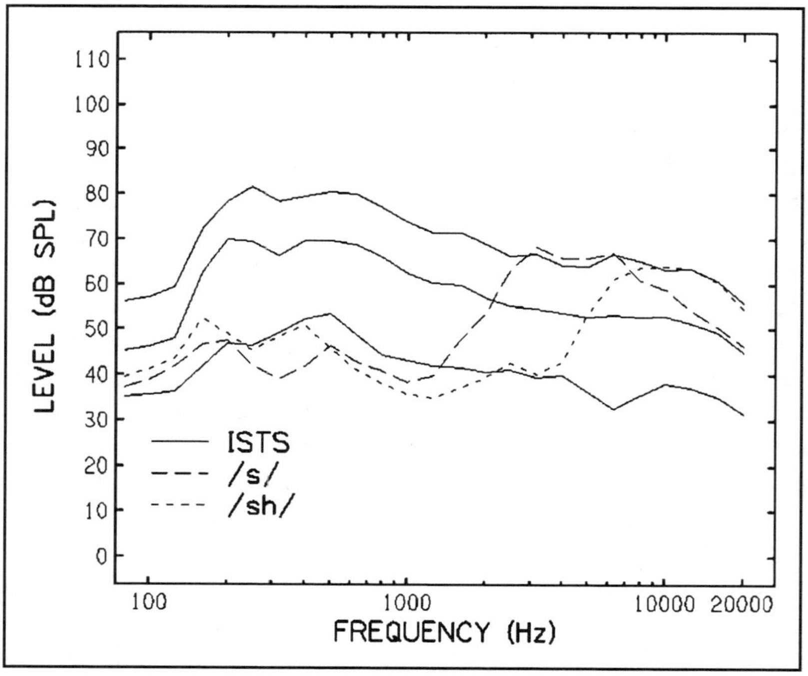

Figure 3–8. Example of the /s/ and /sh/ signal extracted from the ISTS. From the Protocol for the provision of amplification (2014). Reprinted with permission.

For instance, we may want to show a patient how much more of a signal falls above their threshold when aided. Live voice is often used for this purpose. For example, a patient might be shown how much of their spouse's voice they were missing unaided and how much more they hear aided. We can also use this information to counsel a patient that we are not making all sounds audible to them so they will still have some difficulties in some situations. A variety of other recordings that serve this purpose are also available with probe microphone equipment, such as male, female, and child voices produced at various vocal effort levels. Some systems even have speech signals that emulate a patient's own voice with regard to level and frequency shaping. We must emphasize, however, that examining audibility for these speech signals *should not* be viewed as a way to fit hearing aids, or as a guide for adjusting hearing aids (see associated Tips and Tricks). Rather, they can provide useful information for counseling and demonstration purposes, conducted *after* the hearing aids have been programmed correctly using correctly shaped input signals to match validated prescriptive targets.

Earlier, we mentioned the measurement of the effectiveness of the digital noise

TIPS AND TRICKS: Audibility—Just Enough, Not Too Much

Some probe microphone systems calculate the total percentage of audibility. This is commonly referred to as percentile analysis and it can be completed for demonstration signals as well as when completing verification of a validated prescriptive method. Somewhat similarly, other systems calculate the aided Speech Intelligibility Index (aSII) or aided Articulation Index (aAI). Shown in Figure 3–9 is a screen display of the SII following a "fit to target" for the NAL-NL2 for three input levels. Some have suggested that one can use the aided SII to determine when a fitting is "good" or at least "okay." This value will provide some useful information for counseling, but we would hesitate to identify values that could be used to grade a fitting.

We must keep in mind that audibility of *all* speech components is NOT the typical goal of the hearing aid fitting. Full audibility might be achieved by very high levels of gain, amplitude compression and/or frequency lowering. Data have clearly demonstrated, however, that too much gain, frequency lowering or amplitude compression can actually decrease speech recognition even when it also results in more of the speech signal being audible (e.g., Souza, Arehart, Kates, Croghan, & Gehani, 2013, and Davies-Venn, Souza, Brennan, & Stecker, 2009). While audibility is clearly important, *maximum* audibility should not be confused with *optimal* audibility. Consequently, percentile analysis and aAI must be interpreted and used with caution. While they both can provide important information, the "more is better" adage is clearly not always the case with these measures. Observe, for example, in Figure 3-9, that while we had a good match to NAL-NL2 targets (you'll have to take our word for it), even for the 75 dB input, the SII is far from 100%.

Legend, Right			
1		SII: 53%	NAL NL2 - 65 (89) dB - ISTS Signal
2		SII: 36%	NAL NL2 - 55 (85) dB - ISTS Signal
3		SII: 63%	NAL NL2 - 75 (94) dB - ISTS Signal

Figure 3–9. Illustration of the automatic SII (AI) calculation conducted by the probe microphone system following REAR testing. Calculations are conducted for each input level tested.

reduction using a non-speech signal. While it is sometimes important to quantify the exact degree of reduction for different frequencies, this also can be a useful demonstration. By using the noise signals that are available with probe microphone systems, we can show patients in real-time, while they are listening, how noise levels will be reduced with noise reduction processing and how gain will be restored when speech is also presented. This also will reveal the time constants of the noise reduction (just watch the screen to see the action!), which also can be helpful for patient counseling. Real-world noise signals are available on most probe microphone equipment.

Presentation Loudspeaker

To conduct probe microphone measures, it is necessary to have a loudspeaker (or maybe even two) to present the test signals. The preferred location of this loudspeaker differs somewhat among manufacturers. All systems recommend loudspeaker placement relatively near the patient (usually within 1 meter/3 feet). While probe microphone verification should be completed in a relatively quiet room, some noise can be tolerated. In order to obtain an accurate measure, however, the noisier the room, the closer the loudspeaker will need to be to the reference microphone, as we discuss later in this chapter.

Mead Killion and Larry Revit wrote an article back in 1987 titled, "You Want Me to Put My Loudspeaker WHERE?" In this article, they examined optimal loudspeaker placement. Because head shadow can effect signal level, and patients can and do move sometimes during testing, they pointed out that the most reliable measure can be obtained by placing the loudspeaker near the ear being tested (around a 45-degree angle), slightly elevated from the horizontal plane of the ear. For this reason, at least one probe microphone system recommends this angle for testing. Three problems with using this angle, however, is that (1) the loudspeaker (or patient) must be moved to a different position for each of the two ears or two separate loudspeakers must be used; (2) the patient will sometimes want to turn to see the video monitor during testing; and (3) it would not be possible to conduct simultaneous bilateral measures. Consequently, most probe microphone systems forgo the added reliability (about 1 dB) and instead place the loudspeaker directly in front of the patient, sometimes, directly above the video monitor. That is, a 0-degree horizontal and vertical azimuth. At least one other system uses two small and separate loudspeakers that are mounted a few inches from each of the patient's ears. With this high degree of variability in procedures, it is important to consult the user's manual for the specific probe microphone system to ensure the recommended loudspeaker position is used. A typical loudspeaker placement is shown in Figure 3–10.

One other difference across systems is the quality of the loudspeakers. A small, light loudspeaker is commonly used in smaller and more portable systems. While greatly enhancing portability, such loudspeakers typically have limited output. Depending on the system, it may not be possible to test high speech input levels (greater than 70 or 75 dB SPL) without first adding an external loudspeaker with higher output. The addition of a higher output loudspeaker is possible with some smaller probe microphone systems, but not others.

Monitor, Reference, or Regulating Microphone

Each probe microphone system has a microphone at the ear that is used to monitor the test signal. You will hear it referred to as the controlling microphone, reference microphone, regulating microphone, or monitor microphone. This microphone is intended to be near the head and the microphone of the hearing aid. As a result, the regulating microphone usually is located just under the earlobe (Figure 3–11; in this particular case, we maybe could have snugged it up to be a little closer to the ear lobe—something that is easy to adjust). One manufacturer has commonly used a placement just above the ear. The ANSI S3.46-2013 refers to calibration using a reference microphone placed at the ear as the modified-pressure method of equalization, although other types of calibration can be done with a reference microphone. In total, the reference microphone can be used for three different calibration applications:

- Modified-pressure method with concurrent equalization (or just concurrent equalization for short): This measures the stimulus level during the measurement process or to control it

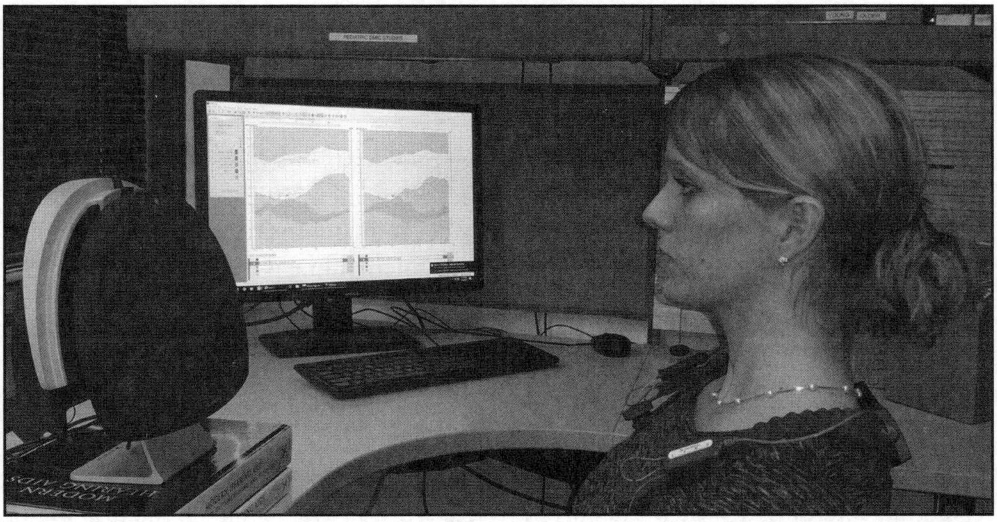

Figure 3–10. Example of patient seated with correct loudspeaker placement for probe microphone measures (e.g., horizontal *and* vertical azimuth of 0 degree).

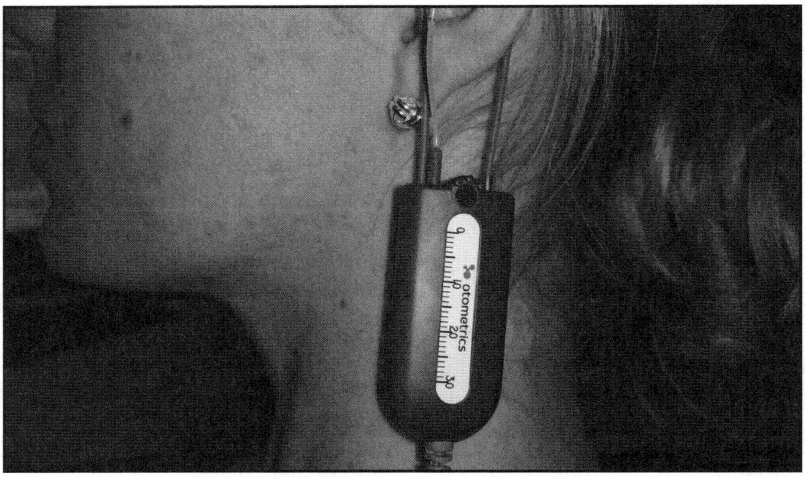

Figure 3–11. Example of typical placement of the reference/monitor microphone—directly below the earlobe.

in the equalization process. Commonly used for all fittings that do not use open coupling.

- Modified-pressure method with stored equalization (or stored equalization for short): The reference microphone is in the test position on the patient and the hearing aid is in place, but equalization is completed with the hearing aid muted. This equalization is stored and then testing begins. Commonly used for open fittings.
- Substitution method of equalization: Equalization is based on data recorded during a prior measurement of the sound field at the position of the patient, but without the patient present. (Note: This method may also be completed concurrently or based on stored data; however, it is rarely used for clinical measures.)

Hawkins and Mueller (1992) reviewed the effects of different placements of the regulating microphone when concurrent equalization was used. The differences were small, especially for the frequencies below 4000 Hz. In general, while the regulating microphone position can affect the frequency response due to body baffle and reflection effects, those differences, for the most part, are accounted for by each individual system. That is, you really don't have to worry about the effects, as long as you place the regulating microphone in the recommended position.

Measurement Microphone

For most probe microphone equipment, the measurement microphone is encased in the same module as the regulating microphone. This microphone is designed so that a silicone probe tube can be attached—hence the name *probe-tube microphone* or *probe microphone*. The probe tube is long enough so that the tip can reach to the patient's eardrum while attached to the microphone—the typical probe tube is about 70 to 75 mm long, with an adapter on the end to allow for attachment to the module. Except for some of the equipment from Fonix, which uses a standard tube that results in a flat frequency response, each probe tube must be calibrated before use. That is, the microphone is equalized for that specific tube, making the tube acoustically invisible. Although this has the disadvantage of an extra calibration step before testing, it has the advantage that different tubes can be used, and the end of a plugged tube can be snipped off, recalibrated, and used again. Of course, tubes should only be reused in the same ear at the same visit to avoid contamination and cross-contamination. Also, with some equipment, cutting the end off and changing the length of the tube could cause some calibration tolerances, and the system will warn you if the tube does not behave acoustically as expected (see later section for specifics on probe-tube calibration).

Signal Analysis

An additional factor that differs across manufacturers is the type of signal analysis used. The analyses differ both with regards to the frequency resolution and the temporal resolution. When a speech stimulus is presented, most systems use a temporal window of 120, 125, or 128 ms. The averaging of these temporal windows occurs over the duration of the stimuli. As mentioned previously, it is common to present the output dynamic range of the speech based on the 99th and 30th percentiles. With regard to frequency resolution, some systems use partial octave analysis (commonly one-twelfth and/or one-third-octave), while others use a Fast Fourier Transform (FFT) which can have a frequency resolution as small as 87 Hz or smaller. One advantage to the greater frequency resolution is that we are able to see very narrow peaks and dips in the frequency response that may be smoothed over using a wider partial octave analysis. Some clinicians may state a preference for the wider analysis band, however, because the representation of a response without narrow peaks will look smoother and prettier. This can be misleading because those peaks are still there! The width of the analysis window also often depends on the test signal. Specifically, whereas narrow windows are sometimes applied for pure tones and steady-state signals, nearly all systems use one-third-octave-wide analysis windows when measuring the hearing aid output for a speech signal to help smooth the multiple fluctuations that occur in natural speech.

Output Display

The display of the testing can be viewed on an external monitor, or with some systems, a screen contained within the equipment itself, or simply the screen of the laptop. Most clinics use a traditional computer monitor for the display, although 42-inch or larger wall-mounted monitors are used in some offices. The larger external displays are great for patient counseling, as the patient becomes more involved with the task at hand (Figure 3–12 is an example). The appearance of the screen usually can be changed to be viewed as a single, full-screen or dual (both ears), side-by-side panels. In some systems, the probe system screen can be viewed in real time with the fitting software, so a single monitor can be used to simultaneously view both fitting and verification. More recently, it has even become possible to view the probe microphone display via a tablet using manufacturer specific Apps. Usually a graphical display is used, but a tabular format sometimes is an option.

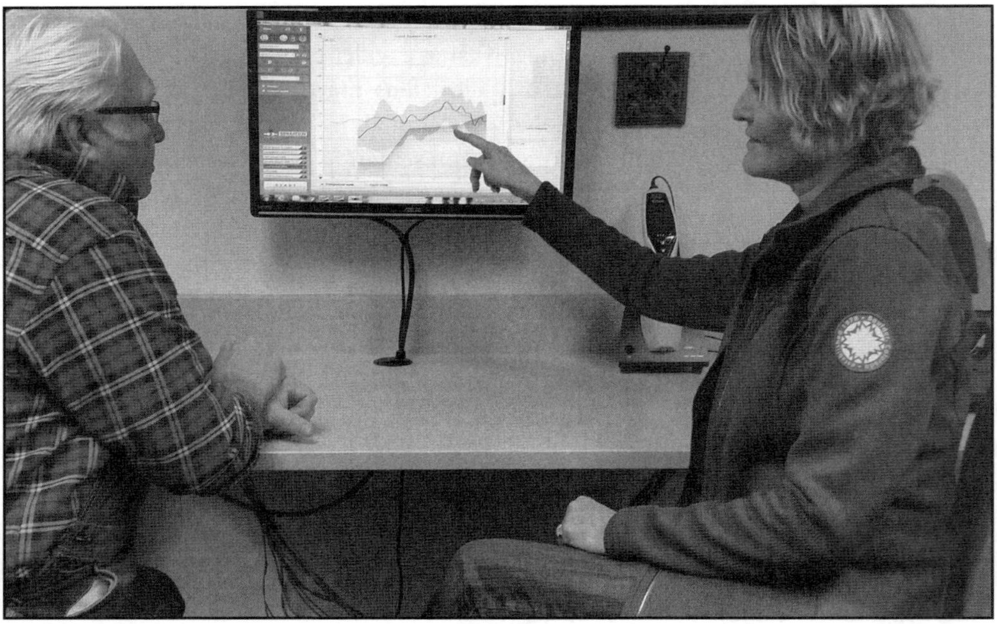

Figure 3–12. Use of a larger monitor to display real-ear findings, which can be useful to facilitate patient counseling.

Monitor Headphones

Although not commonly used, many probe microphone systems have the option of plugging in headphones, so that the audiologist or an interested observer can listen to the output being measured in the ear canal (or coupler during simulated real-ear measurements). "Listening in" can ensure that the processing is smooth, and unwanted distortions are not present, especially useful when frequency lowering is employed. This also can be helpful when troubleshooting patient complaints. It is possible to detect such things as intermittent feedback, and the occlusion effect often will be quite noticeable. One note of caution, however, if the headphones are the loose-fitting inexpensive kind, and the clinician turns the volume up too high, they can provide an additional path for feedback to occur. Consequently, we recommend tighter fitting headphones be used with higher gain open fittings.

Test Procedures and Conditions

Now that we've covered all the components of the probe microphone equipment, it's time to get to work! There are several procedural considerations when conducting probe microphone measures and most of them can influence the test results (see Hawkins & Mueller, 1992, for review). Some "mistakes" can lead to errors of 10 dB or more. It is reasonably easy, however, to follow some simple steps to assure good test validity and reliability.

Introduction to Common Probe Microphone Measures

In Chapter 4, we discuss the different test conditions and measures that can be conducted with the probe microphone equip-

CLINICAL CONCEPT: "Binaural" Analysis with Probe Microphone Measures?

In the promotional advertising from probe microphone manufacturers, you might see mention of *binaural analysis*. First, we believe the term should be *bilateral*, not binaural. Binaural suggests that you are measuring some combined processing of the two ears—such as what we do when we conduct sound-field binaural-aided loudness discomfort measures (see Chapter 6). To assess binaural processing with a probe microphone, however, would require placing the tip of the probe tube somewhere in the low brainstem, around the superior olivary nucleus, which we believe would be an uncomfortable procedure for the audiologist, and even more so for the patient.

So, we are talking about *bilateral* testing.These allow you to hook up a probe microphone assembly to each ear and, at the same time, measure the output in each ear, although we assume that nearly always you will still need to adjust and fit each hearing aid independently. At least one probe microphone manufacturer recommends fitting each ear independently even when in the bilateral analysis mode. This is because bilateral measures create calibration issues related to the reference microphones that will need to be addressed and evaluated in each system before we know that simultaneous hearing aid fitting can be completed reliably—although some unique calibration procedures have been developed. If the patient keeps their head centered and fairly still, you should be okay. These systems do have a slight advantage for the clinician relative to verification of a validated prescriptive method. Rather than moving the assembly to the other ear when you finish the first, you can leave one side hooked up while testing the other. We don't see a specific *measurement* advantage for this type of verification, unless you are using a very long signal presentation, such as the 60-second version of the ISTS—you then might adjust both hearing aids in between measures and test bilaterally.

We should add, however, that with the availability of products having wireless audio data transfer between hearing aids (usually referred to as bilateral or binaural beamforming), there may be an increased interest in bilateral simultaneous measures. Specifically, simultaneous bilateral measurements allow us to quickly confirm that sound transmitted to one hearing aid is being routed to the other, or that signals routed wirelessly from an external source are reaching both hearing aids. Moreover, in the cases when narrow directivity is employed, you can observe how the bilateral processing might impact the output of each ear.

ment. We provide a short introduction here to assist in making sense of the different procedures we will be discussing. The following is a summary of the probe microphone tests included in the ANSI Standard S-3.46-2013. We have also included the primary clinical use of each measure.

- REUR (Real-Ear Unaided Response): SPL as a function of frequency, at a

specified measurement point in the ear canal, for a specified sound field, with the ear canal unoccluded
  - *Primary clinical application: Serves as reference for the calculation of REIG*
- REOR (Real-Ear Occluded Response): SPL as a function of frequency, at a specified measurement point in the ear canal, for a specified sound field, with the hearing aid (and its acoustic coupling) in place and "turned off"
  - *Primary clinical application: Determine the tightness of the coupling in the ear canal*
- REAR (Real-Ear Aided Response): SPL as a function of frequency, at a specified measurement point in the ear canal, for a specified sound field, with the hearing aid (and its acoustic coupling) in place and "turned on"
  - *Primary clinical application: Verification of prescriptive targets, either as absolute values (often referred to as speech mapping), or for the calculation of the REIG*
- REIG (Real-Ear Insertion Gain): Difference in decibels, as a function of frequency, between the REAG and the REUG, taken with the same measurement point and the same sound field conditions
  - *Primary clinical application: Verification of prescriptive targets.*
- REAR85 or REAR90 (Real-Ear Aided Response for an 85 or 90 dB Input). This was previously referred to as Real-Ear Saturation Response (RESR): SPL as a function of frequency, at a specified measurement point in the ear canal, for a specified sound field, with the hearing aid (and its acoustic coupling) in place and "turned on," with the VC adjusted to full-on (or just below feedback if full-on isn't possible). The input signal is sufficiently intense to operate the hearing aid at its maximum output level; usually 85 or 90 dB SPL as noted in the acronym.
  - *Primary clinical application: Determine the real-ear MPO of the hearing aid*
- RECD (Real-Ear Coupler Difference): Difference in decibels, as a function of frequency, between the SPL produced near the tympanic membrane in an occluded ear canal by a coupled sound source having a high acoustic impedance (see ANSI/ASA S1.1) and that which is produced in the HA-1 configuration of the 2-cc-coupler by the same coupled sound source36,37
  - *Primary clinical application: Use with the RETSPL to convert thresholds and thresholds of discomfort from HL to ear canal SPL and to convert output from 2-cc-coupler to real-ear SPL for infants and children*
- REDD (Real-Ear Dial Difference): Difference in decibels, as a function of frequency, between the SPL produced near the tympanic membrane by an audiometric sound source and the hearing level indicated by the audiometer driving the sound source
  - *Primary clinical application: Derive ear canal SPL display of audiometric and prescriptive output data for REAR verification.*

With that brief introduction, we will now review the conditions, techniques, and procedures required to obtain these measures.

Test Environment

In the early days of probe microphone testing, it was fairly common to place the equipment in an audiometric test booth, primarily because audiologists were accustomed to fitting hearing aids in the test booth, going back to the speech testing methods of the 1950s to 1960s, and the popularity of functional gain measures in the 1970s. While it is still acceptable to conduct these measures in the test booth, most audiologists would like to free up this space for other testing, and have established fitting rooms. These fitting rooms typically work well, but there are a couple important points:

- One of the goals of the fitting is determine if we have made soft speech audible. The best way to determine this is to present soft speech that has an input level of 50 or 55 dB SPL. It is possible, if not probable, that if the ambient noise level of some test environments exceed this level (which easily can happen with a loud heating or air conditioning system), the resulting measures will not be valid. Hence, while the test area does not need to be "sound isolated," the room does need to be relatively quiet. An example of how ambient noise can impact the measurement is shown in Figure 3–13. In panel A, the amplified speech—presented at 50 SPL in a quiet room—shows nearly perfect match to the intended targets (crosses). In panel B, you see the results when a low-level noise, such as that of an air conditioner, was added to the room. Observe that the output is clearly altered and the apparent dynamics of the speech signal (i.e., the banana) is compressed as well!
- A second point about the test environment is that the patient should not be seated next to any reflective surface. A common culprit is a wall mirror, which audiologists often have in the fitting room. But any wall or hard surface can generate measurement errors. Softer reflective surfaces, such as well-meaning audiologists can be a problem too, so we need to make sure that we don't stand too close to the patient when the testing is conducted. Sound reflections from nearby surfaces can cause large measurement errors or unusual dips or bumps in the output, especially if stored equalization rather than concurrent equalization is being used (more on that later). With some equipment, standing waves from nearby walls or objects will cause speaker-overdrive errors. We recommend seating the patient so that he is about 2 meters (5 to 6 feet) from any reflective surface. As we mentioned earlier, at least one system conducts a "room calibration" that should help to avoid the situation, or at least alert you that a potential problem exists.

Calibrating the Probe Tube

As we mentioned in our discussion of the measurement microphone, a key player in real-ear measures is the silicone probe tube—we'd be in big trouble without this little $1.50 accessary. Before testing is started, it is necessary to place a new tube on the inlet located on the housing of the reference and measurement microphones. The tube must then be calibrated. The notion is to make the tube acoustically invisible, so that when the tip of the tube is near the ear drum, the measurement is the same as if the microphone itself were in that position. The tubes have natural resonances, and will also roll off the high frequencies, two factors which need to be corrected by the calibration process. While the tubes are machined to be all the same, there can be variances, and we therefore would always recommend doing a new calibration whenever a tube is changed. This usually is for a new patient,

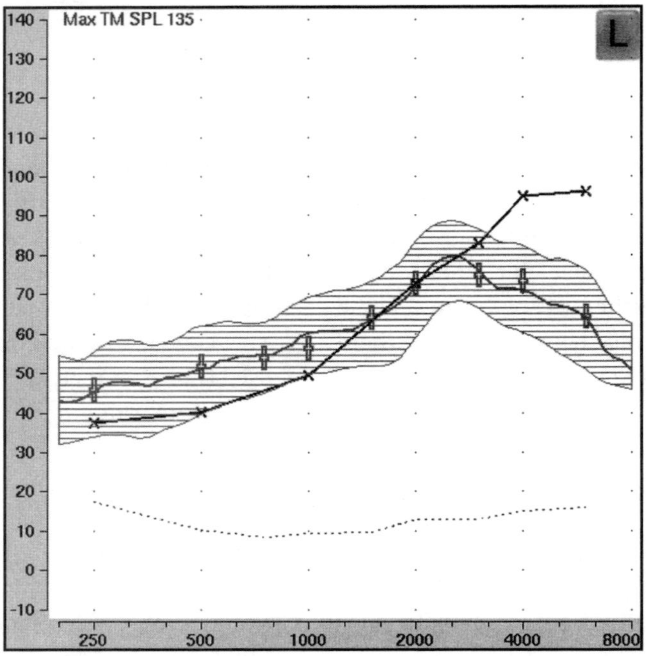

A

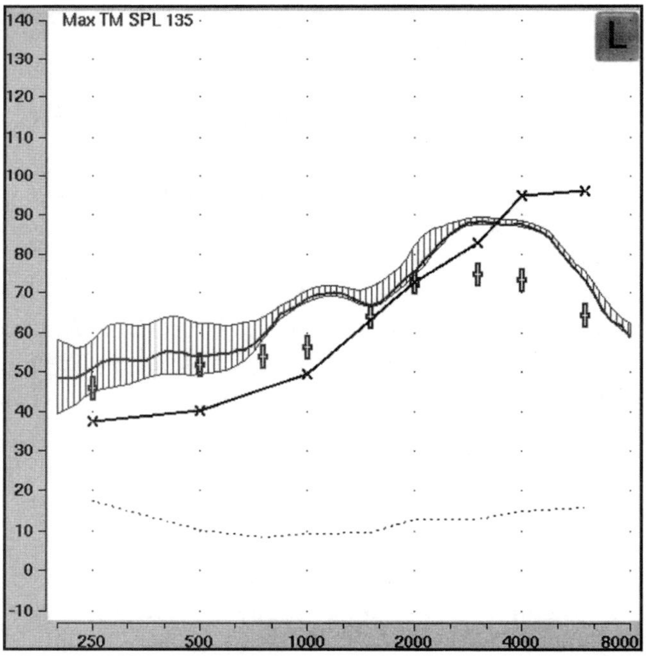

B

Figure 3–13. Measurement results with and without background air-conditioner noise. **A.** The calibrated real-speech signal was presented at 50 SPL in a quiet room. **B.** The same passage was presented but with a low-level (and steady-state) noise in the background.

but if you're fighting gooey cerumen in the ear canal, which plugs the tip of the tube, it could be several times for the same patient.

The probe tubes usually arrive in packs, as illustrated in Figure 3–14A. You simply snap off a new tube. The tubes are around 70 mm long with an adapter on the end. Note from Figure 3–14A, that a movable ring marker has been placed on each tube. The purpose of the marker is to assist in establishing the correct depth placement of the tube tip in the ear canal, which we will discuss in a few pages. It might be tempting to think that the probe-tube manufacturer places the marker at the correct point for testing (e.g., 30 mm from the tip for adult males). This may not be true, however, and certainly isn't for the manufacturer of the tubes shown in Figure 3–14A, which has the marker placed at 35 mm from the tip, a distance which likely would cause a yelp or two from many patients.

To calibrate, place the tip of the tube next to the opening of the reference microphone. Most manufacturers provide a holder/dock for the tube at this location to make the process easier. Once the tube is in place, hold the microphone case with the tube attached at the approximate horizontal/vertical location of where the patient's head will be during testing (see Figure 3–14B). Given that it is a relative measure, the exact distance from the loudspeaker doesn't matter too much, but stay within 3 feet. Some manufacturers recommend facing the reference microphone port toward the loudspeaker, but a grazing angle as shown in Figure 3–14B seems to work just fine too. Once everything is in place, go to the calibration mode of the system and present the calibration signal (predetermined by the manufacturer). For most equipment, you will observe on the monitor the output of the signal that has passed through the tube, which will reveal the acoustic effects we mentioned earlier. At this point you more or less have to have faith that the equipment corrected the variances observed. If you're skeptical, or simply curious, you could go to the fitting screen, present a signal that is equalized across frequencies, hold the probe apparatus in the same calibration position, and you should observe a flat output equal to the input.

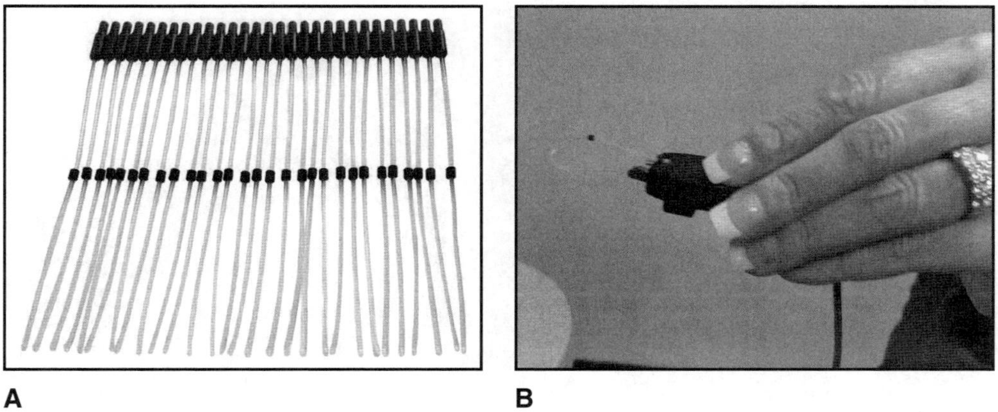

Figure 3–14. A. Typical "pack" of probe tubes as they arrive from the manufacturer. Sleeve markers have yet to be adjusted to correct location. **B**. Probe tube assembly is held in the calibration position.

It is common today to have a right and left probe assembly, which of course means that there are two tubes to calibrate. At least one manufacturer has made this fairly simple, as the probe apparatus can be fixed in a neck yoke, with the tubes fixed at the correct calibration location (see Figure 3-1; the apparatus sitting on top of the loudspeaker). You then can simply hold the yoke at the correct location and both tubes are calibrated simultaneously. The results you will see following this procedure are shown in Figure 3–15. Note that the output falls within the expected range. Although it rarely happens, if it does not fall in this range for a given tube, assume that there is a defect in the tube that will prevent proper calibration, and those tubes get tossed.

Positioning the Patient

To maximize both validity and reliability, it is important to position the patient appropriately relative to the loudspeaker presenting the test signal. Although you might think this would be a simple thing to get right, we have seen the loudspeakers sitting on the floor, pointing at the patient's stomach, or from a shelf three feet above his head. We know of one clinic that placed the speakers at 90 degrees for a monaural fitting, and at a 0-degree azimuth for patient fitted bilaterally! For specific guidance, refer to your probe microphone systems user manual (there are some adjustments needed for special fittings). In general, however, the guideleines are pretty much the same for all manufacturers. Some general rules are:

- The patient should be close to the speaker, not more than a meter (3 feet), referenced to the center of the head (see Figure 3–10). Many audiologists simply attach a string of the desired length to their loudspeaker, and use this for head placement calibration. Many patients do not like to sit this close to something, so repositioning of the patient may be necessary during the testing. For

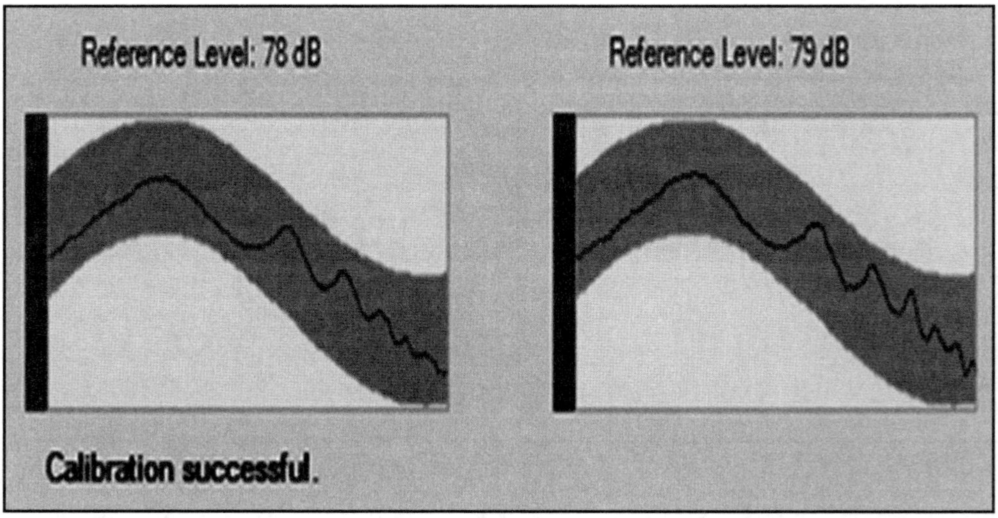

Figure 3–15. Screen display following calibration. Observe numerous resonances and roll-off in the highs, all soon to be automatically corrected. Shaded area is the tolerances.

manufacturers that use a 45-degree angle, an even closer placement may be recommended. For example, the Fonix Company recommends a sound-field speaker placement of approximately 12 inches from the patient's head, at 45 degrees for the most accurate, repeatable measurements. They go on to say, however, that for bilateral testing ". . . it may be more convenient to use a zero degree azimuth. The zero degree azimuth may be slightly less repeatable than the 45-degree azimuth, but within the margin of error for clinical use" (Fonix Operator's Manual, 2012).

- The loudspeaker should also be placed at a vertical azimuth of 0 degree. As we mentioned earlier, this rule seems to be difficult for many clinicians to follow, as we see a lot of stomach and chest testing—probably because the equipment simply was placed on whatever table was handy. If for some reason you were to vary from the recommended 0-degree vertical azimuth, it is best to go higher than ear level rather than lower. In fact, at least one study that we mentioned earlier in this chapter revealed that the test–retest reliability (average standard deviation) was about 0.5 to 1.0 dB better for a 45-degree elevation (Killion & Revit, 1987).

Placing the patient in the correct location initially is important, but keeping him or her in place during the testing is equally important. As discussed earlier, in most cases, we do have a reference microphone active on the test ear, but even so, it

CLINICAL CONCEPT: Close Is Good!

Some patients do not like their "personal space" invaded by a loudspeaker, but keeping the patient close to the test signal is a good idea. Here are three reasons why this is true.

- When testing hearing aids with low compression kneepoints, you'll often want to use a low-level input to obtain the best estimate for gain for soft speech. This input must be above the noise floor of the test room for the equipment to operate properly. As the patient sits closer to the loudspeaker, you improve the signal-to-noise ratio, which allows for testing at lower inputs. We like to be able to test at 50 dB SPL whenever possible, certainly at 55 dB SPL.
- When testing using high inputs (75 to 80 dB or higher), it's possible to overdrive the loudspeaker of the system (some units will abort the run when this happens). This usually isn't a problem if the patient is seated 2 to 3 feet from the loudspeaker, rather than 4 to 6 feet (remember the old half-the-distance rule).
- For loudspeakers that are directly in front of the listener, head shadow can be a problem if the loudspeaker is too close and small head movements can generate errors. For this reason, most probe microphone manufacturers that use a loudspeaker directly in front of the listener suggest a minimum distance, which is usually in the range of 18 to 24 inches.

TIPS AND TRICKS: Getting the Loudspeaker Placed Correctly

As we've mentioned, correct placement of the loudspeaker is critical if you want valid and reliable results. Consider this: A loudspeaker placed too low could result in a measurement that is 6 to 8 dB below what is actually present around 4000 Hz. This in turn will prompt you to increase gain for this region by 6 to 8 dB to match prescriptive targets. The patient leaves the clinic and now turns down overall gain by 8 dB because high frequencies are too shrill. This then means he doesn't have enough gain for the important frequencies of 1000 to 3000 Hz, and decides that hearing aids aren't very helpful—all because he wasn't positioned correctly. Here are three relatively inexpensive items to purchase to improve the quality of your probe microphone assessments:

1. If you have probe microphone equipment with a built-in speaker, a table taller than usual for the equipment can be very useful. We've found that 36 inches works well (height of standard kitchen counter). We will typically place the loudspeaker in a more desirable location if you don't have an external speaker and a wall-mount arm or floor stand.
2. A swivel chair that also has an up-down adjustment (for the unusually short or tall patient) is useful.
3. If you have a system that uses an external loudspeaker we suggest using an adjustable wall-mount arm for your loudspeaker. This makes it easy to place loudspeaker at desired location, and even conduct the testing from the 12-inch, 45-degree location if desired. Minimally you will want a speaker stand that has an easy height adjustment, or as mentioned, a table or counter of the correct height. In a pinch, placing the speaker on a stack of books also will work (e.g., Figure 3–10).

is important that the patient stays in the test position. To illustrate this, observe the test results shown in Figure 3–16. In this case, we used the *stored equalization* calibration technique commonly used with open-fitted hearing aids (see detailed review in Chapter 5). With this technique, the reference microphone is used to calibrate the signal initially and then disabled for all further testing. Consequently, it is assumed that the patient does not move! With the patient seated correctly, we initially fitted him to NAL-NL2 targets, with the hearing aid on the right ear, and those results are shown (lighter line on both charts). Without changing any setting on the hearing aid, we had the patient change his position slightly in two different ways: turn head to the right and turn head to left. These were not exaggerated movements, but simply what we have often observed patients doing during testing—usually to look at the results on the monitor or see what the audiologist is doing. As shown in Figure 3–16, even these slight patient movements can impact the match to target by 5 dB or more (see bottom panel for difference curve)! Notice when turning to the left, the mistake was greater output

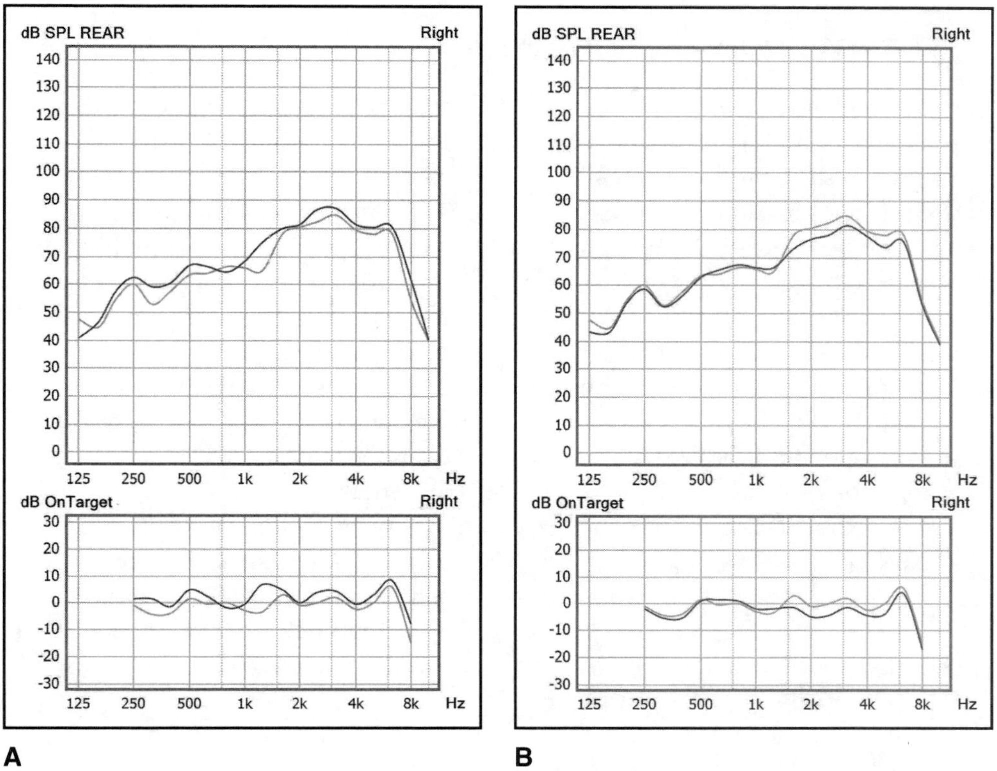

Figure 3–16. Panel **A**: Example of probe microphone results as a function of horizontal changes in the patient's head position, slight turn to the left. The upper curve is the resulting mistake (lower curve is for correct position, patient fit to target). Bottom chart shows difference curve. Panel **B**: Example of probe microphone results as a function of horizontal changes in the patient's head position, slight turn to the right. The lower curve is the resulting mistake (upper curve is for correct position, patient fit to target). Bottom chart shows difference curve.

(head diffraction) and when turning to the right, there was less output (head shadow). What happens with many clinicians is that they then begin to make adjustments based on these invalid measurements, possibly moving away from what would be a perfect fit to target when testing is conducted correctly.

Placement of the Probe Tube

The probe tube has been calibrated to be *acoustically invisible*, so you can think of the tip of the tube as a miniature microphone. The general rule (for reasonably accurate measures through 6000 Hz) is that you would like to have the tip of the probe tube within 5-mm of the TM, and 3 to 5 mm beyond the medial tip of the hearing aid, eartip, or earmold. Although it is important to consider both factors, with most fittings, if you accomplish one, you will also be okay with the other. Unless you have a very deep fitting, if you are within 5 mm of the TM, you probably also will be 3 to 5-mm beyond the tip of the hearing aid/earmold. The 3 to 5-mm position beyond the tip of the hearing aid relates to the fact that that in this region,

TAKE FIVE: Behaviors to Watch For

No matter how carefully you position your patients, they often will do many things to disturb the reliability of the testing. Here are a few to watch out for (modified from Tecca, 1991 and Mueller 2001b):

- The *No-Neck.* This patient will continually scrunch down in the chair making it virtually impossible to position the tube or align the head for testing.
- The *I'm too cool.* Similar to the No-Neck, but with a bit of attitude added to the slouch—often assuming an I'm-in-my-La-Z-Boy posture.
- The *Crane.* The opposite of the No-Neck. This patient sits as straight as possible, craning the neck to the ceiling—only to bring it to a more natural position right in the middle of a test run.
- The *Scooter.* After being seated appropriately close to the loudspeaker, the patient scoots the chair back the moment that you might not be looking.
- The *Professor.* The patient's eyes are glued to the monitor, and leans forward to observe the results even more carefully the moment a curve begins to appear.
- The *Impressionist.* As soon as the test signal begins, the patient turns the test ear toward the loudspeaker.
- The *Motor Mouth.* The patient cannot wait for the test to be completed before commenting on the results, and shouts out "I hear it" as soon as the input signal is presented.

Regardless of which of these patient types you encounter, the *fix* is always the same—indicate where and how he or she should sit, reinstruct, and if you are using stored equalization techniques, recalibrate.

the sound wave is making a transition from the narrow opening from the hearing aid/fitting tip to the larger ear canal, and measures in this region may not be valid. In deep fittings, however, when only a 5- to 7-mm residual distance to the TM remains, we're okay with only 2 to 3 mm beyond the tip. An earlier study by Don Dirks and Gerald Kincaid (1987) provides perhaps the best reference for practicing clinicians. As shown in Figure 3–17, the difference from the true SPL at the eardrum is most often manifested as a high-frequency error—the higher the frequency the greater the error. As can be seen on the graph, at 1 cm (10 mm) from the eardrum, the error for 4000 Hz is only 2 dB, but increases to 4 dB for 6000 Hz, and nearly 10 dB for 8000 Hz. Although we are not likely to get placement wrong by that much (10 mm versus 5mm) very often, the impact on the high frequencies can easily lead to programming errors (e.g., unnecessarily increasing high-frequency gain).

There are four commonly used procedures to help you accomplish appropriate probe placement in adults:

- Visually assisted positioning method (also referred to as the Intertragal Notch Rule or the constant insertion depth

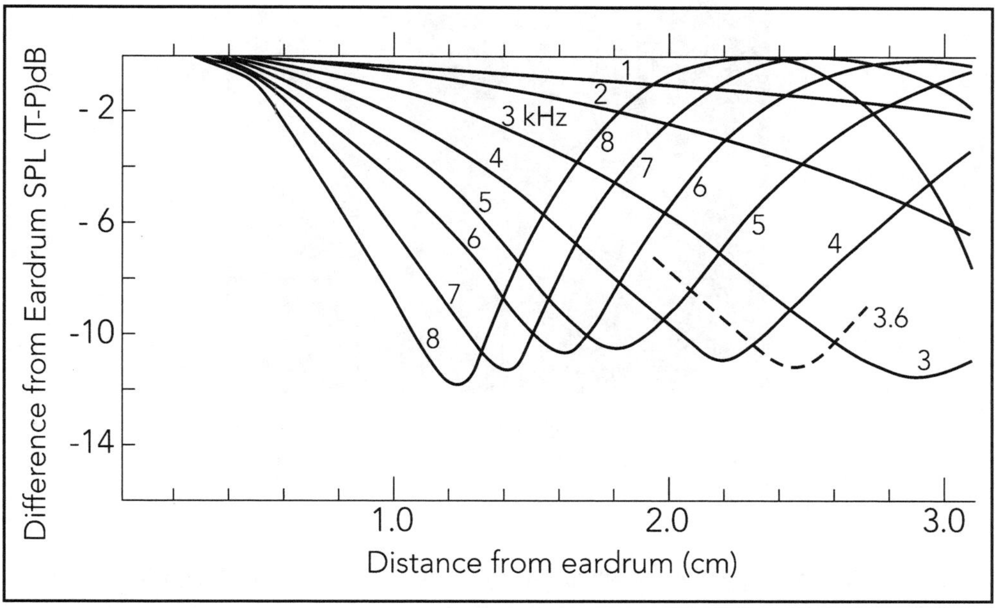

Figure 3–17. Difference between eardrum and probe-measured SPL at eight frequencies as a function of distance of the probe from the eardrum. To determine "measurement error," select a distance from the eardrum (*x*-axis), for example 10 mm (1.0 on this cm chart), then go straight up until you reach the line of a frequency of interest (e.g., 4000 Hz), then observe the point directly to the left of this intersection on the *y*-axis—for this example that would be about 2 to 3 dB. That would be your measurement error. From Dirks and Kincaid, 1987. Reprinted with permission from Wolters Kluwer Health, Inc.

method). We know that the average ear canal is about 25 mm long and the average distance from the opening of the ear canal to the intertragal notch is 10 mm; a total of 35 mm. As discussed earlier, most probe tubes come with an adjustable sleeve that can be moved along the tube. So if we put the probe tube sleeve marker 30 mm from the tip and slide the tube down the ear canal until the marker is at the intertragal notch, we should be about 5 mm from the TM. Figure 3–18 shows the probe placed for testing, with the sleeve marker located at the intertragal notch. If the tube does not have a sleeve, use a marker pen to indicate the distance. If it is obvious that a person has a short ear canal (usually a petite female), or there is a shorter-than-average distance between the intertragal notch and the opening of the ear canal, place the marker at around 25 to 27 mm. This method is not recommended for infants and children, as the dimensions of their ears are of course smaller and quite variable. However, a depth of 20 to 25 mm is recommended if you do attempt to apply this method in children. One company has mm printed on the probe-tube itself, so if your vision is good enough, this could also serve as a handy guide (look cloely at the tube in Figure 3–18).

- Geometric positioning (earmold or hearing aid as a guide). This is the

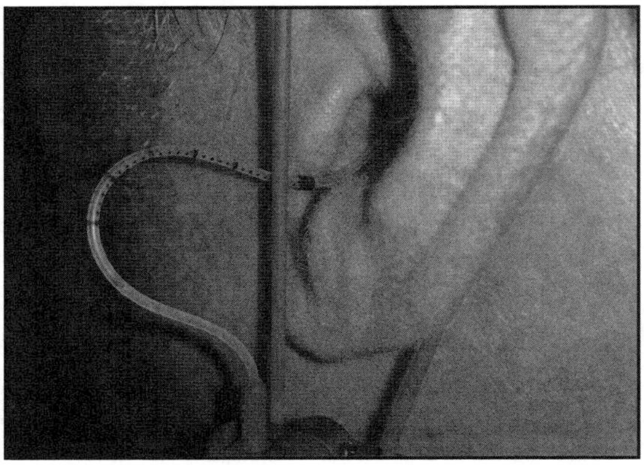

Figure 3–18. An example of the probe placed for testing, with the sleeve marker located at the intertragal notch.

method that many people use when conducting measurements with children. Position the probe tube along the inferior portion of the child's earmold or custom hearing aid, extending the tip of the tube 2 or 3 mm beyond the tip of the earmold (hearing aid) and then place the sleeve marker equal to the inferior lateral portion of the earmold (hearing aid). This should result in the marker being placed in the region of the intertragal notch. When used with adults, have the tube extend 5 mm beyond the hearing aid/earmold (Figure 3–19). A shortcoming of this approach is, however, that for adults with a relatively short fitting tip and a long ear canal, this approach will not get you within 5 mm of the TM, and you could be underestimating true ear canal SPL for the higher frequencies. How deeply the earmold/tip/dome fits in the canal is important for this technique.

- Acoustic Positioning (standing wave notch). By observing standing waves in the ear canal, the distance between the probe-tube tip and the eardrum can be predicted fairly accurately. First, the examiner finds the position of the tube in the ear canal where a 6000 Hz warble tone is at its minimum, which will be close to 14 to 15 mm from the eardrum for most adults. The tube then can be further inserted a known distance to reach the desired point;

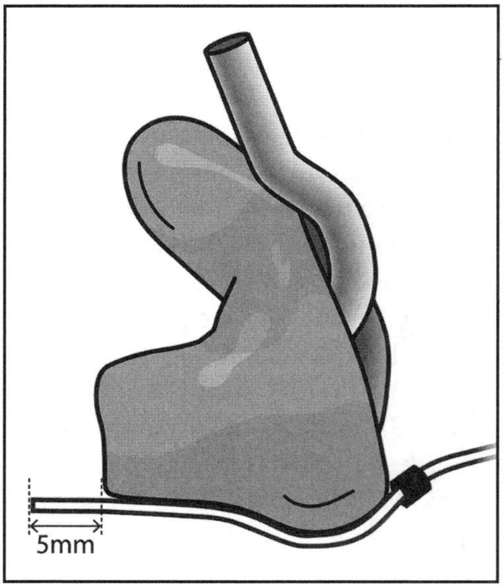

Figure 3–19. An example of using the earmold as a guide in determining the location of the sleeve marker on the probe tube.

that is, an additional insertion of 8 mm would place the tube approximately 6 mm from the tympanic membrane. This procedure was first suggested by Sullivan in 1988, and more recently reviewed by Storey and Dillon (2001). The method also can be used in a more indirect manner: Simply monitor the output in the range above 6000 Hz to assure that no notch is present. The visibility of this notch will vary from system to system, depending on the degree of smoothing of the measured output (more on this in Chapter 7; see Figure 7–1 for examples).

- Acoustically Assisted Positioning. Essentially a combination of the two methods above. First, the visually assisted positioning method is applied. Then, as a second step, the acoustical positioning method is applied to increase accuracy.
- Bump-and-pull. This method is used on occasion, although often not intentionally. In fact, if you haven't ever done the bump-and-pull, we are guessing that you are new to probe microphone measures, or you haven't been placing the probe tube deep enough. Using this approach, the probe tube is gently slid down the ear canal until the tip of the tube bumps the patient's TM. Don't worry, they'll tell you when you are there. Warn them in advance that they might feel a little tickle. Once you obtain the patient's response, pull the tube back a little, and you know you are deep enough. This method is *not* recommended for infants and children or highly excitable patients (or for any real patient for that matter!). However, it actually is a very handy method when you are by yourself and want to do a quick probe measure on your own ear.

Tips and Tricks: Probe Placement and Video Otoscopy

We've mentioned the importance of a before and after view of the ear canal when doing probe placement. You can add some modern-day equipment to make this task easier and more interesting. At least one probe microphone manufacturer includes video otoscopy as an option. This provides an excellent view of the probe placement, and your patients can enjoy the view with you if you like. An example is shown in Figure 3–20, although it's difficult to see the exact tip of the tube in this view, but you know you are close. What you can see, however, is a very nice looking malleus! The view is much better in color (maybe in our next book).

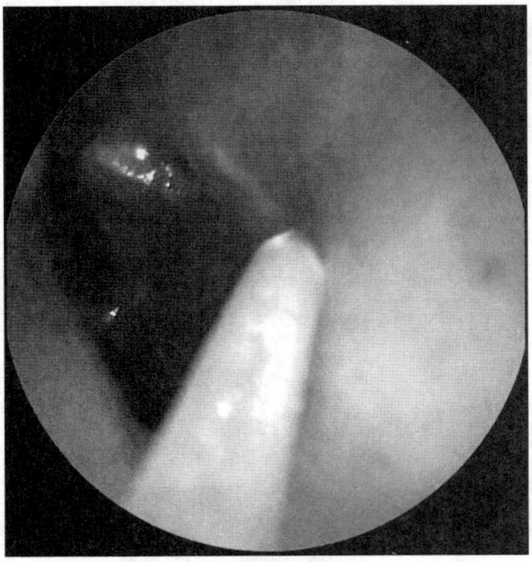

Figure 3–20. Using video-otoscopy to assist with probe tube placement.

TECHNICAL TIP: Keeping the Tube in Place

Probe tubes tend to be a little bouncy, and there are times that just when you have them placed perfectly, they will pop back. Probe microphone manufacturers have developed gadgets that are designed to hold the probe in place. Some audiologists like them, other audiologists get rid of them. Other tricks include: (1) putting the tube in a small rigid *U* device or other specific holding device provided by the manufacturer (Figure 3–21), (2) slipping the probe behind the wire/cord that is holding the probe assembly in place (if an under-the-ear assembly is being used—see example of this in Figure 3–18), (3) adding some lubricant to the middle of the tube (being careful not to plug the end of the tube), which helps the tube adhere to the skin of canal, stay in place, and minimize slit leaks, and (4) using retention clips to secure the probe housing cable underneath the patients chin and across to the opposite shoulder, and/or, using another module to hold the module and probe tube in place should the patient move.

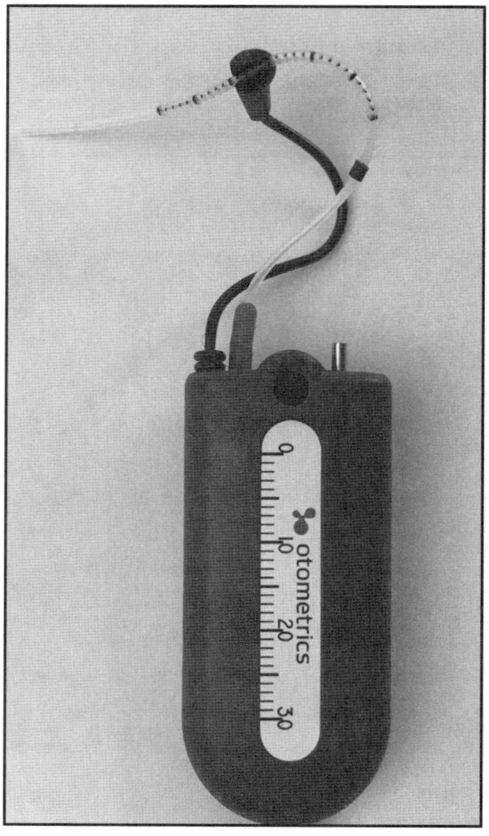

Figure 3–21. Example of probe-tube holder as part of reference microphone assembly. Holder can be used to keep probe in rigid position. Also shown is tube with printed mm-markers on the tube. Photo courtesy of Otometrics (2017).

Comparisons of the first three methods in adult listeners suggest they are roughly equivalent for the average patient (Dirks, Ahlstrom, & Eisenberg, 1994). However, for the higher test frequencies (4000 Hz and above), patients with long ear canals (>25 mm) can demonstrate slightly higher (and more accurate) levels using the standing wave notch method.

We need to mention that with all of these methods, you would first start with a good otoscopic exam, and then take another peek into the ear canal after the tube has been placed. There are times, often because of a cerumen-induced detour, the probe tube will curl, and the actual depth of the tip is not as deep as you would predict from the location of the sleeve marker.

Quick Summary

Here is quick summary of what to remember for the test setup:

- Select a quiet room with low ambient noise and away from the hustle and bustle of the clinic/office.

CLINICAL CONCEPT: Probe Depth and Verification Strategy

As discussed in Chapter 4, there are two similar, but different ways to verify your hearing aid fitting using probe microphone measures: REIG, and the REAR. We bring this up now, because the method selected does have some impact on probe-tube placement. Here is why. If you use the REAR for verification, you will be looking at an absolute measure of ear canal SPL. It is critical therefore that the probe-tube tip is deep enough, so that high-frequency signals (at least through 4000–5000 Hz) are measured accurately. With the REIG, however, *if* you use a measured real-ear unaided response, then you are calculating a relative difference from two measures (the REAR minus the REUR). In this case it is not as critical that the probe tube is deep (within reason), but more important that the tip is the same place for both measures. For example, if the tip is somewhat shallow, and a 5 dB mistake at 4000 Hz is made (output 5 dB less than it should be), if the tube is kept in the same location, this mistake will be made for both the REUR and the REAR, and the calculated REIG will be the same as if the tube had been deep for both measures (Hawkins & Mueller, 1992). Yes indeed —two wrongs can make a right!

For a variety of good reasons that we will discuss in the next chapter, the REAR procedure is currently the more popular technique. However, it usually is easier to see if you have the wrong depth when using the REIG procedure and a measured REUR (because of the REUR measure; we have a general idea of what the REUR should look like with a deep placement), and it is easier to make a mistake regarding probe depth when measuring REAR. Therefore, it is particularly critical that we really pay attention to probe depth for the REAR in order to avoid providing too much high-frequency gain (a short placement will underestimate true gain, and the prudent audiologist will compensate for this by programming more gain—which really wasn't needed)!

- Select a sturdy office swivel chair that can be adjusted for height.
- Seat patient approximately 2 meters (at least 5 to 6 feet) away from any reflective surface. Remember that you too are a reflective surface, so move back when you do actual measure.
- Position patient relative to the loudspeaker at the angle and distance recommended by the manufacturer (usually directly in front—0-degree horizontal azimuth—at a distance of 0.5 to 1 meter—1.5 to 3 feet).
- Place the loudspeaker presenting the test signal at, or slightly above, the vertical azimuth of the patient's head.
- Place the reference microphone relatively close to the opening of the ear canal.
- Place the tip of the probe tube measurement microphone so that it is within 5 mm of the TM.
- Instruct the patient to sit still and to look forward during the testing.
- Sit back and enjoy the science aspect of fitting hearing aids (the *art* part is yet to come)!

In Chapters 1 and 2, we discussed the importance of selecting a well-researched prescriptive method, and then assuring that the hearing aid output matches these prescriptive targets in the patient's ear canal. Of course, these measures must be valid and reliable. In this chapter, we described many considerations, techniques and procedures to assure that accurate results are obtained, and that these real-ear findings provide meaningful information regarding the quality of the fitting. Armed with this background and procedural information, it is time to start doing some testing.

4 The Essential Measurements

Always do the right thing. This will surprise some people and astonish the rest.
—Mark Twain

If you've read our previous chapters, you probably have already deciphered that when we're talking about the fitting of hearing aids, we believe that "the right thing" is careful real-ear verification. You also might have picked up on the fact that although probe microphone measurements are part of every Best Practice document, they often are not used by practicing audiologists. So indeed, as Mark Twain suggests, your routine use of these procedures might surprise, or even astonish, a few of your colleagues—but don't let that slow you down. We will do our best in this chapter to provide you with clinically relevant protocols that will lead to verified fittings, and long-term improved patient outcomes.

In Chapter 3, we introduced you to the basic probe microphone equipment and measures, and some of the techniques important for collecting valid and reliable information. We also briefly described some of the most common clinical probe microphone measures. In this chapter, we discuss each one of these probe microphone measures in greater detail. Some of the measures we'll discuss are used in the clinic more routinely than others, so note that the length of our discussions does not reflect how commonly each measure is currently used, or how much we believe you *should* use a given test. For example, although still used routinely by some clinicians, real-ear unaided gain (REUG) and real-ear insertion gain (REIG) are used far less often for verification—if at all—when compared to the REAR. However, we believe there are two main reasons for providing a full discussion of each measure. First, clinical practice is ever changing, and the underlying reasons for doing things in a particular way also often change. Therefore, it is important to understand multiple ways to perform each type of measurement. Second, understanding all available measures gives us a better understanding of the measures we do use. In almost every case, there is a trade-off in the information we have when we make a measure. For example, REAR measures allow us to view frequency-specific audibility, whereas REIG measures allow us to easily visualize frequency-specific gain. Knowing what we are gaining or giving up when we choose a particular measure can be informative. Such underlying information is important for interpreting results, even if we don't routinely complete the measures.

A Bit of History

When clinical probe microphone measures were first introduced (early 1980s) the Prescription Of Gain and Output (POGO) and

Libby 1/3 prescriptive fitting methods were at the peak of their popularity, and a revised National Acoustic Laboratories (NAL) procedure (NAL-R) was just being published. All three of these methods were verified using functional gain, but insertion gain could be substituted easily, so manufacturers included calculation of these prescriptive targets as part of the probe microphone equipment software.

Audiologists, frustrated with the tedious and unreliable functional gain procedure

POINTS TO PONDER: Automated Real-Ear Verification?

Currently, closed-loop self-verifying hearing aids are available from only a few manufacturers. However, we predict that in the relatively near future, most hearing aids will "autofit" to the desired prescriptive targets after the clinician enters thresholds, appropriately places the probe tube and the reference microphone from the probe microphone system, and places the hearing aid to the ear. Several automated methods have already been introduced. As we describe later in this chapter, integrated probe microphone and hearing aid fitting systems that automatically fit to targets have been available for more than a decade—in some cases, as a unified system from a single manufacturer, in other cases, as a partnership between a hearing aid manufacturer and a probe microphone manufacturer with the systems interacting through Noah, or other means. Because this combination uses two existing and proven methods, we have little doubt that such systems can provide a reliable fit much more quickly than can be done by hand (a skilled clinician is still necessary to assure positioning, probe microphone placement, etc.). Why haven't they caught on yet? The big hurdle in the past was that these systems often locked the audiologists into a single probe microphone system and brand of hearing aid. However, it is a hurdle that can, and we think, will be overcome.

More recently, hearing aids that can fit themselves without the need for probe microphone equipment have been introduced, although there are some concerns regarding their reliability and validity. So, why a whole chapter on probe microphone verification if it will become automated? Two reasons: First it is important to understand basic verification so that we can troubleshoot and treat problems that may arise. More importantly, basic verification procedures are the foundation for all the advanced verification techniques that we describe in more detail in the second half of this chapter. Indeed, we look forward to the automation of basic verification techniques. If a computer can help us do a part of our job more quickly and accurately, we should let it! Doing so frees up valuable clinical time for tasks that only a highly trained professional can perform, including, (1) advanced verification techniques, (2) quantification of hearing aid outcomes, and (3) using pre-fitting measures, outcome measures, and patient input to individually optimize hearing-aid fittings and maximize patient outcomes (through better counseling!).

they had been using, soon developed a fascination with matching real-ear results to prescriptive targets on a computer monitor. To do so, it was necessary to conduct a calculation called the real-ear insertion gain (REIG), which is derived by measuring the real-ear unaided gain (REUG) and subtracting it from the real-ear aided gain (REAG). That is, REAG minus REUG equals REIG, and, of course, REAR minus REUR also equals REIG. Confused? Don't be. These are just some of the measures that are clinically conducted using probe microphone equipment, and these measurements—and the acronyms used to identify them—will be much clearer by the time you reach the end of this chapter.

As you can see from the preceding paragraph, it is difficult to talk about real-ear testing without getting into the acronyms that are the vital components of probe microphone lingo. Some people cringe when they come upon acronyms, but they do provide an easy way for us to talk to each other—eating a SPAM sandwich, buying SCUBA gear, or flying under the RADAR just wouldn't be the same without them.

The first ANSI standard regarding probe microphone measures was published in the late 1990s (S3.46-1997), and, among other things, helped to define the procedures and clarify some of the already common acronyms (ANSI, 1997). Deciding on the appropriate terminology, however, was apparently not an easy task. In 1986, Dave Preves was quoted in the *The Hearing Journal,* as stating:

> An Acoustical Society of America study group will meet this month [May 1986] to begin discussing the standardization of real-ear measurement terminology.

As you see from the 1997 date of the ANSI reference, more than ten years passed before the standard was published. Like good wine, standards take time to reach maturity.

While waiting for the phantom standard to emerge, some people published papers and book chapters using the terminology that was rumored to be part of the standard and that already was being used in journal articles (e.g., Mueller, 1990; Schweitzer, Sullivan, Beck, & Cole, 1990; Mueller, 1992a). These terms were accepted and were commonly used by manufacturers, researchers, and clinicians. For the most part, the terms in the probe microphone standard were similar to what was then well-known terminology. In fact, it's now been 30 years since those acronyms were first suggested, and very little has changed in the current and revised probe microphone standard ANSI, 2013(S3.46–R2013).

Term Ends in a "G" or an "R"?

As we go through the terminology, it's important to remember that, if a measure represents *SPL in the ear canal,* the term ends in an "R" for Response—for example, the REUR. If a measure represents *a difference value* (e.g., the input has been subtracted from the output), the term ends in a "G" for Gain—for example, the REUG. This difference is often confusing. Here's an example. If we were to say to audiologist Dr. Michael Valente: "Hey Mike, what's your REUG at 3000 Hz?" He would reply, "17 dB." (he knows this because he has measured his REUG several times). But what if we were to ask, "Hey Mike, what's your REUR at 3000 Hz?" There is no way he could answer this question because he would have to know the input level that was used to measure the REUR. If the input was 50 dB SPL, then the answer would be 67 dB SPL; if the input was 60 dB, then the answer would be 77 dB, and so on. Consider also, that gain is *always* a difference value (e.g., REIG), so the REIR term, beloved and used by many in the 1990s, no longer exists (see related Technical Tip—later in this chapter).

At this point, we have briefly mentioned several probe microphone test procedures. It is now time to discuss how and when to use each of these procedures in the everyday fitting of hearing aids. The definitions that we use for each term are taken from ANSI Standard (S3.46–R2013) Methods of Measurement of Real-Ear Performance Characteristics of Hearing Aids.

Real-Ear Unaided Response (REUR)/Real-Ear Unaided Gain (REUG)

Definitions:

- *REUR: SPL as a function of frequency, at a specified measurement point in the ear canal, for a specified sound field, with the ear canal unoccluded*
- *REUG: Difference in decibels between the SPL as a function of frequency at a specified measurement point in the ear canal and the SPL at the field reference point, for a specified sound field, with the ear canal unoccluded*

When the REIG was commonly used for verification, the REUG was the first measure conducted in the probe microphone verification process because, at the time, the REUG was the preferred method for calculating the REIG. That is, it served as the baseline for determining gain in the ear (although it is possible, and some even say preferred, to use the *average* REUG, which is readily available on probe microphone equipment). If you, like most clinicians in the U.S., verify performance using the REAR (e.g., speech mapping), the REUG is of little interest, and typically not used at all in the fitting decision—more on that later in this chapter.

Figure 4–1 shows the average REUG for adults, and Table 4–1 shows values for key frequencies (from Seewald, Cornelisse, Richert, & Block, 1997). Prior to the days of

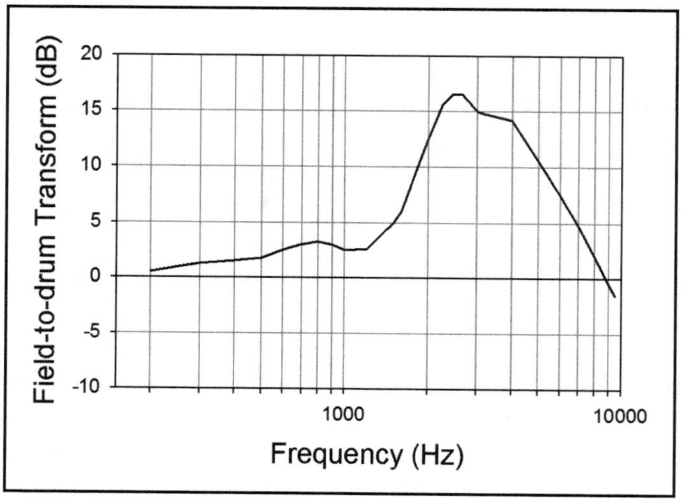

Figure 4–1. Average real-ear unaided gain (REUG) also referred to as the free field-to-eardrum transformation.

Table 4–1. Average REUG Values in Adult Listeners for Key Frequencies

	Frequency (kHz)									
	.25	*.5*	*.75*	*1*	*1.5*	*2*	*3*	*4*	*6*	*8*
REUR (dB)	1.0	1.8	3.0	2.6	5.1	12.0	15.4	14.3	7.3	1.8

Source: From Seewald et al. (1997).

KEY CONCEPT: Keeping it Simple

As we introduce each procedure, we provide a definition of the measurement, but if those definitions sound a little too "ANSI-standard-like" for you, you might appreciate the following:

- REUG: The patient's "natural" amplification—that is, what he brings to the clinic with him
- REOG: What we do *to* the patient before we do something *for* him; that is, when the hearing aids are turned off, what are the attenuation properties of the hearing aid or earmold/ear tip?
- REAR: The output provided by the hearing aid
- REAG: The gain provided by the hearing aid
- REIG: The gain the patient has when he/she leaves the clinic that he/she didn't have when he/she entered the clinic.
- REAR-85 (RESR): The real-ear maximum output of the hearing aid

probe microphone equipment, the laboratory measure of the REUG was referred to as *free-field to eardrum transfer function.* This term is important because it reminds us that the resulting measure depends on several factors. In clinical parlance, it is sometimes simply called the *ear canal resonance.* Although the resonance of the ear canal is nearly always the primary factor, the concha and pinna can also contribute significantly. And, depending on the type of equalization system used for the input signal (e.g., modified pressure, stored, or substitution), the head, neck, and torso can also alter the measurement by a small degree.

Much of the basic research studying the acoustic effects of the external ear was conducted by E.A.G. Shaw with cadavers, and his 1974 article is a good summary of his work. From Shaw's work, in Figure 4–2 we illustrate the average contributions of the head, torso, neck, concha, pinna flange, ear canal, and eardrum. The eardrum is included because middle ear impedance can influence this measure. The data from Shaw clearly show the peak of the ear canal resonance around 2500 Hz, and the peak from the concha just above 5000 Hz. Observe that the combined effect (the curve labeled T in Figure 4–2) is very similar to what we display in Figure 4–1. The individual REUG will change based on the geography of the individual's ear. If we consider basic acoustics and resonance, we know that the

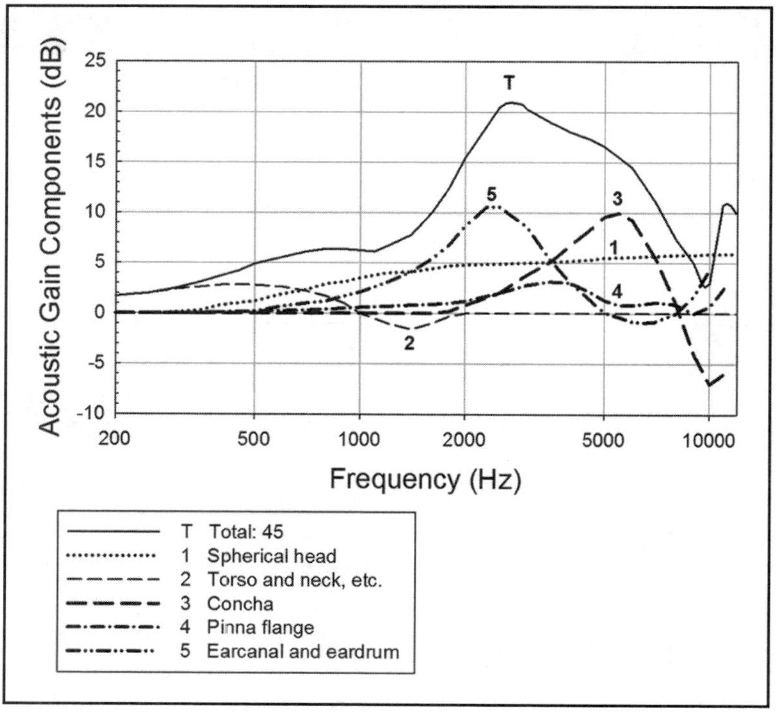

Figure 4–2. The average pressure gain contributed by the different components of the outer ear in man, with stimulus in the horizontal plane at 45-degree azimuth. From Shaw, 1974. Reprinted with permission from Springer Science and Business Media.

peak frequency of the ear canal resonance is higher or lower depending on the size of the ear canal. People with small ear canals might have a resonance peak as high as 3500 Hz or higher. People with large ear canals often have resonance peaks as low as 2000 Hz, or even lower. Similarly, the size of the concha will have an effect. A person with a somewhat smaller ear canal (moving this peak higher) and a somewhat larger concha (moving this peak lower) might have an REUG with one single peak around 3000 to 3500, as the two acoustic components have merged.

Figure 4–3 shows the REUG variability that's commonly observed in the clinic. This figure shows the REUG of eight patients. Note that several patients have an REUG very similar to average, but not all of them do. In fact, the frequency region of the peak of the response varies from near 2000 Hz to 4000 Hz. The maximum intensity at the peak varies from about 14 to 24 dB, and you see peak frequencies as low as 2500 Hz and as high as 4000 Hz.. The teaching point here is that the actual measured REUG might not look like the expected/average REUG.

Now it's time to move on to a discussion of hearing aid fitting. If you're using the REIG for verification, the REUR (either measured or average) is always subtracted from the REAR. In general, REAR curves tend to be relatively smooth. So it's common that bumps in the REUR become dips in REIG and that dips in the REUR become bumps in the REIG. An example of this is shown in Figure 4–4.

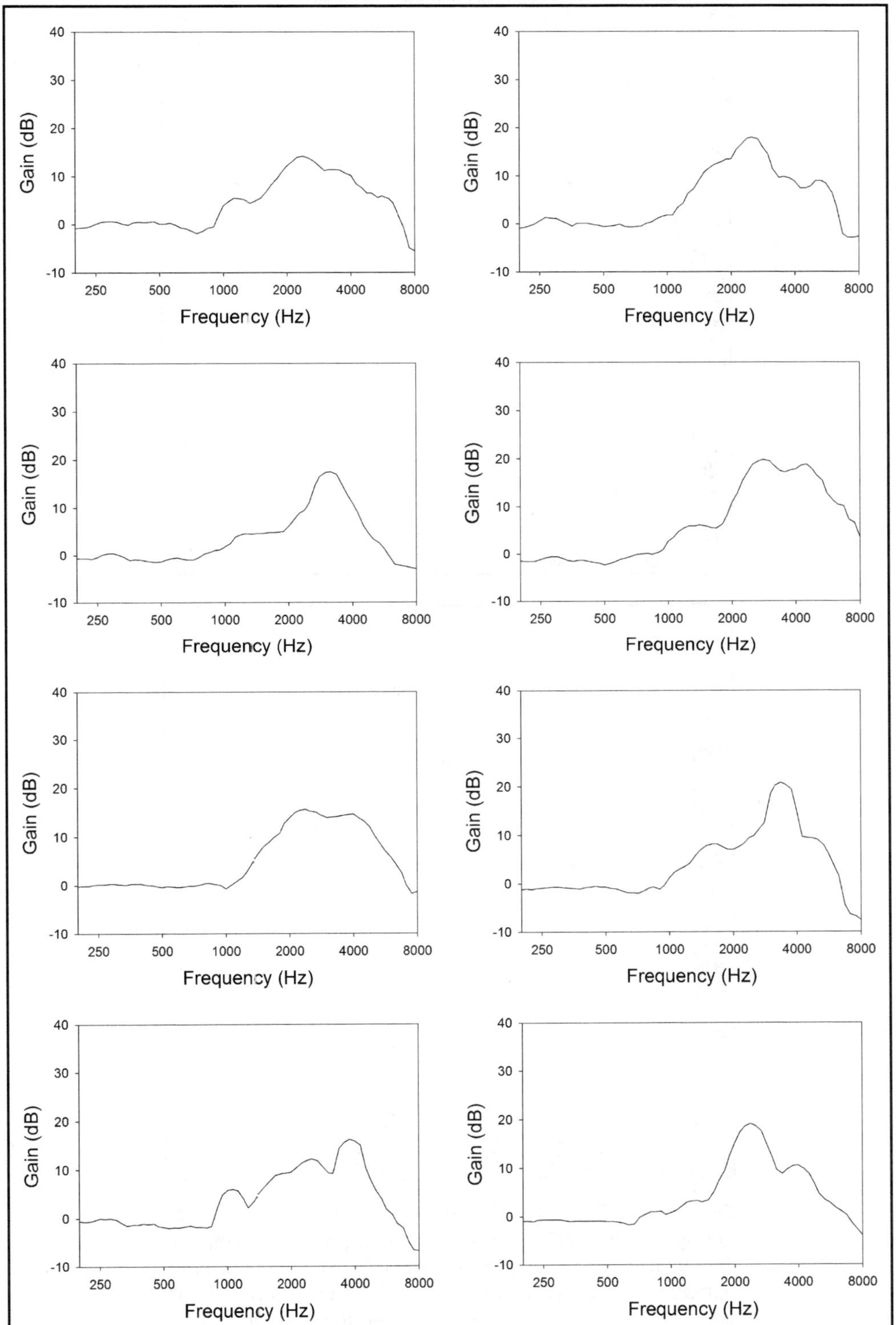

Figure 4–3. Measured REUG from eight patients.

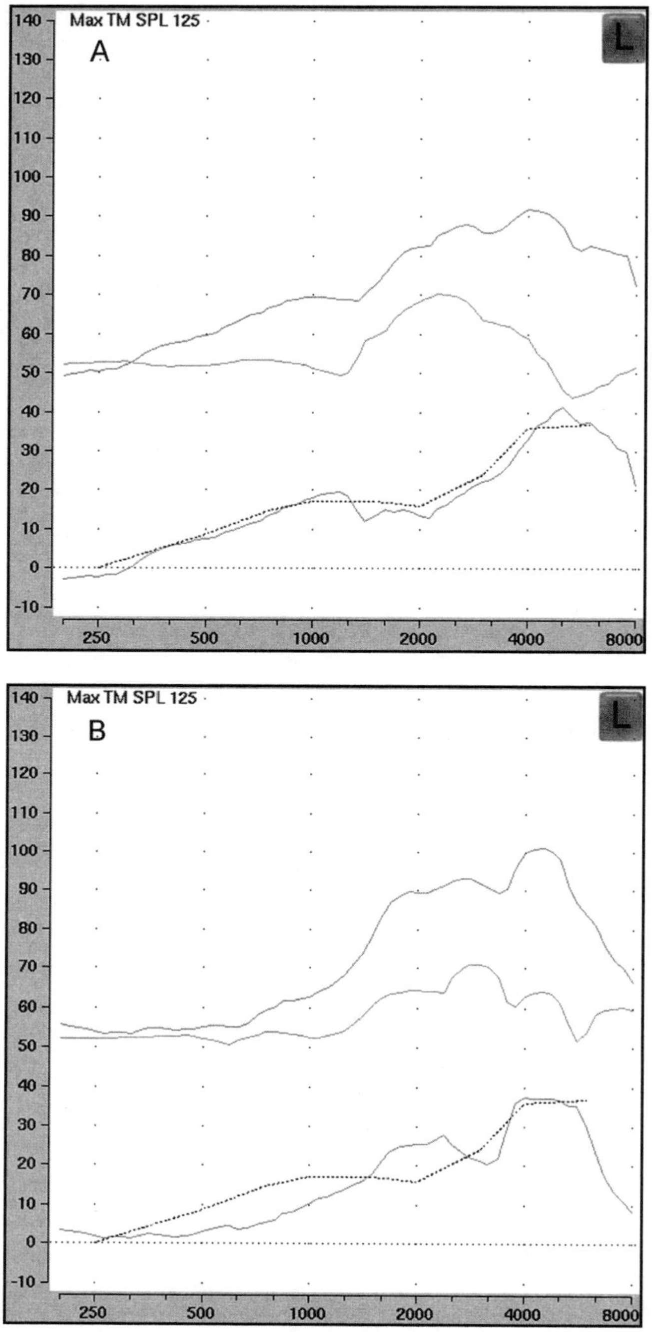

Figure 4–4. Examples of how the REUR impacts the match to target. **A.** The REUR is fairly average (*middle curve*), and the resulting REIG is a good fit to the NAL-NL2 target (*bottom curve*). **B.** The same hearing aid to a different individual with an atypical REUR (*middle curve*). Note the poor fit to NAL-NL2 target (*bottom curve*).

Figure 4–4A shows the results of a mini-BTE RIC with a stock closed dome fitted to an individual with a downward sloping hearing loss. Note that the individual's REUR is fairly average and that the resulting REIG is a good fit to the NAL-NL2 target (65 dB SPL real-speech input). Figure 4–4B shows what happened when we fitted the same hearing aid (no changes to the programming) to a different individual with very similar hearing loss. We entered the same audiogram to show a one-to-one comparison. The difference, however, is that the second patient doesn't have a typical REUR. This unusual REUR has a significant effect on the calculated REIG and, depending on your fitting philosophy, how the hearing aid will be programmed. Observe that we no longer have an REIG target match (although we might have an REAR target match; those values are not displayed). This is because the REAR is very similar for both patients—many of the factors that make REURs differ are no longer in play when the input signal is fed through a BTE (microphone above the ear) and the ear canal is plugged with an earmold. Also, consider that these REUG differences are not revealed during audiometric testing, as the ear canal is plugged with an insert earphone.

In Figure 4–4B, the REUR of the patient is probably not a typical finding, although it occurs often enough to warrant discussion. Most probe microphone systems have an average REUR or REUG stored in memory, and you can compare the patient's measurement to average. In Figure 4–5, we show a measured REUR compared to average; the darkest line is average. Note, in this case, we see with the measured REUR has a distinct peak just above 2000 Hz (ear canal resonance) and a second peak around 4000 Hz (concha effects). This REUR is 5 dB or more greater than average in the 2000 Hz range, which means that *if* you are using the REIG for verification and *if* you use the measured REUR shown here, you will need to program 5 dB more gain into the instrument for this frequency range than if you use an average REUR. Likewise, you will need 5 dB less gain around 3000 Hz, where this person's REUG is about 5 dB less than average.

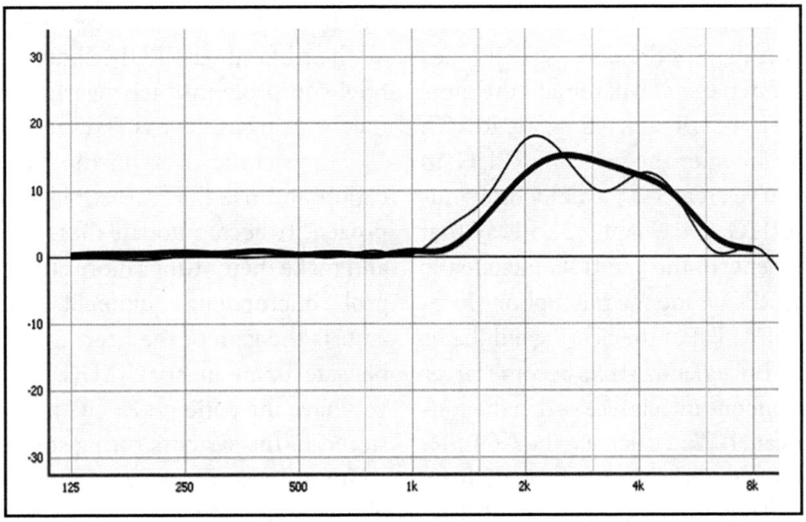

Figure 4–5. Average REUR (*darkest line*) compared to a patient's REUR. Note the higher resonance but at a lower frequency.

If this logic seems correct to you, then you are a good candidate to verify using the REIG and individually measured REUR. If it seems a bit strange, you probably will be happier using average REUR, or the soon-to-be-explained REAR. The arguments for choosing to use the average REUG versus the individually measured REUG are provided in the following section, and in one of our Clinical Concepts.

Because REIG bumps and dips usually are unsightly, and the goal of the fitting is to obtain gain that is a good match to the NAL-NL2 target, if you use the REIG for verification, it is common to try and make the REAG resemble the REUG more closely so that the REIG has a smoother appearance and is a closer match to the target gain curve. With today's hearing aids with multiple channels and sophisticated programming features, doing so is usually fairly easy, although you may end up with a rather unusual looking REAR (which of course is what the patient "hears").

Some prescriptive fitting methods in manufacturer's software allow you to enter the patient's REUG, and if these values are different than average, the desired 2cc-coupler gain is influenced accordingly. Note, we said "2cc-coupler gain"—the *desired REIG* (i.e., the REIG gain targets) will remain the same because they are not affected by the REUG.

When you enter the patient's REUG, in essence, you've created a partially individualized CORFIG (see Chapter 3). Recall that the components of the CORFIG include the REUG, the RECD, and the microphone location effects (MLEs) of the hearing aid that is being fitted (in general, MLEs become larger as the microphone inlet is recessed in the concha or ear canal). You calculate the CORFIG by subtracting the RECD and the MLE from the REUG. Therefore, the bigger the REUG, the more positive the CORFIG. The CORFIG is added to the REIG to obtain desired 2cc-coupler gain, so the bigger the REUG, the bigger the desired 2cc-coupler gain.

On the surface, correcting the CORFIG for the patient's REUG seems like a reasonable thing to do if you want to fit the REIG to a prescriptive target. Although understanding the concept is important, it is certainly not worth investing too much time entering these values into the fitting software because you can easily make these adjustments during the fitting while conducting speech mapping.

There are times when this correction for an unusual REUG can result in some rather bizarre desired 2cc-coupler values or REARs. Unusual desired values commonly occur when you have a patient with little or no hearing loss at 2000 Hz and his REUG (we say "his" because the patient is usually a male with a big ear canal) is 10 dB or so larger than average at 2000 Hz. By correcting for the unusual REUG, you end up with a large increase in the aided speech spectrum for a region where he may have normal or near normal hearing. For such cases, the use of average REUG values will provide a more desirable REAR spectrum. Well, desirable to our way of thinking. If you really believe that how a person's ears have shaped speech all their life (their REUR) should influence how you program their hearing aids, then maybe using average *isn't* desirable.

Some clinics rely on the REIG verification and use the "measured REUG" approach. To accommodate these audiologists and make their fittings more efficient, some probe microphone equipment automatically adjusts the gain of the hearing aid to compensate for an unusual REUG. That is, once you have the patient's REUG measured, it's stored in the system's fitting software. This communication between the probe microphone equipment and the manufacturer's fitting software occurs in the automated real-ear systems we described earlier. It's

CLINICAL CONCEPT: Measured or Average REUG?

Whether to use the measured or average REUG has been a topic of discussion since the early days of probe microphone measures (e.g., Mueller, 1989, Revit, 1991). In general, we prefer using the average REUG rather than the measured, for REIG calculation, and we've mentioned examples of why the measured REUG can cause some problems, most notably bizarre REARs. But one could, at least in theory, build a case to support the use of the measured REUG. If a person has always listened to speech through a "different" amplifier (his unusual REUR), it might be in his best interest to modify the amplified signal to match that speech spectrum. By correcting for the unusual REUG, the REAR will have a spectrum more similar to what the patient is used to. Moreover, if we do examine the individual REUG, we're more apt to apply desired prescriptive gain—again, this assumes that gain is the verification tool, not ear canal SPL at the eardrum. Consider that, if the hearing aid doesn't provide significant gain where the REUG has an unusually large peak, and the earpiece is occluding and eliminates the REUG (for hearing aid fitting purposes), and the patient doesn't have much hearing loss at this frequency, it's possible that the patient's audibility will be worse using the hearing aid than if the patient simply used his REUG.

As early as 1991, Larry Revit was writing about the pitfalls of using the measured REUG and was advocating simply using an average value. This notion was based in part on the fact that prescriptive methods are referenced to sound field thresholds, yet we typically use earphone thresholds for target calculations. If you're interested in using average values, note that most probe microphone units offer this option, although few data exist for average REUGs for infants and children.

actually a pretty amazing thing to sit back and watch the match happen on the fitting screen, and this approach is a real timesaver.

Measurement of the REUG

- Calibrate or equalize the probe microphone system.
- Position the patient appropriately.
- Position the probe tube at the correct depth in the ear canal.
- Present a calibrated signal to the open ear.
- The input-level of the signal is not too critical—the REUG will remain the same across a wide range of signals. It makes sense, however, to use a signal within the range of typical hearing aid gain verification—50 to 80 dB SPL. We usually use 65 dB SPL.
- Theoretically, the type of signal doesn't matter, especially for the REUG, but the visualization of the REUR will be easier if the signal has equal level across frequency. Therefore, we recommend displaying the REUG or REUR for a test signal that is displayed as a flat frequency response in the sound field without a hearing aid or patient present. If you use a shaped signal such as speech, considerable experience is

TECHNICAL TIP: The REUG and TM "Perfs"

Earlier in the chapter, we discussed how the REUG depends heavily on the size of the ear canal because the ear canal resonance is the primary factor. So what happens when a TM perforation occurs and the volume now includes a portion of the middle ear cavity? As you might likely expect, the usual resonance around 2700 Hz is gone because the ear canal volume is much greater than it typically is. The concha effects, however, remain the same, and you tend to have a curve with two large peaks separated by a valley around 2500 to 3000 Hz. Although the primary clinical purpose for conducting the REUG is to obtain the values for calculating the REIG, observing the configuration of the REUG can also provide useful information regarding the status of the middle ear. Now, you might say, "Wouldn't you already know that there was an eardrum perforation from your otoscopic exam?" Maybe. But some perforations are difficult to visualize, especially if you don't have years of experience. If you see many patients with hearing aids and routinely do probe microphone measures (including REURs), there's a pretty good chance that you'll detect a TM perforation, previously unknown to both you and the patient. If you're simply doing an REAR for verification, you may be fooled into thinking something bizarre is going on with the hearing aid. For more information on the effects of middle ear pathology on the REUG, see the review by deJonge (1996).

needed to recognize the typical REUR shape, and what deviations from that shape look like if the probe microphone manufacturer does not display it on the screen. Some equipment, however, will display the speech-input REUR as an REUG, which is how the REUG in Figure 4–5 was obtained.

- Observe the recorded REUG (or REUR if you are in that display mode).

Clinical Applications of the REUG

- Primary: To serve as a baseline for the calculation of the REIG; this value will be subtracted from the REAG.
- Secondary: To provide reference for REOG testing
- Secondary: To correct 2cc-coupler data to derive an individualized 2cc-coupler fitting target
- Secondary: To assist in determining if the tip of the probe tube is at an appropriate depth (e.g., notch effect discussed in Chapter 3)
- Secondary: To detect abnormal middle ear conditions such as a perforation of the eardrum (unusual peaks and dips in response)
- Secondary: With the SPL-O-Gram fitting approach, it can be used for conversion of sound field audiometry from dB HL to dB SPL (Pumford & Sinclair, 2001).

TIPS AND TRICKS: Test Signal for the REUR

An REUR is an REUR is an REUR, and for the most part, the signal that you use does not change the effect measured. However, if you are interested in observing the individual characteristics of the REUR and how a given patient's REUR differs from average, then it's best to use a signal that has the input equalized across frequencies. If you use a real-speech signal, where the spectrum is rolling off in the higher frequencies, it is difficult to visualize the average REUR reference shape, as shown in Figure 4–5. If, however, you simply view the REUG, then the familiar pattern should be present regardless of the input signal used. The availability of the REUR versus REUG display feature using real speech seems to vary somewhat among manufacturers.

The Real-Ear Occluded Response (REOR) and Real-Ear Occluded Gain (REOG)

Definitions:

- *REOR (Real-Ear Occluded Response): SPL as a function of frequency, at a specified measurement point in the ear canal, for a specified sound field, with the hearing aid (and its acoustic coupling) in place and "turned off"*
- *REOG (Real-Ear Occluded Gain): Difference in decibels between the SPL as a function of frequency at a specified measurement point in the ear canal and the SPL at the field reference point, for a specified sound field, with the hearing aid (and it's acoustic coupling) in place and "turned off"*

The REOG is a measure of how the hearing aid or earmold has changed the REUG and the degree to which the hearing aid or earmold is serving as an earplug. Although some research has attempted to relate individual REOG values to speech understanding in background noise (e.g., Chasin, Pirzaniski, Hayes, & Mueller, 1997), the primary clinical application is to observe the sound inflow caused by an open fitting, purposeful venting, or slit-leak venting. For example, if you have a patient with normal hearing at 500 Hz and want to know whether the combined effects of slit leak and a pressure-relief vent allow 500 Hz signals to pass to the TM without attenuation, the REOG will give you this information (e.g., an REOG of 0 dB will show that sound is passing through without attenuation). You can, therefore, use repeated REOG testing to ensure that vents are sized appropriately, to monitor the acoustic effects of vent modifications, and to help predict potential feedback problems (we assume that "inflow" values are predictive of "outflow").

With today's common use of open fittings, the REOG will quickly reveal whether the fitting is truly open, partially open, or not open at all, and the REOG or REOR is a helpful way to select the most appropriate dome or tip for a patient, as exemplified in Figure 4–6. The top curve is the patient's REUR. The curve immediately below that is the patient's REOR for an open fitting

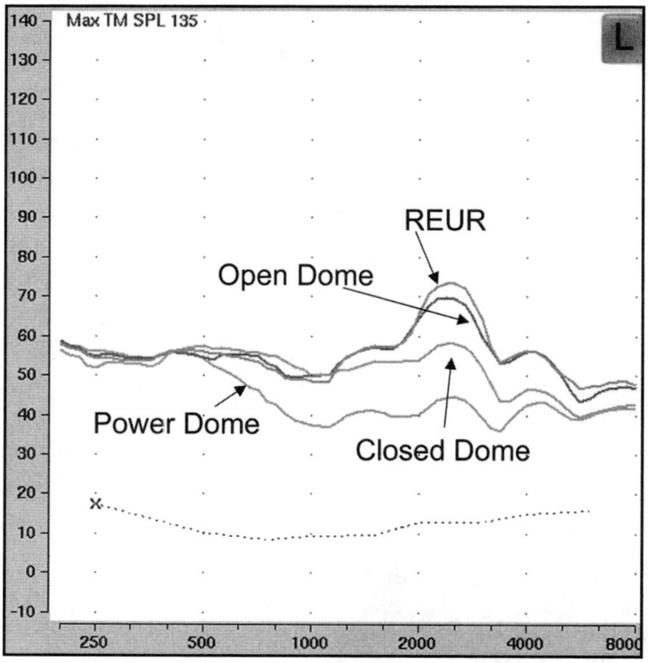

Figure 4–6. Example of REOR for different canal occlusions. The top curve is the patient's REUR. The curve immediately below that is the patient's REOR for an open fitting tip. Note that the REOR is not identical to the REUR because the eartip changes the volume of the ear canal causing a slight shift in the resonance peak. The next lower curve is the REOR for a closed fitting dome. The bottom curve is for a tighter fitting, a double-dome tip. Although there is no attenuation for 500 Hz and below, it's clear that 10 to 15 dB of attenuation is present in the mid-high frequencies.

tip. Note that this tip truly is open, because the REOR is nearly identical to the REUR. You can see they are not completely identical, however, because the presence of the eartip changes the volume of the ear canal causing a slight shift in the resonance peak. The next lower curve is the REOR for a closed fitting dome. For the closed dome, the ear canal resonance and concha effects are missing, but the fitting isn't tight enough to provide attenuation. That is, the output is not less than the input signal. The bottom curve is for a tighter fitting, a double-dome tip. Although there still is no attenuation for 500 Hz and below, we now see that above that level, 10 to 15 dB of attenuation is present. Indirectly, these REORs also give us useful information regarding feedback, as the difference between the open and closed fittings provides a rough idea of how much extra gain before feedback is possible.

In general, the REOG is determined by three factors:

- The degree that the earmold or hearing aid fills the concha, reducing concha effects (although, this won't be a factor if the canal is completely closed, even if the concha is left open);

- The degree that the earmold or hearing aid fills the ear canal, altering ear canal resonance; if the canal is closed, a new resonance will be present based on the shortened length of the tube (i.e., the ear canal) and that now the tube is closed on both ends, rather than open on one end. These two factors will move the residual ear canal resonance to a point that it no longer plays a part in the amplified signal. Clinically, we often say that patients have "lost" their ear canal resonance, although at some higher frequency, it is still there.
- The degree that the earmold or hearing aid attenuates sound; earmolds and custom hearing aids can act as an earplug, which will attenuate sounds mostly in the higher frequencies—unless it is a *very* tight fit, when low frequencies also will be reduced. This attenuation can be 10 to 20 dB with a relatively tight fitting, and, therefore, negative REOGs are common.

Considering the three preceding factors, it is understandable that an REOG can take on many different forms. If it is an open fitting, the REOG may look similar to the REUG. If it is a closed and tight fitting, the REOG will be 20 to 30 dB less than that for an open fitting. As we mentioned earlier, although we state that the concha effects can be a REOG factor, with a closed fitting (tight fitting CIC, for example), even if the concha effects are present, they will not impact the REOG because they don't have a pathway to the measurement point at the TM.

Given that we normally are interested in openness of the fitting, the acoustic effects of venting, or modification of venting, it seems reasonable to routinely conduct an REOG whenever hearing aids are fitted. We find it particularly useful when fitting custom instruments with venting

TAKE FIVE: The REAOG?

Yes, you read that correctly—not the REOG, and not the REAG, but the REAOG, which is the abbreviation for the real ear aided-to-occluded gain. The value is derived by subtracting the REOG from the REAG. This allows you to determine how much of the REAG exceeds the sound that is simply reaching the eardrum naturally. Consider that in a very open fitting, where the REOG is similar to the REUG, the REAOG will be very similar to insertion gain. If you have a very tight fitting, where the REOG will be near 0 dB, or may even have negative values, the REAOG will be much larger, even if the REAGs are equal.

The REAOG is not a term from the ANSI standard, and not a term you'll see very often. So why should you care about it? One application might be for looking at the benefit obtained from directional or noise reduction technology. We know that the greater the amount of the hearing-aid processed signal, the greater the benefit of these features (this is why the DI for open fittings typically is only about 1/2 of that for a closed fitting). It seems reasonable that the REAOG could be used to help predict the degree of benefit of this type of signal processing—the larger the REAOG, the larger the benefit.

CLINICAL CONCEPT: REOG and Insertion Loss

You will read in some papers that the REOG is used to determine *insertion loss.* Over the years, the term insertion loss has been used in different ways regarding hearing aid measurement; only in one of these definitions is the REOG directly involved. In short, insertion loss is not typically defined as the REOG and here is a brief description of the three uses of the term

- In some cases, insertion loss has been used to describe the difference between coupler gain and real-ear (or manikin) gain (Erickson & Van Tasell, 1991). This concept is related to the CORFIG, which, as we mentioned earlier, is calculated by subtracting the RECD and the MLE from the REUR. In the case of the CORFIG, if real-ear gain for a closed earmold is compared with coupler gain, there indeed will be "insertion loss" in the higher frequencies for some hearing aid models, especially those with a poor microphone location, such as BTEs.
- In the early days of probe microphone measures, it was common to verify hearing aid performance via the *in situ* response, which we now refer to as the real-ear aided response, or REAR. It was observed that the *in situ* response was greater than insertion gain (what we now call the real-ear insertion gain, or REIG) and that difference was referred to as insertion loss. In other words: REAR minus REIG = insertion loss. The REIG is calculated by subtracting the real-ear unaided response (REUR) from the REAR; therefore, insertion loss by this definition was simply the REUG (real-ear unaided gain). What if the REUG is not totally lost when the earmold plumbing tip is placed in the ear canal, as it is with most open-canal (OC) fittings? Is it still okay to subtract the REUG and use REIG calculations. The simple answer is yes—for a review of these effects on open fittings, see Mueller and Ricketts (2006).
- The third use of the term insertion loss relates to our discussion of the REOG, which nearly always falls below the REUG and often is negative (lower than the input signal). It is tempting to subtract the REOG from the REUG and think of this as insertion loss. Because the REUG in the high frequencies is usually around 15 to 17 dB and the earplug effect of the hearing aid plumbing or the custom instrument often results in an REOG of −10 to −20 dB in the highs, the UG-OG difference can be quite large. This calculation has led some to conclude that, in a closed fitting, the amplifier must add as much as 40 dB of extra gain to compensate. Why is this logic wrong? This amount of insertion loss would apply only if the patient never turns on the hearing aid—more on this later.

and when fitting mini-BTE instruments using non-custom eartips that are at least partially occluding—the REOG values will help determine when the eartip needs to be more open or more closed. In these cases, very little extra time is required; simply run a quick curve with the hearing aid muted before turning on the hearing aid and conduct the REAR. It is also sometimes useful to run an REOR when you have an unusual REAR—what you think is the result of the amplified signal might actually be the direct signal (more on this in Chapter 7).

Now that we have talked about what the REOG *does* measure, it is important to mention what it *does not* measure:

- The REOG does not measure the occlusion effect. The occlusion effect is related to sound pressure levels in the ear canal generated by a bone-conducted signal (usually one's own voice). The REOG, unless it is reasonably similar to the REUG (e.g., a very open fitting), is a rather poor predictor of whether the occlusion effect is present (for one thing, some people, because of their voice quality and other characteristics, have little or no occlusion effect for their own voice regardless of how tightly the ear is plugged). In the absence of an occlusion effect, a patient's REOG could still range anywhere from 0 to −30 dB. For example, if the canal portion of a custom instrument is very shallow (allowing considerable venting), the REOG will be at or near 0 dB in the low frequencies, and there probably will not be a significant occlusion effect (especially if the patient's primary occlusion effect is below 500 Hz). Compare this to a very different fitting where the canal of the custom instrument fits tightly and terminates in the bony margin of the ear canal (e.g., a deep-fitted CIC). This will produce an REOG of approximately −20 to −30 dB, but again, there probably will not be a significant occlusion effect (for review, see Mueller, Bright, & Northern, 1996, Mueller 2003b). In further contrast, consider a shallow, tight-fitted ITC with little venting. We have seen the fitting of these instruments resulting in an REOG of −20 dB and an occlusion effect of more than +20 dB.
- The REOG does not predict required hearing aid gain, nor can it be used to assist in predicting real-ear gain. Consider these two cases: Patient A has an REOG of −10 dB, and Patient B has an REOG of −30 dB. At first glance you might say, "Patient B needs more gain because he has more insertion loss." It's important to remember, however, that once the hearing aid is turned on, sound has a new pathway to reach the TM (through the hearing aid), and the negative REOG differences (the differences that exist below the 0 dB gain point) have been equalized. What have not been equalized are the effects that the insertion of the hearing aid had on the REUG, but those effects are taken care of by the way the insertion gain is calculated. Hence the REOG is not a player in gain selection, except indirectly—if the REOG is similar to the REUG, we know we have a very open fitting and will have to consider the loss of gain in the low frequencies. Although initially it may seem counterintuitive, it is common that the patient who starts off with the least SPL at the TM with the hearing aid turned off will have the most SPL with the hearing aid turned on.

TECHNICAL TIP: Vent-Associated Resonance— Using the REOG for Detection

One clinical application of the REOG is to detect when vent-associated resonance is present and when that resonance adversely affects the real-ear gain. Although bothersome, vent-associated resonance is a fairly rare occurrence, especially with the common use of today's fitting tips. However, it can be very annoying to the patient, and the problem often is misdiagnosed by the clinician. Vent-associated resonance, which can be 10 dB or higher, is observed as increased gain in the 500 to 600 Hz region and frequently occurs when the vent diameter is 1 mm to 2 mm. The patient may complain that his voice sounds "hollow" or "booming," and the clinician might implement treatment strategies for the occlusion effect, which will not solve the problem. Because vent-associated resonance is an acoustic event, not an electroacoustic event, it is present with the hearing aid turned off—the measurement procedure for the REOG.

As we mentioned, a vent-associated resonance usually happens with a medium-size vent, and the reason that a medium-size or larger vent normally is employed in a custom instrument (ITE or ITC) is that the patient has limited hearing loss and little hearing aid gain programmed in the low frequencies. Hence, the people for whom vent-associated resonance is the most bothersome are the very people who are the most likely to have it. If the patient has hearing loss in the low frequencies and 10 dB or so of hearing aid gain is present, then the 10 dB of vent-associated resonance gain is less noticeable (adding decibels will at most result in a 3 dB increase). It is also possible the output of the hearing aid is phase-reversed with the input, and in this case, the gain shown in the REOG might not be as great as it will be when the hearing aid is turned on (because of cancelation due to the phase interaction of the "through the vent signal" versus the "through the hearing aid signal"). So it's always good to observe both the REOG and the REAG/REIG.

Figure 4–7 shows an example of vent-associated resonance for a custom instrument with a 2-mm vent. In the REIG, observe the peak just above 500 Hz, which, for this patient with normal hearing for this frequency range, is undesirable. Had the REOG findings not been available, the audiologist programming the hearing aid probably would have tackled this problem by turning down gain for this frequency region,—which probably already was adjusted to a low level. If we look at the REOG, however, we see that the origin of much of this output—10 dB or so—is from the vent resonance, and not produced by the hearing aid amplifier.

Measurement of the REOG

- Calibrate or equalize the probe microphone system.
- Position the patient appropriately.
- Position the probe tube at the correct depth in the ear canal.

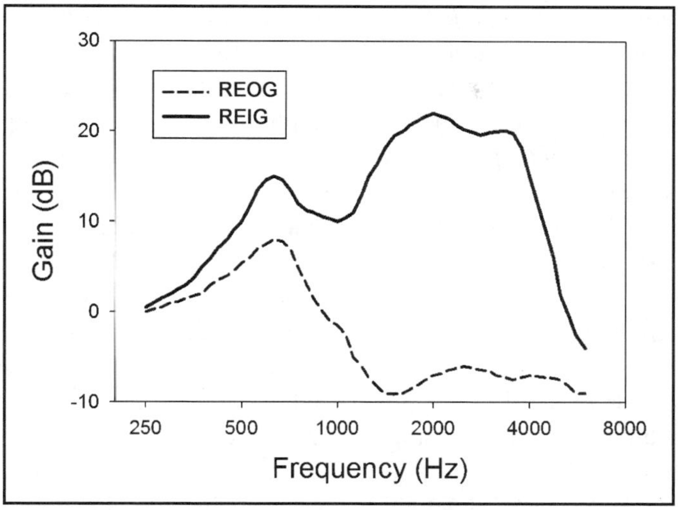

Figure 4–7. Example of vent-associated resonance for a custom instrument with a 2-mm vent. The "bump" near 500 Hz in both the occluded responses (hearing aid turned off) and the insertion responses (gain with hearing aid turned on) indicate the resonance characteristics.

- Place the earmold and/or custom instrument in the ear, but do not turn on the hearing aid.
- Present a calibrated signal, typically the same as used for the REUR.
- The input-level of the signal is not too critical; the REOG will remain the same across a wide range of signals. An input level the same as used for the REUR is typical.
- As with the REUG, the type of signal doesn't matter. In order to see effects clearly, we strongly recommend either (1) displaying REOG (this allows for easiest visualization); (2) displaying REOR in response to a test signal that is displayed as a flat frequency response in the sound field without a hearing aid or patient present, or if you are using a shaped signal such as real speech; or (3) displaying REOR and REUR on the same screen.
- Observe the recorded REOG (or REOR if you are in that display mode).

Clinical Application of the REOG

- Primary: To determine overall tightness of the fitting
- Secondary: To select appropriate eartip or earmold
- Secondary: To identify direct sound versus amplified sound in the REAR
- Secondary: To detect vent-associated resonance
- Tertiary: To estimate the occlusion effect, but only if REOG closely resembles REUG

Rear-Ear Aided Response (REAR)/ Real-Ear Aided Gain (REAG)

Definitions:

- *REAR: SPL as a function of frequency, at a specified measurement point in the ear canal, for a specified sound field, with the hearing aid (and its acoustic coupling) in place and "turned on"*

- *REAG: Difference in decibels between the SPL as a function of frequency at a specified measurement point in the ear canal and the SPL at the field reference point, for a specified sound field, with the hearing aid (and its acoustic coupling) in place and "turned on"*

Of all the measures we make using probe microphone equipment, the most important—and fortunately the easiest to understand—is the REAR. As the ANSI definition states, the REAR is simply the output in the ear canal with the hearing aid in place and turned on—more or less an ear canal measure of what we have been assessing with a coupler since the 1940s. It doesn't matter if the input signal is a swept tone or real speech or if the input level is 50 dB or 80 dB SPL, the measurement is still referred to as the REAR. Today, when audiologists use an input of real speech or some speech-like signal, there is a tendency to refer to the process as "speech mapping," and we agree that this term does sound a bit cooler than REAR, but it really is just an REAR, or a series of REARs.

As we discuss later in the chapter, there are a variety of uses for the REAR regarding the assessment of hearing aid special features and the collection of general information on ear canal-aided output. For the moment, however, we will limit our discussion to the two primary uses: verification of prescriptive targets using the REAR values themselves and verification of prescriptive targets using the REIG, which is calculated using REAR values. Currently, the most popular way to verify a validated prescriptive hearing aid fitting procedure using a probe microphone is the REAR. It is certainly our preferred method because of several advantages we discuss in the remainder of this section.

Using the REAR to verify the fitting is quite logical, as everything is referenced to ear canal SPL, and we can easily visualize the portion of the speech signal that is audible for individual patients in their own ear. The SPL-O-Gram format means that louder outputs indeed fall *above* softer outputs. If you're new to using an SPL-O-Gram, the common "upward sloping" audiogram takes some getting used to because it seems upside down compared to the traditional HL audiogram, but it's well worth the effort. In fact, when viewing most any chart, about the only people who think big numbers should be on the bottom and small numbers should be on the top are audiologists!

Shown in Figure 4–8 is a typical fitting screen using the REAR for verification. The example here is for a real-speech 65 dB SPL input—the complete verification process would also include a soft and loud input signal (e.g., 55 and 75 dB SPL). The HL audiometric thresholds and the patient's LDLs have been converted to ear canal SPL using the REDD. This conversion is done automatically by the probe microphone equipment. Some equipment will use the patient's own RECD for this conversion if it is entered to provide a more accurate reflection of the patient's true threshold in dB SPL and for calculation of prescriptive targets. This calculation, however, also depends on the transducer used for the hearing assessment. In this example, we are looking at the NAL-NL2 fitting targets. The shaded area represents the amplitude range of the amplified signal (30th to 99th percentiles), with the LTASS the dark line near the middle. The goal, accomplished very nicely here, is to make the LTASS equal to the prescriptive targets. The amplitude range of the amplified speech signal also provides some

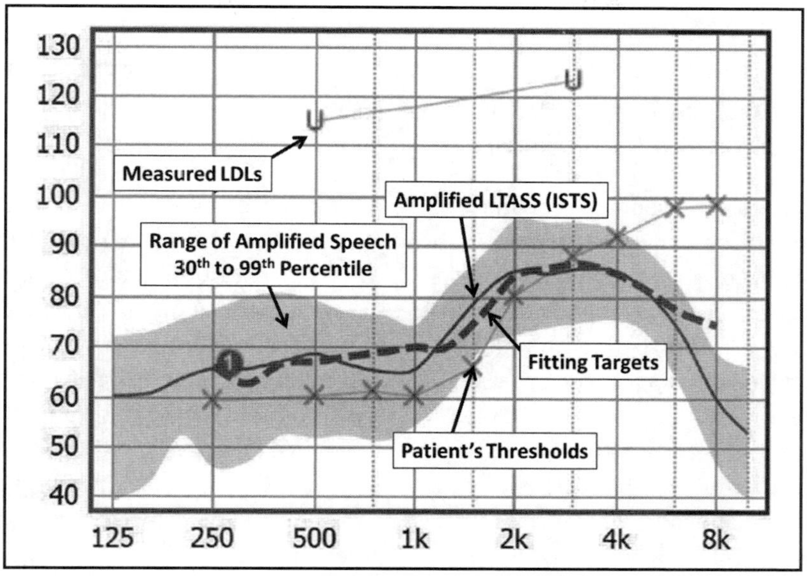

Figure 4–8. Example of typical REAR fitting screen. Thresholds are converted from dB HL to dB SPL in the ear canal. The amplified speech (65 dB SPL input) is shown both as the average LTASS and as the range (30th to 99th percentile). The patient's thresholds, LDLs, and fitting targets also are displayed.

insights regarding compression; note that the range is smaller for the higher frequencies, where compression is the greatest (e.g., 500 Hz versus 4000 Hz).

Here are a couple of important points to consider when using the REAR to verify prescriptive targets:

- First, as we discussed in Chapter 3, the placement of the probe tip is very important. Because the measure is the absolute ear canal SPL, and poor probe-tip placement (shallow rather than deep) tends to mostly influence high frequencies; a less-than-ideal placement can significantly alter the recorded values, which in turn could prompt the audiologist to change the overall fitting. Figure 4–9 shows an example of how even minimal changes can influence the outcome. The top curve is a near-perfect match to the REAR targets for the patient with a moderate hearing loss. This measure was taken with the probe tip at the preferred location—within 5 mm of the patient's TM. The lower curve was obtained with the tube pulled back 2 to 3 mm. Notice that the lower curve on the chart falls 3 dB or so below the original curve in the higher frequencies. This output was obtained with the tube still at a reasonable deep location (6–8 mm from the TM), a common mistake if one isn't careful. But what if the tube would have been a little more shallow (as you will see in Figure 7–1)? This would give the appearance that there was not enough high-frequency gain programed, and would probably lead to increasing gain up to 10 dB in the highs to match target. Now, the patient leaves the clinic with excessive gain in the highs, which will no doubt prompt him to turn

TAKE FIVE (or Ten): REIG Versus REAR for Verification—A Little History

When clinically friendly probe microphone equipment was introduced in the early 1980s, there was some discussion about whether the preferred verification measure was the REAR (then referred to as the *in situ response*) or the calculated insertion gain, soon to be called the REIR, now the REIG. The Madsen equipment, for example, originating in Europe, defaulted to the *in situ* setting. Audiologists by far, however, favored the REIG, for several reasons:

- All the popular prescriptive methods had gain targets.
- REIG is essentially the same as functional gain, which was a common verification procedure at the time,
- It's just simply a lot easier to talk about fitting hearing aids using gain terminology.

So insertion gain became the preferred method of prescriptive target verification for the next 20 years or so. The exception for some audiologists was for pediatric fittings where the DSL prescription was used, as this fitting method did not have REIG targets (see Chapter 2).

In the early 2000s, two factors converged that started to move audiologists toward using the REAR, rather than the REIG for target verification. First, the NAL-NL1 had just been introduced, and unlike previous versions of this fitting algorithm, REAR prescriptive targets were now available. A second contributing factor was that the equipment company Audioscan introduced the Verifit®, which had a calibrated real-speech signal that could be used with the NAL-NL1 targets, which had been converted to ear canal SPL for the NAL-NL1 LTASS and were displayed on the fitting screen. Other probe microphone manufacturers soon followed with similar ear canal SPL fitting methods, and verification using the REAR rapidly grew in popularity. In their 2010 survey, Mueller and Picou asked dispensers who routinely use probe microphone measures what their primary method of prescriptive target verification was: Of the responses, 78% said the REAR and only 22% said the REIG. We suspect that even fewer audiologists are using the REIG today.

That said, using the REAR as the verification approach does have two possible limitations. First, as we discussed in Chapter 3, with the REAR, it is not as obvious when the probe tube is not deep enough as it is in the REUR measure. Second, since REAR targets are for a response instead of gain, it is sometimes unclear how much gain there is or how much should be present. As we discuss later in this chapter, and again in Chapter 7, this uncertainty can create particular issues in the low frequencies for open fittings.

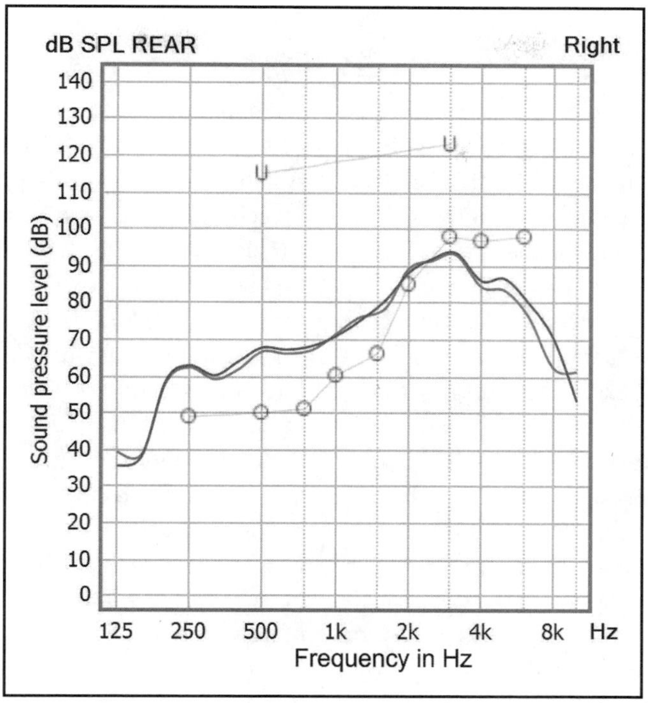

Figure 4–9. Example of how probe placement can impact measures REAR values. The top curve is a near perfect match to the REAR targets for the patient with a moderate hearing loss; the measure was taken with the probe tip at the preferred location—within 5 mm of the patient's TM. The lower curve shows the high-frequency effects of simiply moving the probe-tip back a couple mm.

down overall gain, and we now have less audibility throughout the speech range—not a good outcome.

- A second consideration is to ensure that the input signal used corresponds to the targets on the fitting screen. That is, the fitting targets must be calculated using the LTASS being used for testing, which is why it is important to use a calibrated signal. This is why, with some probe microphone equipment, the on-screen targets will change if the input signal is changed, or for some display modes or with some inputs you will not see any fitting targets at all (which is certainly better than providing incorrect ones).

Test Protocols for REAR Verification of Prescriptive Targets

When using the REAR for verification, there are a couple of things to consider related to the level of the input signals: what levels to use, and in what order to use them. First, we'll talk about the best input levels to use. As we have said many times, we want to obtain measures for soft, average, and loud speech. Soft speech is considered to be 50 to 55 dB SPL, average is 60 to 65 dB SPL, and loud is 75 to 80 dB SPL. So we could select three inputs with a 30-dB range (50 to 65 to 80 dB SPL), or only a 20-dB range (55 to 65

TIPS AND TRICKS: Special Features On or Off?

Hearing aids have several special features that, depending on the type of test signal, interact with the REAR measure. The most notable one is *digital noise reduction,* because if you are using an input signal that the hearing aid classifies as noise, the signal will be reduced, and the subsequent output will not represent the gain that the patient will have when listening to speech. This was a big problem when digital noise reduction was introduced, as most input signals used at that time indeed were classified as noise by the hearing aids. This led to the cry that "you can't do probe microphone testing with digital hearing aids," which pleased more people than it should have (see Mueller, 2001a). Fortunately, this issue was solved in the short term by using only short bursts of noise, and it was permanently solved shortly thereafter when most all probe microphone systems provided a real-speech or speech-like signal (see Chapter 3 for a review of these test signals). Now that we have these speech signals, we certainly recommend conducting verification with features such as directional technology and noise reduction activated. Given that they will be activated for the patient's everyday use, we want to determine how the hearing aid will function for the use condition—it is likely that there will be no effect, but if there is, we want to know about it. One possible exception to the "everything activated" philosophy is frequency lowering. We discuss evaluation of frequency lowering later in this chapter.

to 75 dB SPL). Both of these two options are popular, and some clinics use a combination of the two. Although the 50 to 65 to 80 dB SPL gives us a larger range of measures, there are limitations with this approach. In some offices, ambient noise makes it difficult to test at 50 dB SPL, and the loudspeaker of some probe microphone equipment tends to overdrive for the 80 dB SPL speech signal. For these reasons, we tend to prefer the 55 to 65 to 75 dB SPL approach. Because most of the products today have WDRC with kneepoints of 50 dB SPL or lower, we have found that, if the output for the 55 dB SPL input is okay, the output for the 50 dB SPL input is probably okay, too. And if the output for the 75 dB SPL input is okay, the output for the 80 dB SPL input is probably close enough. We are referring to fittings that have been already programmed reasonably close to a prescriptive method. Note that for the manufacturer's proprietary fittings, as shown in Chapter 1, which are essentially linear, bigger mistakes would be likely.

After you decide which three input levels to use, the next decision involves the ordering of the verification levels—what level to do first?. The goal is to obtain a target match for all three levels as efficiently as possible. The main thing that leads to inefficiency occurs when the programming for one input level messes up the output for a different input level that you already programmed. In which case, you have to go back and forth trying to obtain the best match, or compromise. We can't think of a good reason for starting with loud, so let's eliminate that choice. A case can be made, however, for starting with either soft or average.

- Starting with soft: Most products have a kneepoint around 50 dB SPL; therefore, compression will have a minimal effect on the soft level. We then can adjust overall gain (may be labeled "gain for soft" or "gain for 50 dB input" or something similar in fitting software) until we reach our desired targets. Using this approach, the next input presented will be loud. At this point, we no longer change gain but now alter the kneepoints/ratios for the WDRC until a match is obtained (this is typically labeled "gain for loud," "gain for 80 dB input," or something similar in the fitting software). This second adjustment should have little or no effect on the gain for soft already programmed. If the WDRC system is relatively linear (as opposed to curvilinear), then the output for the 65 dB input should be fairly close to prescriptive target, as it falls midway between the 55 and 75 dB SPL inputs. If not close enough, changes in "gain for 65 dB SPL" must be made, and the 75 dB input needs to be rechecked.
- Starting with average: Although starting with the soft input may be the best choice for some hearing aid brands and models, there are two good reasons to start with average for other brands and models. First, depending on the patient's hearing loss and the compression system of the hearing aids being fitted, it may not be possible to obtain a precise fit for all three inputs (we talk about this more in Chapter 7). Typically, the hearing aid will simply not allow enough compression to meet all three targets, and you end up underfitting the soft targets and overfitting the loud targets no matter what you do. In some of these systems, adjusting gain for loud does indeed affect gain for soft. In such a case, we argue that it is best to start with average inputs. If you are only able to match targets for one input level it is likely best to match gain for average input levels and then adjust MPO settings to make sure that loud sounds do not exceed discomfort levels. That is, if you use a hearing aid for which you effectively cannot increase the compression ratio after the initial fitting, all you can do is program average correctly and then measure soft and loud to see how far off they are.

  The second and better reason to start with average is the case where your manufacturer typically gets the compression right when you enter the thresholds into the fitting software and select the "correct" prescriptive method. In this case, you adjust overall gain to obtain a good fit to average targets and then simply verify that your match to soft and loud are correct. In some cases, you can do this with no additional adjustments for soft and loud inputs—now *that* is time-efficient!

Using the REAR for Overall Assessment of Audibility

As we mentioned, probe microphone equipment converts audiometric thresholds and LDLs to the SPL-O-Gram format (using average or measured REDD corrections), as illustrated in Figure 4–8. In the absence of prescriptive targets, this approach does provide a general "window of acceptability" for the fitting. It is fairly intuitive that, if the goal of the fitting is to make soft sounds audible, then the REAR for the soft speech

CLINICAL CONCEPT: Choosing the Best Prescriptive Procedure in the Software

We know of at least one manufacturer who uses different compression characteristics if you select NAL-NL2 versus their proprietary fitting, and indeed, you will be much better able to match NAL-NL2 targets if that is what you initially select. But on the other hand, we have noticed that, for some manufacturers, the prescriptive method you need to select to obtain a match to the correct compression parameters may have a different name than the method to which you are fitting. It might seem strange that you get a better match to the compression parameters you need for an NAL-NL2 fit when you select the manufacturer's proprietary fitting method or one that's labeled "NAL-NL1," but we have seen both happen. In particular, compression release times may vary substantially from one software-fitting algorithm to another (and are not adjustable within a given algorithm). Consequently, it may be worth experimenting a bit with your favorite manufacturer's software to see if one of their built-in prescriptive methods leads to a close match to the compression parameters being prescribed by your chosen prescriptive method. If you find one, you can apply the "average input first" procedure we described and save a little time in the long run!

inputs must be above the threshold curve. And, if we want to ensure that loud inputs are not too loud, the REAR for high inputs (swept tones) must be below the top LDL curve. This method lacks the preciseness of a validated prescriptive fitting; however, Mueller and Picou (2010) report that about one-third of audiologists who routinely use probe microphone measures, use this general approach rather than match specific targets. It does at least provide some basic evidence regarding audibility of speech and certainly is better than not conducting probe microphone measures at all, but there are some important limitations. For example, making soft speech audible is, of course, important, but what percent of the 30 dB range of soft speech should be above the patient's threshold? Is it 100%? 50%? Is 25% good enough? And, in a downward sloping hearing loss, when do you concede that the hearing loss is so great that it may not be possible, or perhaps even desirable, to make soft speech audible? 70 dB? 80 dB? 90 dB? And how should the required percent of speech that needs to be audible change as a function of hearing loss? The goal of fitting a hearing aid is rarely to make all of speech audible. Patients reject such fittings as far too loud and/or having poor sound quality. By the time you try to sort all of this out and make all of the necessary decisions, you might as well be using a prescriptive method that already has researched these very factors, such as the NAL-NL2 or DSL v5, which is what we recommend in the first place.

Measurement of the REAR (Assuming a 3-mm Effective Vent Size or Smaller)

- If necessary, calibrate the probe tube (not all systems require this step).

- Position the patient appropriately.
- Position the probe tube at the correct depth in the ear canal.
- Place the earmold and/or custom instrument in the ear, with hearing aid programmed to desired starting point (e.g., manufacturer's implementation of a validated fitting method for the patient's hearing loss).
- If necessary, calibrate/level the reference microphone (not all systems require this step).
- Activate the hearing aid with all special features on, with the possible exception of frequency lowering, depending on fitting goals.
- Present a calibrated real-speech or speech-like signal; use an input level consistent with fitting protocol (see previous discussion).
- Observe the recorded REAR; if fitting to prescriptive targets, make programming changes to obtain the desired output.
- Once target has been met, conduct testing at next input level. Continue until target match and verification is obtained for soft, average, and loud inputs.

Clinical Application of the REAR

- Primary: To obtain output match to desired prescriptive fitting targets
- Primary: To obtain general information regarding aided audibility
- Secondary: To calculate REIG (see next section)
- Secondary: To assess special features (e.g., directional, noise reduction, frequency lowering, etc.)
- Secondary: To assess assistive listening technology

Real-Ear Insertion Gain (REIG)

Definition:

- *REIG: Difference in decibels, as a function of frequency, between the REAG and the REUG, taken with the same measurement point and the same sound field conditions*

As we have already discussed, the clinical application of the REIG is to verify prescriptive fitting targets. The REIG is not a measurement per se, but rather a calculation based on two other measures that we've already discussed: the REUR subtracted from the REAR or the REUG subtracted from the REAG. Consider that when we talked about using the REAR for verification in the preceding section, we were looking at placing the amplified speech signal at a desired SPL in the ear canal. With the REIG, we're looking at the *gain* that is needed to accomplish the same task. When we assess the gain the patient has with the hearing aid, we have to consider the gain that he first had with his open ear—which takes us back to the REUR.

While the REUG is more or less ignored when we verify with the REAR, when comparing REIG findings to prescriptive targets, the patient's REUG can have a huge influence (assuming a measured REUG is used). When we first started conducting probe microphone testing in the mid-1980s, the hearing aid technology at the time had little insertion gain above 3000 Hz. Audiology students often would ask, "How can I obtain more insertion gain at 4000 Hz?" The answer was always the same: "Find a patient who has an REUG of 0 dB at 4000 Hz!" A bit absurd, yes, but the point is that you can nearly always predict the goodness of the REIG as soon as you've measured the REUG. For example, let's say that Patient A and Patient B both have an identical 50 dB hearing loss at 3000 Hz, and we're conducting probe microphone testing using a 55 dB input. We'd like to see about 30 dB of insertion gain for this soft input signal. Patient A has an REUG of 10 dB at 3000 Hz, and Patient B's REUG is 25 dB for this frequency. What might very likely happen is that on our first measure following the manufacturer's first fit, our REIG for Patient A is exactly what we want, so we deem it a good fitting; whereas for Patient B, we are 15 dB below our fitting target, so we deem it a bad fitting. Yet, the REAR for the two fittings might be exactly the same! So was one really a good fit and the other a bad fit if speech was placed at the same ear canal SPL for both patients?

It's these types of questions that generate interesting lunchtime discussions among audiologists fitting hearing aids (see last page of chapter), especially if one favors REAR speech mapping and another favors the REIG approach. The earlier example had two patients with quite different REUGs, and indeed if your patient has an unusual REUG, you will end up with a considerably different fitting when the REIG is used rather than the REAR for a target match. But in general, for average REUGs, you would expect the match-to-target results to be similar.

Shown in Figure 4–10 is the same patient who was fitted in Figure 4–8. Note that we previously had a very good fit to target when the REAR was used. When we now look at the same patient in the REIG mode, we still see pretty good match to target, although we are lacking 5 to 7 dB of gain in the 3000 Hz region. This is no doubt a reflection of how this patient's ear canal and residual volume differs from average. If this bothers you, it would be easy to add in some gain here, except that then you would be 5 to 7 dB over target for your REAR. This is why it's usually best to pick your favorite verification mode and stick with it (although going back and forth does satisfy one's curiosity).

TAKE FIVE: The REIR Didn't Make the Cut

In the early days of probe microphone testing, when insertion gain was measured, it was referred to as the real-ear insertion response (REIR). If we talked about gain at a specific frequency, we referred to it as real-ear insertion gain (REIG). As pointed out in the standard (correctly, of course), insertion gain is gain, and therefore cannot be a *response*. It's always an REIG. This was a good change because calling it a response tended to get one thinking that it indeed was a "response" with related bumps and dips, rather than a "difference curve." When looking at the REIR (now the REIG), audiologists would often say, "I need to get rid of that 'bump' right there," when in fact it really wasn't a "bump in the frequency response" but only an area where gain was greater, which often was caused by a dip in the unaided response (REUG), and had nothing to do with the REAR, which might have been very smooth. The bottom line is that, while most probe microphone measures do have an acronym containing an "R" at the end, REIG is always REIG. Don't be surprised, however, to see the acronym REIR used in literature prior to the release of the ANSI 1997 standard.

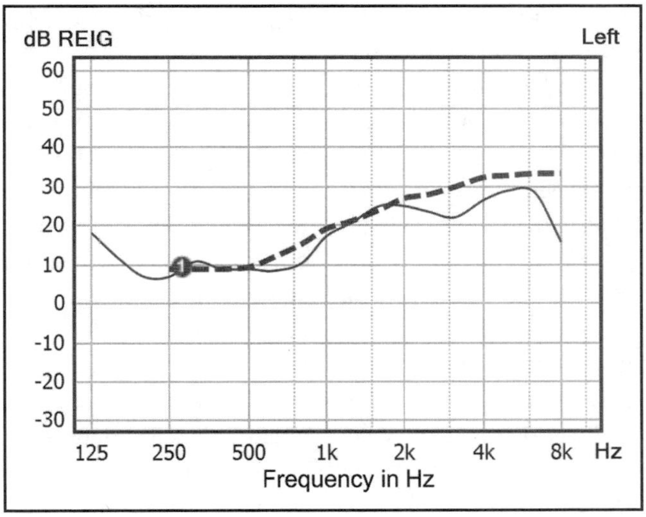

Figure 4–10. Example of an REIG calculation following a near-perfect match to REAR targets.

Real Speech and REIG Calculations

Logically, you would use real speech for REIG calculations (REAR minus the REUR); however, some probe microphone equipment limits the type of input signal that can be selected when insertion gain calculations are conducted, compared to those available when speech mapping is selected. That is, the signal for the REIG measures does not include a speech-type signal. This is a problem because some special features, such as digital noise reduction, will now interact with the REIG measurement. It is possible, however, even with this

TIPS AND TRICKS: How Close Is Close Enough?

It is unfortunate that prescriptive targets are often displayed as a single value because they really represent a range for an acceptable fitting. The single target value, often displayed for the dispenser and patient to see, encourages some people to try to attain a level of preciseness that may not be necessary. As we discussed in Chapter 2, background research with the development of the NAL-NL2 revealed that +/−3 dB of target (a 6 dB window) is satisfactory for the preferred listening level of about 60% of patients. Each office or clinic must establish its own rules for what is close enough, but given the lack of preciseness in threshold measurement (5 dB steps), the common use of average correction factors, and the variability of applying average prescriptive targets to individual listeners, a +/−3 to 5 dB deviation from REIG or REAR targets certainly seems acceptable. At least one manufacturer does provide a vertical bar, rather than a single point representing an acceptable range for the fitting target.

equipment, to conduct measures for REIG calculation using your favorite speech signal. You can simply conduct the REUR and the REAR in the speech mapping mode, and then use a cursor to calculate the REIG (i.e., the different between the two curves) if the equipment does not automatically do the subtraction.

As with the REAR, the REIG can be used to verify several different hearing aid features. It's probably easier to conduct these measures using only the REAR, but if the REIG is used for verification, then it may be easier to continue to use this same reference when observing the effects of digital noise reduction, adaptive feedback, and other dynamic hearing aid signal processing.

Reliability of the Measures

When probe microphone measures were first introduced, there was some concern regarding the reliability of these measures and how this reliability might vary from machine to machine. All research findings on this topic, however, have been encouraging. For example, Mueller and Sweetow (1987) found that REIGs measured on three different systems were very similar, and Hawkins and colleagues (1991) provided test–retest data, showing results that certainly are adequate for clinical work. As shown in Table 4–2, they found that the 95% confidence intervals (CIs) were 2 to 3 dB at 3000 Hz and below and 4 to 5 dB at

TECHNICAL TIP: Placement of Probe Tube for REIG Measures

As we discuss in detail in Chapter 3 and in the previous REAR section, placement of the tip of the probe tube in the ear canal is critical. When in doubt, "deep" is usually the best approach, particularly when attempting to accurately match prescriptive gain targets at 4000 Hz and above. There is some forgiveness, however, when REIG values are used for verification. If you use a measured REUG, then it also is important that the probe-tube tip is the same place for both the REUR and REAR measures—but it doesn't really have to be deep (within reason). That is, if your probe is a little too shallow for the REUR, and is also a little too shallow for the REAR, the resulting REIG will be as accurate as if a deep placement had been used for both fittings—one of the few times that two wrongs make a right! This is illustrated in Figure 4–11 (adapted from Mueller, 1992a). The reference in this graph is 0 dB, the REIG that was obtained with the probe tip deep for both the REUR and REAR measures. What is shown are three common mistakes that could be made with probe-tip placement: REUR shallow/REAR deep (upper curve), REUR deep/REAR shallow (lower curve), and both REUR and the REAR conducted with the probe tip shallow. Notice that errors of 5 to 8 dB are present in the higher frequencies when the two measures were obtained at different distances from the TM. But when both measures are obtained at the same shallow point, the results are essentially the same as if both had been conducted with the probe tip at a deep location.

Table 4–2. Mean Signed Test–Retest Differences, Standard Deviations (SDs), and 95% Confidence Intervals (CI) for the Real-Ear Unaided Response (REUR), Real-Ear Aided Response (REAR), and Real-Ear Insertion Gain (REIG) Measures

	Frequency (kHz)								
	.25	*.5*	*.75*	*1*	*1.5*	*2*	*3*	*4*	*5*
REUR									
Mean	0.3	0.3	0.4	0.0	−0.2	0.0	0.1	0.4	2.0
SD	0.7	1.3	1.8	1.0	1.1	1.4	1.6	2.7	1.9
95% CI	1.4	2.6	3.6	2.0	2.2	2.8	3.2	5.4	3.8
REAR									
Mean	−1.3	−0.6	−0.6	−0.4	−0.2	−0.2	−0.3	−0.4	−0.2
SD	*	*	*	1.6	1.4	1.7	2.0	2.7	3.0
95% CI	*	*	*	3.2	2.8	3.4	4.0	5.4	6.0
REIG									
Mean	1.4	0.9	−0.9	−0.4	0.1	0.1	−0.3	−0.8	−0.6
SD	*	*	*	1.7	1.5	1.6	2.0	2.2	2.5
95% CI	*	*	*	3.4	3.0	3.2	4.0	4.4	5.0

Note. *Values not reported due to variable leakage around earmold resulting in inflated test–retest variability.
Source: From Hawkins et al. (1991).

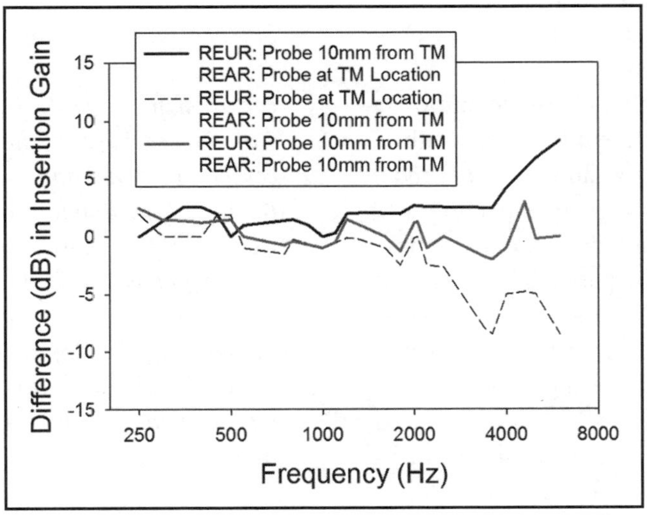

Figure 4–11. Examples of error (differences in insertion gain) resulting from changing the probe tube placement between REUR and REAR measures. The zero line represents the measure conducted with a deep placement of the probe tip for both the REUR and REAR. Adapted from Mueller,1992a.

4000 and 5000 Hz. As expected, the mean test–retest differences for the REAR/REIG were a little higher (because now we have the variable of hearing aid or earmold insertion), but these values were still respectable with CIs of 2 to 3 dB below 1000 Hz, 3 dB in the 1000 to 2000 Hz region, and 4 to 6 dB at 3000 Hz and above. Similar findings were reported by Valente et al. (1990), and we certainly would expect findings as good or better with today's equipment.

Calculation of the REIG (Assuming Limited Venting)

- If necessary, calibrate the probe tube (not all systems require this step).
- Position the patient appropriately.
- Position the probe tube at the correct depth in the ear canal.
- If necessary, calibrate/level the reference microphone (not all systems require this step).
- Measure the REUR and store (or use the average REUR in your probe microphone system).
- Place the eartip or earmold and/or custom instrument in the ear, with hearing aid programmed to desired starting point (e.g., manufacturer's implementation of a validated fitting method for the patient's hearing loss).
- Activate the hearing aid with all special features on, with the possible exception of frequency lowering, depending on fitting goals.
- Present a calibrated real-speech or speech-like signal; use an input level consistent with fitting protocol (see previous REAR discussion).
- Observe the calculated REIG; if fitting to prescriptive targets, make programming changes to obtain the desired output.
- Once target is met, conduct REAR testing (with subsequent REIG calculation) at next input level. Continue until target match and verification is obtained for soft, average, and loud inputs.

Clinical Application of the REIG

- Primary: To obtain gain match to desired prescriptive fitting targets
- Secondary: To assess special features (e.g., directional, noise reduction, etc.)
- Secondary: To estimate aided thresholds (see example in Chapter 5)

Real-Ear Aided Response for an 85 dB Or 90 dB Input (REAR85 or REAR90)

Definition:

- *SPL as a function of frequency, at a specified measurement point in the ear canal, for a specified sound field, with the hearing aid (and its acoustic coupling) in place and "turned on," with the VC adjusted to full-on (or just below feedback if full-on isn't possible). The input signal is sufficiently intense to operate the hearing aid at its maximum output level. Usually 85 or 90 dB SPL as noted in the acronym. Previously referred to as Real-Ear Saturation Response (RESR).*

This measure became part of the ANSI standard in the latest revision, but the use of the RESR term (and the measurement) dates back to the early days of probe microphone testing. As the definition states, this test is conducted with the volume control (VC) "full-on" (or just below feedback) using an 85 or 90 dB SPL input signal. You can think of it as conducting the 2-cc coupler OSPL90 measure in the real ear, although this is only partially true, as the measurement is taken with the hearing aid's maximum output adjusted for the patient, which often will not be the maximum. In other words, we want to create a "worse case" measure in the clinic to ensure that there isn't excessive aided loudness in the real world. If the patient's hearing aid does not have a VC, then the programmed use–gain is the level used for conducting the measure. The clinical application of conducting this measure is twofold: to ensure that the hearing aid's maximum output does not exceed the patient's comfort levels and to ensure that the maximum output does not exceed safe levels.

The general use of the REAR85 or REAR90 in clinical practice is to verify that the MPO, that was set based on the unaided LDL measures, is appropriate. Refer back to Figure 4–8 and you see that the patient's LDLs have been converted to ear canal SPL and are displayed on the fitting screen (normally we only test LDLs at two frequencies). We can think of these as the REAR85/90 targets—targets in the sense that we don't want to exceed these levels. If our unaided LDLs (in HL) during the initial audiometric evaluation were conducted carefully (see Chapter 6), and we then used these values (converted to 2cc coupler using the RETSPL) to program the hearing aid's MPO, there should not be any surprises during the REAR85 testing. In fact, it's common that the REAR85/90 values are well below the upper level, simply because the output is being limited by the WDRC, rather than the AGCo or some other type of output limiting. But, if there are peaks in the output, these can be handled by using the channel-specific output limiting controls in the software.

A concern that has been associated with this measure since it was first introduced is the potentially high levels of sound that can be present in the ear canal while conducting this procedure. In a worst-case scenario, a linear power hearing aid with a coupler output of 135 to 140 dB SPL could be driven to its maximum if the VC is set to "max" and the input is a pure tone. If the residual ear canal volume is small (e.g., deep earmold, small ear canal), the output in the ear canal could be 150 dB SPL or higher. This raises the concern of acoustic trauma during the test procedure, or the procedure could trigger tinnitus. We assume that a prudent dispenser will ensure that levels of 150 dB are never delivered to a patient; however, it could happen. Probe microphone equipment does have safeguards for this, as you can set the maximum output measured by the system to a specific value (e.g., 120 dB SPL), and it will shut down the input signal when this output is reached.

If you do choose to conduct REAR85 measurements, it is important to remember that the input signal can influence the results significantly—the spectrum level of the output at a particular frequency using a broadband signal will be lower than the total rms output, as illustrated in Figure 4–12. Observe the difference between the output for swept tone and the speech signal, both presented using an input of 85 dB. The question then becomes, do you want to set the maximum output of the hearing aid for the most common signals the patient hears (broadband signals like speech), or do you want to set the maximum output of the hearing aid for the occasional narrow-band signals the patient hears? A conservative approach is to adjust the maximum output of the hearing aid using pure-tone inputs, as many signals that the user experiences do have narrow-band spectra and will drive the hearing aid output close to this level (see Stelmachowicz, 1991).

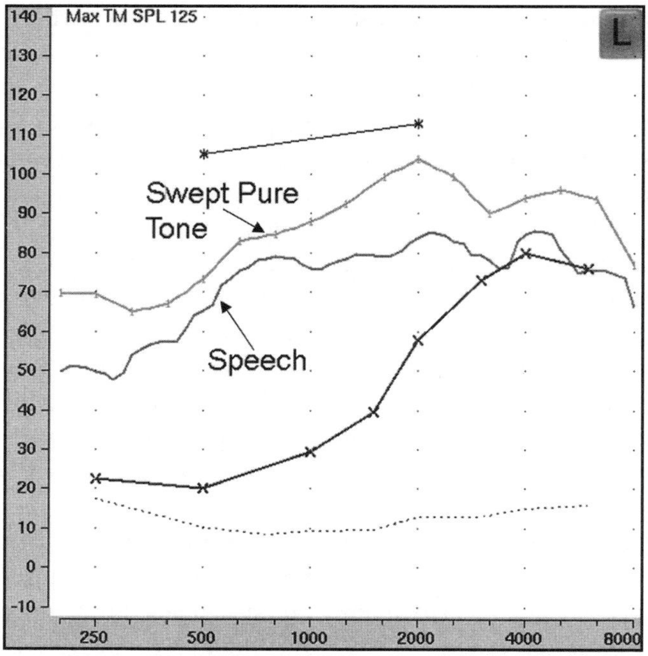

Figure 4–12. Example of the output of a hearing aid for both a speech signal and a pure-tone sweep of the same input level.

Measurement of the REAR85/90

- If necessary, calibrate the probe tube (not all systems require this step).
- Position the patient appropriately.
- Position the probe tube at the correct depth in the ear canal.
- Place the eartip or earmold and/or custom instrument in the ear, with hearing aid programmed to desired starting point (e.g., manufacturer's implementation of a validated fitting method for the patient's hearing loss).
- If necessary, calibrate/level the reference microphone (not all systems require this step).
- Activate the hearing aid with all special features on, with the exception of frequency lowering. Frequency lowering must be deactivated in order to measure an accurate REAR85/90 in response to tonal signals.
- If patient has a VC, adjust to full-on, or just below feedback. If patient does not have a VC, conduct testing at use-gain settings.
- Present a calibrated swept pure tone (or tone pips) of either 85 dB or 90 dB SPL.
- Observe the recorded real-ear MPO; make programming changes to obtain the desired output.

Clinical Application of the REAR85/90

- Primary: To ensure that MPO doesn't exceed patient's LDLs
- Primary: To ensure that MPO is safe
- Secondary: To ensure that MPO is not unreasonably low, unnecessarily restricting headroom

TECHNICAL TIP: Setting the VC for the REAR85/90 Measure

As mentioned in the definition for the REAR85/90 measure, the hearing aids should be set to full-on if possible. Although we like to follow rules laid out in standards, there may be times when this one can be broken. The primary purpose of doing this testing is to ensure that the MPO of the hearing aid will not exceed the patient's LDLs. We understand that if the patient is using a hearing aid with a VC, it's certainly possible that she may be listening to something soft with the VC turned up when a sudden loud sound occurs. But what if the patient doesn't have a VC, as is the case for approximately 25% of fittings? Does it make sense to turn the hearing aid to full-on gain for this testing when we know that the patient will never have the gain at this level in the real world? We don't think so. For these patients, we propose doing the testing at the patient's use-gain setting.

Real-Ear Coupler Difference (RECD)

Definition:

- *RECD: Difference in decibels, as a function of frequency, between the SPL produced near the tympanic membrane in an occluded ear canal by a coupled sound source having a high acoustic impedance (see ANSI/ASA S1.1) and that produced in the HA-1 configuration of the 2 cm^3 earphone coupler by the same coupled sound source*

In our discussion of the RECD in this section, we'll be tossing out some other commonly used correction factors—we talked about them in Chapter 2, but in case you are new to all this, here is a quick review. There are basically four different corrections that are commonly applied related to hearing aid fitting and probe microphone measures (Figure 4–15 illustrates the relationship between these measures):

- Coupler Response for Flat Insertion Gain (CORFIG): The difference between hearing aid gain in the coupler vs. gain in the real ear
- Real Ear Coupler Difference (RECD): The difference between hearing aid output in the coupler vs. output in the real ear
- Reference Equivalent Threshold in SPL (RETSPL): The difference between HL (audiometric dial setting) vs. output in a 2-cc coupler
- Real Ear Dial Difference (REDD): The difference between HL (audiometric dial setting) versus output in the real ear

The RECD is a new addition to the ANSI probe microphone standard, and as you can see by the caveats in our associated Tips and Tricks, there is considerable concern about the measure being conducted correctly. Although this procedure was not in the standard until recently, the RECD has been a common measurement conducted with children since the late 1980s (e.g., see Feigin, Kopun, Stelmachowicz, & Gorga,

1989). If you fit hearing aids to infants and children and do not own probe microphone equipment, the ability to conduct this procedure alone justifies the purchase. If we know a child's RECD, we have information that will assist us in selecting the appropriate hearing aid output and in predicting the output in the child's ear (OSPL90 + RECD = Predicted Real-Ear MPO, or 2-cc coupler + RECD + MLE = Predicted Real Ear Output). Moreover, on the day of the fitting, the majority of the patient-specific hearing aid adjustments can be made in the 2-cc coupler, reducing the time and cooperation required from the child. Matching hearing aid gain to validated prescriptive targets in a coupler by applying average or individually measured RECDs can also be useful with some adult patients (assuming a closed coupling system for the hearing aid). We have all seen difficult-to-test patients who are unable to sit quietly motionless for enough time to adjust the hearing aid to REAR targets. A short RECD measure greatly lessens this time and will typically result in an accurate fitting. In some cases, we are even unable to measure RECDs. Fitting the hearing aid in a coupler with an age-specific average RECD value in these cases will typically result in a fitting that is considerably closer to the desired real-ear targets than simply applying a manufacturer's first fit.

TIPS AND TRICKS: Three RECD Caveats

The current ANSI standard for real-ear measurements (ANSI S3.46–2013) has three caveats to the measurement of the RECD:

- Caveat 1: The HA-1 configuration of the 2-cc earphone coupler is described in ANSI/ASA S3.7 and excludes any coupling tubing.
- Caveat 2: If the coupled sound source is the same for both the ear canal and the coupler SPL measurements, and if the magnitude of its acoustic impedance is significantly higher than the magnitudes of the acoustic impedances of the ear canal and of the 2-cc coupler, the RECD will be a measure of the magnitude of the acoustic impedance of the ear canal relative to that of the 2-cc coupler, independent of the coupled sound source. Otherwise, the SPL difference between the ear and the coupler is dependent on the coupled sound source utilized in its measurement.
- Caveat 3: Because the HA-2 configuration of the 2-cc coupler described in ANSI/ASA S3.22 contains 25 mm of 2-mm inside diameter (i.d.) tubing plus 18 mm of 3-mm (i.d.) tubing, which in most cases will be different from that in the individual earmold or eartip used for the ear canal measurement, its use for the coupler portion of RECD measurements will result in a different coupled sound source for the two measurements. The resulting RECD will not be a measure of the magnitude of the acoustic impedance of the ear canal relative to that of the 2-cc coupler. For this reason, its use in the determination of RECD is strongly discouraged.

AUDIOID: Who Was Bobby Boyle?

In general, the value of the RECD relates to the increase in dB when the volume of a cavity (such as is an ear canal) is reduced—that is, how much smaller is that cavity when compared to a 2-cc coupler (which we are thinking is very close to 2 cc). We usually use the rule that if the volume is reduced by one-half, the SPL output will increase by 6 dB. This is referred to as Boyle's Law. Who is (was) Boyle? Robert Boyle, an Irishman, constructed, with the help of his assistant Robert Hooke, an air pump in his private laboratory within his house in Oxford, England. With this device, he carried out numerous experiments, among them careful measurements of the elasticity or the "spring" of air. Using knowledge he gained from some colleagues (Boyle probably didn't discover Boyle's Law), Boyle quantified that when he compressed a volume of air and the volume decreased, the pressure increased. He published his work in 1662, two years before the immensely successful launch of Kronenbourg's 1664 beer.

CLINICAL CONCEPT: The ANSI Standard RECD and Past Clinical Practice

In the past, the two different uses for the RECD (application for hearing aid fitting, adjustment of threshold for calculation of accurate prescriptive targets) were somewhat in conflict. Specifically, because the primary application was hearing aid fittings in children, the hearing aid was being fitted with a specific plumbing (tubing and venting) in a BTE earmold. Conversely, thresholds were measured with insert earphones in the absence of this plumbing. A common recommendation of the time was to assess the RECD using the child's earmold, and to be most accurate, consider re-measuring thresholds through the individual's earmold as well. Furthermore, many probe microphone systems measured and referenced the RECD to the HA-2 coupler. The advantage of this method was that it allowed the clinician to fit the hearing aid in the coupler before the child arrived (for closed earmolds/ eartips). As pointed out in the notes from ANSI S3.46-2013, however, this was problematic since the plumbing assumed in an HA-2 coupler (a stepped bore horn) rarely reflects what the patient is actually fitted with, and impedance issues also were a factor. In order to address these issues, the new standard recommends measurement using an insert transducer that is calibrated relative to the HA-1 coupler, a considerably different measurement than the RECD calibrated in an HA-2 coupler. In other words, the plumbing effects are removed from the RECD, and it reflects only the acoustic differences between the ear and a 2-cc coupler. Consequently, the same RECD can now be applied when correcting individual thresholds for target calculation as when fitting a hearing aid in the coupler. The plumbing is then accounted for when the hearing aid is programmed by attaching the hearing aid with all plumbing (e.g., the earmold and tubing) to an HA-1 coupler. Overall, we agree this standard should improve consistency and accuracy across clinical fittings that apply the RECD; however, some equipment requires that we have the earmold in hand when programming the hearing aid. Consequently, introduction of the new standard had a considerable impact on clinical practice in some clinics, particularly those that were fitting hearing aids using an HA-2 coupler before obtaining the earmold.

In order to circumvent this issue, at least one probe microphone manufacturer allows for fittings to validated prescriptive targets in an HA-2 coupler using an HA-1 referenced RECD. This fitting is accomplished using a HA-2 to earmold simulator correction factor that is applied by the probe microphone manufacturer. This procedure has the advantage of not requiring the patient's earmold prior to fitting to targets, as well as being a very repeatable measure (ensuring that the hearing aid earmold is oriented correctly in an HA-1 coupler and well-sealed with putty takes considerable care). When fitting with this procedure, the match to target on the HA-2 coupler will be very similar to that obtained in an HA-1 coupler using standard tubing and an unvented earmold (and consequently in the ear of the patient using REAR procedures). Of course, the accuracy of using this HA-2 based fitting procedure will be lessened when the earmold tubing is shorter or longer than assumed by the correction factor and when there is any venting introduced.

The earliest RECD data was from Sachs and Burkhard (1972), who determined the eardrum pressure developed by insert receivers on 11 ears. In an attempt to improve existing normative data with a greater number of infant ears, a collaborative study was conducted between the University of Western Ontario and Boys Town National Research Hospital. The completed RECD measurements were on 392 children between 1 month and 16 years old (Bagatto, Scollie, Seewald, Moodie, & Hoover, 2002). These measures were completed using either acoustic immittance eartips (141 ears) or personal earmolds (251 ears). A reanalysis of these data was used to generate age-specific RECD normative data for infants up to 36 months of age (Baggatto et al., 2005). In Table 4–3, we show average values for different age groups, obtained from different data sets. These newer RECD values have been implemented into the DSL v5.0 prescriptive gain calculations used by many probe microphone systems. It is common for a probe microphone system to display the measured RECD of a given patient, compared to average values (Figure 4–13). In Figure 4–13, you see the average RECDs displayed on the top, with the measured RECDs below.

The measured RECD also can be used routinely with adults to refine the fitting. The results of one large study reported that adult RECD standard deviations are 3.1 dB for 1000 Hz, 3.5 dB for 2000 Hz, and 5.4 dB for 4000 Hz (Saunders & Morgan, 2003). Hence, entering the patient's RECDs rather

Table 4–3. Estimated Real-Ear to 2-cc Coupler-Difference (RECD) Transformations as a Function of Age and Audiometric Frequency*

	Frequency (Hz)								
HA-1 Coupler	***250***	***500***	***750***	***1000***	***1500***	***2000***	***3000***	***4000***	***6000***
0–12 months	5.4	9.8	10.0	13.0	14.4	14.5	18.5	21.6	22.4
13–24 months	7.3	10.2	9.9	12.6	13.7	14.2	16.1	18.5	15.5
25–48 months	4.0	8.5	8.7	11.8	13.2	13.2	15.5	16.2	15.4
49–60 months	2.8	8.0	8.5	9.8	11.9	12.7	14.0	15.0	14.8
>60 months	2.2	4.6	4.3	6.3	7.7	8.8	11.2	13.1	13.7
HA-2 Coupler	***250***	***500***	***750***	***1000***	***1500***	***2000***	***3000***	***4000***	***6000***
0–12 months	5.5	9.7	9.6	11.9	11.6	10.5	16.2	19.4	17.8
13–24 months	7.4	10.1	9.5	11.5	10.9	10.2	13.8	16.3	10.9
25–48 months	4.1	8.4	8.3	10.7	10.4	9.2	13.2	14.0	10.8
49–60 months	2.9	7.9	8.1	8.7	9.1	8.7	11.7	12.8	10.2
>60 months	2.3	4.5	3.9	5.2	4.9	4.8	8.9	10.9	9.1

Note. *Values for individuals >60 months were derived by Seewald, Ramji, Sinclair, Moodie, and Jamieson (1993) at the University of Western Ontario. Values for individuals <60 months were derived by applying age group data reported by Feigin et al. (1989) to the values of Seewald et al. (1993). HA-2 coupler values were derived by applying an HA-1 to HA-2 coupler transformation (Seewald et al., 1993) to the HA-1 coupler values.

Source: Bess, F. H., Chase, P. A., Gravel, J. S., Hedley-Williams, A., Seewald, R. C., Stelmachowicz, P. G., & Tharpe, A. M. (1996). Amplification for infants and children with hearing loss. Reprinted with permission from *American Journal of Audiology*, *5*(1), 66.

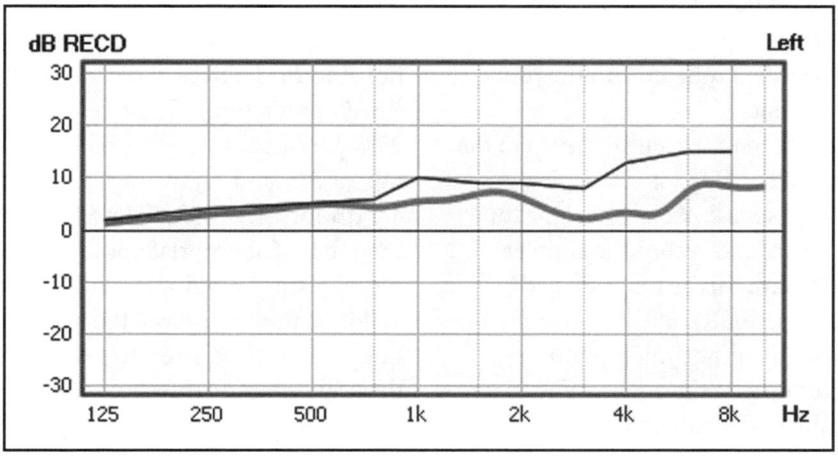

Figure 4–13. The average, age-specific, RECD values (*top line*) relative to a measured RECD (*bottom line*).

than using average values will add preciseness to the threshold measures and, in turn, increase the accuracy of the calculated prescriptive targets.

In 1994, Moodie, Seewald and Sinclair described an RECD procedure that utilized insert earphones, a HA-2 coupler, and the child's own earmold. Even with the recent standard, we expect this method is still commonly used in some clinic protocols. Specifically, the procedure they described is as follows:

- Conduct appropriate calibration and configure the software of the probe microphone equipment for RECD measurements (this procedure will vary depending on manufacturer of the probe microphone equipment).
- Connect the insert earphone to the loudspeaker output terminal of the probe microphone equipment using a matching phone plug.
- Thread the probe tube through the calibrator adapter plug so that the tip of the tube extends no more than 3 mm above the surface of the plug.
- Place the calibrator adapter plug into the microphone port of the HA-2 2-cc coupler.
- Connect the probe tube to the probe microphone.
- Connect the insert earphone tip to the tubing of the HA-2 2-cc coupler.
- Deliver a speech-weighted signal of 50 dB SPL, and record the coupler output. Save this as the "unaided" measure (REUR).
- Remove the probe microphone apparatus from the coupler and place the tube in the patient's ear with the probe tip at the appropriate depth.
- Place the patient's earmold in patient's ear.
- Attach the insert earphone tip to the tubing of the earmold (the length of the earmold tubing should be appropriate for BTE hearing aid use).
- Deliver a speech-weighted signal of 50 dB SPL, and record the real-ear output. Save this as the "aided" measure (REAR).
- Either automatically or through software command, the probe microphone equipment will calculate an "REIG," which in this case is not an REIG, but an RECD. What will be displayed is the coupler output subtracted from the real-ear output for all test frequencies.
- Positive values are added to the OSPL90 to predict the RESR and subtracted from ear canal SPL targets to determine appropriate 2cc-coupler output. By also adding the MLE to the RECD, values can be used to predict real-ear SPL for other inputs of interest.

This procedure has been used successfully for several years and has been found to be a highly accurate predictor of real-ear output. Using this approach, Seewald, Moodie, Sinclair, and Scollie (1999) compared the predicted REAG and RESR to the respective measured values for 14 children fitted with BTE hearing aids (head diffraction and MLE effects were included for the REAG prediction). Their results showed a 95% confidence interval of +/−2.3 dB for the REAG and an average error range of 4.4 dB for the RESR. These findings illustrate that, if appropriate probe microphone measures are employed with infants and children, the certainty of the hearing aid fitting is probably greater than the certainty of their audiometric thresholds.

Using RECDs for Open Fittings?

As we mention in our related Tips and Tricks sidebar, a handy use of the RECD is to con-

CLINICAL CONCEPT: Factors Complicating The RECD Measurement

We now have a standard describing an RECD procedure, but as we just noted, there have been several variations of how these measures were conducted over the years. These differences complicated the precise description of the measurement, hence the need for the standard. A description of some of the complicating factors follows, including two that still apply.

These factors no longer apply:

- If the measurement was conducted using the patient's own hearing aid (which is one approach that had been suggested), MLEs become part of the RECD (assuming the testing is conducted in the sound field; if direct audio input is used, then the MLE is not included). If a given prescriptive fitting approach (such as DSL v5 or NAL-NL2), or a manufacturer's software that already includes average MLEs, and it allows you to enter the patient's RECD, then it's possible that the MLE would be added twice. Recall that the CORFIG is calculated by the formula: REUG – RECD + MLE, which assumes that the MLE is not part of the RECD.
- The MLEs for a hearing aid tested by using a moderate input level are not the same as the MLEs when the hearing aid is in saturation. One of the uses of the RECD is to predict the output of the hearing aid when it's in saturation, yet the hearing aid REAR measurement often is conducted using a 60 dB input.
- If the patient was fitted with a WDRC instrument, then it is necessary to consider the effects of WDRC on the MLE. That is, if a 60 dB signal at 4000 Hz becomes a 70 dB input because of an MLE of 10 dB (CIC fitting), the increase in output will not be proportional if the input signal is compressed (e.g., if the compression ratio is 2:1, the MLE will now yield only a 5 dB change in output).
- If a HA-1 coupler is used, then the RECD will be different than if an HA-2 coupler is used.

These factors still apply:

- If an inset earphone is used, the output impedance effects need to be the same as for the patient's hearing aid. If a foam plug is used, the placement depth in the ear canal should approximate the depth of the patient's hearing aid or earmold.
- Even when depth is controlled, the RECD using a foam tip will be somewhat different from the RECD using the patient's earmold. Correction factors for this recently have been suggested (Moodie et al., 2016)

duct a verification-to-target procedure in the coupler. That is, if you know how the patient's real ear differs from a coupler, you can do the entire fitting in the coupler. This is not just a pediatric application, it works even better for adults (as it easier to obtain a valid RECD). But, and this is an important "but," this only applies *when you are doing a closed fitting*. With adults, this isn't very often. Back in 2009 (Mueller, 2009), many clinics reported doing 75% open fittings, and that value is certainly higher today, as feedback systems have improved, and open fittings have become more routine. Moreover, most "closed dome" fittings using manufacturer's tips aren't really all that closed. The problem, of course, is that you can't use a measure conducted with a closed fitting (the RECD) to predict ear canal SPL for an open fitting. Let's talk about that a bit. You, of course, are immediately thinking of the leakage of low frequencies, but it's more than that. Consider that with an OC fitting that is truly open, the patient retains all or most of the natural ear canal resonance (with a closed fitting this is not the case). This REUG boost is primarily in the 2000 to 3000 Hz range. The remaining average ear canal resonance is often around 15 dB or so, so is this a *free* 15 dB of gain for our patients? Sound too good to be true? It is. Remember the advantages of a closed deeper fitting—the increased SPL when we make the residual ear canal smaller (Boyles law). With an OC fitting, we do not obtain this advantage, which can amount to 10 dB or more, depending on how deep the earmold goes into the ear canal. So, we have one advantage for open, another for closed, and we need to know the net result of the interaction.

The relationship between closed and open fittings was studied by Mueller and Ricketts (2006) and is displayed in Figure 4–14. By conducting probe microphone measures on real ears and changing only the earmold (open versus closed), they were able to identify the differences between the fitting methods. This figure represents a difference curve; above the 0 dB line indicates an advantage for the OC fitting. Observe that on average, this advantage is about 5 dB in the region of the ear canal resonance. There are individual variations depending on the patient's open ear resonance (how much do they have to lose?) and the size

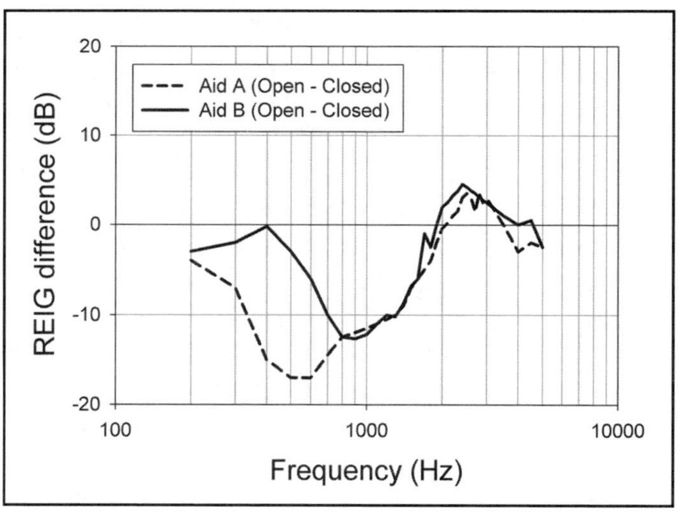

Figure 4–14. Difference in average insertion gain for two mini-BTE hearing aids measured using an open and closed fitting tip. Earmold tubing and hearing aid settings were unchanged. Adapted from Mueller and Ricketts, 2006.

of the ear canal (smaller ear canals will be impacted more by a closed earmold). We need to point out that the *individual* closed versus open difference in the high frequencies is considerably greater than shown in this chart. This is because the differences occurred at different frequencies for different people—individual differences of around 10 dB were common.

As expected, the closed earmold made a large difference in the average gain in the lower frequencies, especially for hearing aid A; hearing aid B did not have much amplifier gain for the very low frequencies. This shows just how much gain really is leaking out with the OC fitting, and again, why RECD corrections for this type of fitting don't work.

Measurement of the RECD

The approach described by Moodie, Seewald and Sinclair (1994) really needs only minor modifications that mainly relate to calibration details to be in line with the current ANSI standard. Our modified version of these instructions follows:

- Connect an insert earphone or RECD transducer to the probe microphone equipment.
- Configure the software of the probe microphone equipment for RECD measurements and conduct appropriate calibration of the transducer referenced to an HA-1 coupler (this procedure will vary depending on manufacturer of the probe microphone equipment).
  - One method is to attach the transducer via foam insert eartip to the HA-1 coupler. Another is to attach the transducer to the individual's earmold, with all venting blocked and putty the earmold to the HA-1 coupler. A broadband speech-weighted or pink noise signal is typically used for calibration.

  Note: At least one probe microphone manufacturer currently calibrates the transducer in an HA-2 coupler (without an insert eartip or earmold) and then applies a correction so that the measure is referenced to an HA-1 coupler. We assume that this procedure is applied to improve reliability compared to attaching a transducer to an HA-1 coupler. Some systems also use a 0.4-cc coupler and connector adaptor to allow the transducer to be easily coupled to the coupler, and then automatically provide an equivalent HA-1 referenced RECD for compatibility with other equipment and fitting software.
- Place the probe tube in the patient's ear, with the probe tip at the appropriate depth.
- Remove the transducer from the HA-1 coupler (with earmold or foam insert attached) and insert it in the patient's ear.
- Deliver the same signal used in calibrating the transducer in the HA-1 coupler through the loudspeaker and measure the output in the ear. The difference between the coupler and real-ear values is the individual's RECD. These values are typically calculated automatically by the probe microphone system.

Clinical Application of the RECD

- Primary: To predict hearing aid output in the ear canal when 2cc-coupler values are known

TIPS AND TRICKS: Application of RECD for Real-Ear Equivalent Verification

When considering young children or other difficult-to-fit patients, one important use of the RECD is the simulated REAR. Once you measure an individual's RECD, a fitting procedure that accurately reflects verification in the real ear can be completed using the following steps:

- Configure your probe microphone software for a simulated REAR and enter the patient's thresholds and LDLs and identify the validated prescriptive fitting method you plan to use.
- Measure or enter the patient's RECD.
- If a BTE instrument is being fitted, attach the patient's earmold or eartip with the tubing length size appropriate for the patient and all plumbing configured as it will be for the patient. Attach the earmold or ear shell (in the case of a custom hearing aid) to an HA-1 coupler using putty. As noted earlier in this chapter, at least one probe microphone system will allow you to use a BTE and an HA-2 coupler and will automatically apply an HA-2 to earmold simulator correction factor.
- Adjust hearing aid gain in the coupler to match prescriptive targets. Typically, this will use methods that are very similar to REAR verification procedures.

Although this procedure typically yields fittings that are equivalent to those measured in the real ear, there is one considerable limitation related to venting. Specifically, larger vents must be wholly or partially plugged to avoid uncontrollable feedback that occurs because of the reflective surfaces within the hearing aid test box. Therefore, it's not possible to use this procedure with open fittings—in addition to the feedback issue, it's also very difficult to accurately simulate an open fitting using a coupler, although a standard open coupler is currently under development.

- Primary: To determine desired OSPL90 and coupler output settings
- Primary: To apply when programming the hearing aid in the coupler to equivalent real-ear targets (only for *closed* fittings)
- Secondary: To individualize REDD corrections so as to provide a better estimate of hearing thresholds for calculation of real-ear prescriptive targets

Real-Ear Dial Difference (REDD)

Definition:

- *REDD: Difference in decibels, as a function of frequency, between the SPL produced near the tympanic membrane by an audiometric sound source and the hearing level indicated by the audiometer driving the sound source.*

Note: The REDD can be used to convert hearing level (HL) behavioral measures obtained with an audiometer to ear canal SPL for comparison to the measured real-ear quantities described in the standard. The REDD is specific to the audiometer and sound source used in its measurement.

A final probe microphone term that you may not be too familiar with is the REDD, a term has been in use since 1995 (Mueller, 1995). The REDD is another calculation that was just added to the current ANSI standard. The primary purpose of the REDD is to allow you to plot SPL-O-Grams—the REDD is added to the HL thresholds (and LDLs if available) to obtain a plot of these values in ear canal SPL. Most of today's probe microphone equipment will do this calculation and plotting for you using average or measured REDD values. Consider that the REDD is really a combination of two other correction factors, the RETSPL, which takes us from the audiometer to the 2-cc coupler, and the RECD, which then takes us from the 2-cc coupler to the real ear—RECD + RETSPL = REDD. For example, the average RECD for an adult at 3000 Hz is around 9 dB, and the RETSPL for insert earphones is 3 dB (we'll assume that the audiometer is appropriately calibrated). So we would expect the average REDD at 3000 Hz for insert earphones to be around 12 dB (9 + 3 = 12). RETSPLs are somewhat different for insert versus supra-aural earphones, and the REDDs will then be slightly different also.

It is not too difficult to measure individual REDDs, but very few people do it. For one thing, it does require that your audiometer and probe equipment are located fairly close to each other, if you have an integrated system, no problem. If you'd like to try it, see the step-by-step procedure outlined by Mueller (2001b). If your equipment is not in close enough proximity, another easy way to obtain individualized REDDs is to measure the individuals RECD and add the RETSPL.

TAKE FIVE: Remember the RETSPL

We've talked about the RETSPL before, but because it is a component of the REDD, we'll do a quick review. These correction factors allow us to convert HL values to 2-cc coupler SPL. This correction factor isn't directly related to probe microphone measures, but it certainly relates to hearing aid selection and verification. Most clinics today have their audiometer calibrated by a local Special Instruments Dealer (SID) that is probably a member of NASED (National Association of Special Equipment Dealers). Today's audiometers nearly always can be calibrated within 0.3 to 0.5 dB of the ANSI standard values, so usually you can assume that the values listed in ANSI S3.6-1996 are reliable RETSPLs for you to use (in this maze of acronyms, it's important to remember that audiometers have RETSPLs, people don't). In addition to REDD calculations, a common clinical application of RETSPLs is to convert LDL values to 2-cc-coupler values when considering the appropriate maximum output of a hearing aid (see Chapter 6).

Clinical Applications of the REDD

- Primary: To convert HL hearing thresholds to ear canal SPL
- Secondary: To convert HL LDLs to ear canal SPL

If you're somewhat new to hearing aids, all these terms and correction factors can be a little confusing. When do you add what to what to get . . . whatever? If you start to get the sense you're sometimes going in circles, you're correct. Several years ago, Larry Revit put together a chart to simplify things, and called it the "Circle of Decibels" (Revit, 1997). We think it's still helpful today, and have included it here in Figure 4–15.

Now that we have reviewed all the specific probe microphone measures, it is time to talk in a bit more detail about how you can use this ear canal information in your everyday fitting of hearing aids, which is included in Chapter 5. As we have said before, the use of this testing is limited only by your imagination, but to help you out a little, in the following chapter, we provide examples of several uses for probe microphone testing in your daily practice. At this point, we hope that at the least you have a good understanding of all the basic measures—why some terms end in an "R" and others in a "G." We'll close this chapter with a transcription of a lunchtime conversation among a group of audiologist who just finished their morning hearing aid fittings. If

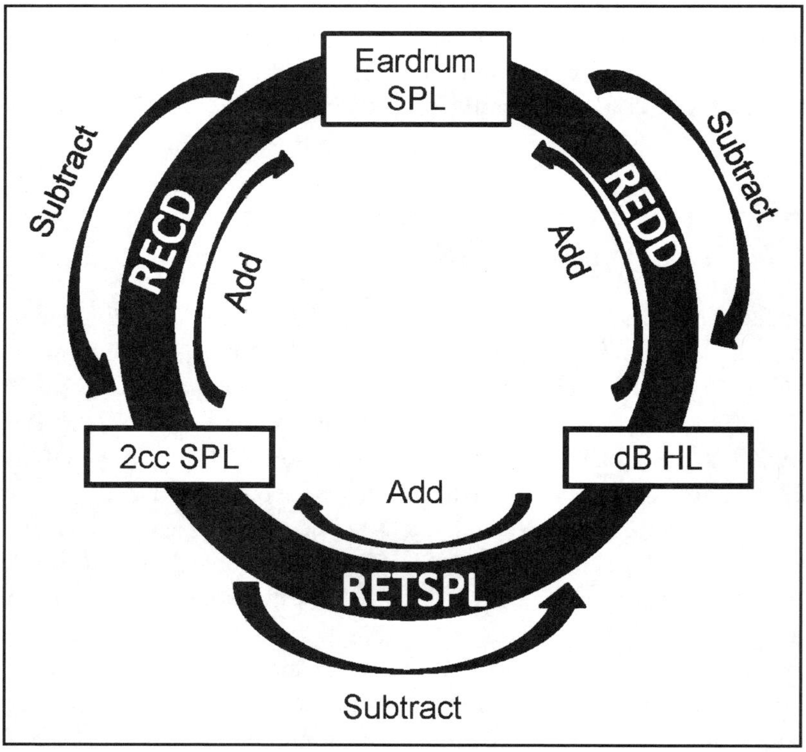

Figure 4–15. The Circle of Decibels showing the formulation of correction factors from dB Hearing Level (HL) 2-cc coupler and eardrum SPL measures. Adapted from Revit, 1997.

it all makes sense to you—we think you've got it!

Todd: You should have seen the patient I had this morning. His UR was 28 dB at 3K!

Ruth: Todd, Todd. You mean his UG was 28 dB. If you used a 50 dB input, his UR would have been 78 dB, not 28.

Todd: Yeah, well, okay you're right. But anyway, when I put in the open earmold tip for his OC fitting, the OR actually was –2 dB, so I guess the tip was more occluding than I thought.

Fred: Very interesting Todd, but sounds like you're talking about his OG, not his OR. If you're using a 50 dB input, the OR would have been 48 dB.

Gus: Could someone pass the ketchup please?

Peter: I see an OG like that sometimes for my OC fittings too. How did your speech map results turn out?

Todd: I didn't do speech mapping, I did insertion gain, and my match to NAL-NL2 was pretty good.

Fred: You mean your match to the REIR? I'd think with a UG that big, the REIR would have a dip at 3K.

Gus: Fred. I hate to tell you, but we dumped the REIR term 15 years ago. Gain is always gain, which is always a difference. The term is REIG, not REIR.

Fred: Okay, sorry, that REIR thing just sort of slipped out by accident. I switched to speech mapping several years ago, so I use the AG for verification and don't think much about insertion gain anymore—oops, should I have said the AR rather than the AG?

Ruth: Well Fred, that was just a little "oops." We still use both the AG and AR terms, but usually when we do speech mapping, we indeed use the AR for verification.

Todd: So am I the only one who is still verifying hearing aids using the IG?

Gus: Well, insertion gain measures are still pretty popular in places like the U.K., but in the U.S. you are indeed in a small minority.

Ruth: I still do REIG calculations for some patients with open fittings when the low-frequency speech map results look strange.

Peter: I can't remember the last time I used the IG. The beauty of speech mapping is that you don't have to worry about those nasty bumps and dips in the patient's UG.

Gus: I rarely use the REIG, but when I do REIG calculations, I simply use the average UG, and then you don't have those problems.

Todd: What? You can do that? Isn't that cheating?

Fred: Okay folks, the party is over. Looks like our 1:00 patients are here.

Gus: Hey wait, doesn't anyone want to talk about RETSPLs?

5 Verification and Assessment of Fittings and Features

A good intention, with a bad approach, often leads to a poor result.
—Thomas Edison

Now that we have reviewed all the specific probe microphone measures, it is time to talk in a bit more detail about how you can use this ear canal information in your everyday fitting of hearing aids. In this chapter, we offer step-by-step guidelines for conducting most all the measures you will encounter, for as Thomas Edison said, a bad approach often leads to a poor result, even if your intentions are good. A prime example of this is the all-too-common use of a "live voice" input for programming gain and output. While the dispenser who thinks that Mary's hearing aids should be programmed for Bob's voice probably has good intentions, the outcome of this approach is dubious at best. As we have said before, the general use of speech mapping and probe microphone measures is limited only by your imagination, but to help you out a little, in the following section, we provide examples of several uses for probe microphone testing in your daily practice.

Verification of Prescriptive Targets Using the REAR (Speech Mapping)

We begin this section with the most common, and most important, probe microphone measure conducted by audiologists —verification of prescriptive targets using speech mapping. We use the term "verification," but this has the unstated implication that a fair amount of adjustment is also required. It is very unlikely that the manufacturer's software-derived setting will be an acceptable match for even one input level, and certainly not all three (see Sanders et al., 2015, and our discussion in Chapter 1). The process, of course, begins with selecting a validated fitting algorithm (e.g., NAL-NL2 or DSL v5) and ensuring that these real-ear targets are available with your probe microphone equipment (which should not be a problem unless your equipment is quite dated). The task then becomes measurement-tweaking-measurement-tweaking until you obtain a close match to the desired output. We talked quite a bit about this procedure in Chapter 4, and we offered a general protocol when we introduced the REAR, so let's go directly to the application of the REAR to fitting and verification.

Test Protocol

- Enter patient's audiogram and measured LDLs. If a conductive loss is present, enter bone conduction thresholds (conductive losses impact calculated targets). The LDLs will impact targets for the DSL, not the NAL.

- Select your choice of validated prescriptive method in the probe microphone fitting software, and also select appropriate variables that could influence target calculation (e.g., adult versus child, gender, experience, transducer type, tightness of fitting, unilateral versus bilateral fitting—not all choices are available with all manufacturers or all fitting methods).
- Program hearing aid to desired fitting algorithm using manufacturer's software control process (again, select appropriate patient and fitting factors).
- Select appropriate speech or speech-like signal (e.g., shaped real speech, ISTS).
- Place the probe tube in the ear at an appropriate depth, mute the hearing aid, and fit it to the patient's ear.
- After the hearing aid is fitted (physically), unmute the instrument and begin testing using the first input level in your personal protocol (see discussion of test order in Chapter 4). Adjust frequency-specific gain to achieve a reasonable match to target.
- Continue until a match is obtained for all three input levels. We suggest a final check of all levels to ensure that programming for one did not significantly impact another.

Sample Findings

Figure 5–1 is an illustration of REAR verification using the ISTS input at three levels: 55, 65, and 75 dB SPL. Although it might be interesting to see the entire amplitude range

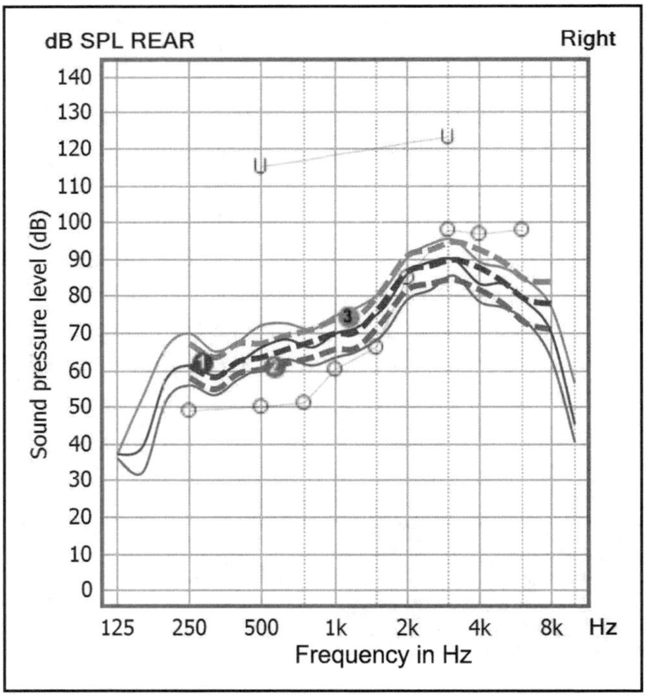

Figure 5–1. Example of REAR measures obtained with ISTS stimulus, with match to NAL-NL2 fitting targets, shown for three input levels (55, 65, 75 dB inputs).

of the amplified signal (e.g., the "banana"), when plotting all three curves together, doing so becomes a bit too much information, so only the LTASS is shown here. This patient has a fairly typical hearing loss, although he does have a rather substantial drop at 4000 Hz (to 80 dB HL, which might not be obvious on this type of plot). We have done a quite good job of matching targets—about as good it gets when you look at all three inputs. At first glance, you might be questioning whether we have enough audibility at 4000 Hz—we address that in an associated Clinical Concept. Or you might also question whether frequency lowering should be activated above 3000 Hz. That is probably a patient-specific decision, but could be considered in this case. Notice that in the 1500 to 3000 Hz range, the LTASS range is now about 10 dB for the inputs that differed by 20 dB (55 to 75 dB), suggesting a compression of the speech signal of about 2:1. We suspect that this hearing aid has a fairly short release time because otherwise, you probably wouldn't see this degree of compression (e.g., while the fitting software may say 2:1, effective compression may be only 1.3:1 or so for real speech for WDRC with slower release times). If you use the protocol of fitting to soft inputs first and if the compression has a slow release, it may not be possible to match the prescriptive targets for the 75-dB input, even with WDRC set to max, (which is usually 3:1 or 4:1).

Fitting Tips

- We recommend conducting speech mapping with all special features activated. The exception to this is frequency lowering, which should be turned off unless the specific purpose is to measure the lowered signals (see the Frequency Lowering section later in this chapter).
- We mention in the preceding section that the fit to target can be influenced by the release times of the WDRC. We know that at least one manufacturer uses fast release times if you select NAL-NL2 in the fitting software and long release times if you select its proprietary fitting. If your goal is to fit to the NAL-NL2 targets and you can get there from different starting points, we advise starting off with the manufacturer's NAL algorithm, rather than their proprietary default setting.
- When viewing the REAR output, especially if it is on a small monitor, and the range of the graph is large, it's difficult to visualize the mismatch to target. A small visual difference can be 10 dB. To assist with this, we have found it handy to view the "on target" display that also is available with some systems. This provides a difference curve for all inputs tested. An example of this is shown in Figure 5–2. As you can see, for this patient we are pretty darn good for all three inputs, with some small errors in the low frequencies.

Verification of Prescriptive Targets Using Insertion Gain (REIG)

As we have discussed, while the majority of audiologists (at least in the U.S.) use the REAR for verification, some audiologists still prefer to stick with an old friend, insertion gain. Because this is just a different approach to accomplishing the same thing, much of what we have said about REAR verification also applies. As shown in Chapter 4, for a given hearing aid programmed to specific gain and output levels, you expect to see the same good or poor match to prescriptive targets with either approach.

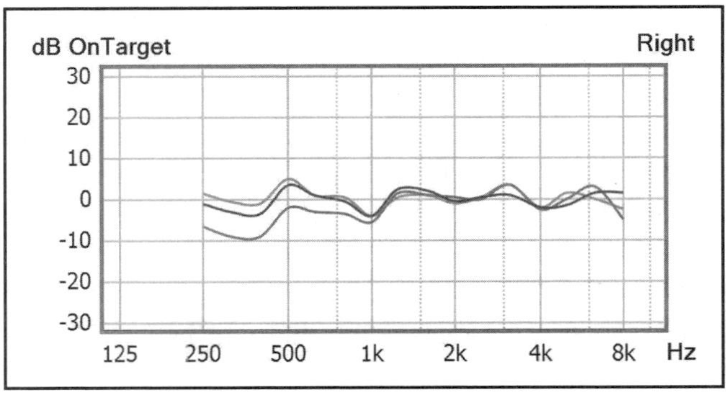

Figure 5–2. Example of view of "difference curves" which can be used to assess match to target for different input levels.

CLINICAL CONCEPT: How Much Gain Is "Enough Gain" in the High Frequencies?

We all agree that audibility is a good thing, but there are times when making things too audible can have a negative effect. We talked about this back in Chapter 3, but it's important enough to bring up again here. Observe that the patient in Figure 5–1 has a hearing loss that drops significantly at 4000 Hz (80 dB HL, about 95 dB in ear canal SPL). Also observe that the target for the LTASS for the NAL-NL2 fitting is below his threshold at the frequency, even for the 75 dB input signal. This bothers some audiologists, and they will be tempted to make speech in that area as audible as possible—maybe to the limits of the hearing aid if feedback is not an issue. As you can see by the targets, the developers of the NAL-NL2 obviously don't think this is a wise move, and we agree with them. Here are three reasons why (also see Mueller, 2017):

- First, it's important not only to consider the LTASS, but also to view the entire range of amplified speech. Because the peaks of the speech signal fall about 12 to 15 dB above the LTASS, it may indeed be the case that some speech information is audible. An example of this is shown in Figure 4–8. If we had only displayed the LTASS, it would have appeared that average speech was not audible for either 3000 or 4000 Hz. However, with the percentages displayed (shaded area) we see that indeed speech was audible for both of these frequencies.
- All patients have a preferred level of loudness. Adding more highs will add to that overall loudness level, and if the overall fitting was appropriate prior to adding the highs, speech will now be too loud. This result will prompt the patient to turn down overall gain, reducing audibility for the 1500 to 3000 Hz range, where audibility is more important than 4000 Hz. The key is to use the total signal loudness as effectively as possible by providing

the greatest audibility for the most important speech frequencies.

- There is a point, referred to as *effective audibility,* where increased audibility doesn't lead to an increased understanding of speech. The NAL-NL2 targets have attempted to account for this issue in the algorithm.

The preceding points are particularly true for downward sloping configurations, but apply to some degree for all types of hearing loss. Our comments, however, are based on fittings for adults with acquired hearing loss—the fitting philosophy might be quite different for infants and children.

The exception is a patient with an unusual REUG. If in this case the measured REUG is used, rather than using the average REUG for calculation of the REIG, then the match to target will vary from the REAR match, roughly by the difference between average and measured REUG.

Test Protocol

- Enter patient's audiogram and measured LDLs. If conductive loss is present, enter bone conduction thresholds (conductive losses impact calculated targets). The LDLs will impact targets for DSL, not the NAL.
- Select your choice of validated prescriptive method in the probe microphone fitting software, and also select appropriate variables that could influence target calculation (e.g., adult versus child, gender, experience, tightness of fitting, and unilateral versus bilateral fitting—not all choices are available with all manufacturers, or all fitting methods).
- Program hearing aid to desired fitting algorithm using the manufacturer's software control process (again, select appropriate patient and fitting factors).
- Select appropriate speech or speech-like signal (e.g., shaped speech, ISTS).
- Place the probe tube in the ear at an appropriate depth and conduct the REUR, or enter average REUR (our recommendation). *Note:* the input level for the REUR doesn't matter; it will be subsequently adjusted to correspond to the REAR levels selected.
- Mute the hearing aid and fit it to the patient's ear.
- After the hearing aid is physically fitted, unmute the instrument and begin testing using the first input level in your personal protocol (see discussion of test order earlier in this chapter). Adjust frequency-specific gain to achieve reasonable match to target.
- Continue until match is obtained for all three input levels. We suggest a final check of all levels to be sure that programming for one didn't significantly impact another one.

Sample Findings

Figure 5–3 shows the findings for REIG verification for a patient with a downward sloping hearing loss (same patient as shown for REAR verification in Figure 5–1), fitted to NAL-NL2. Keep in mind when viewing REIG, that now soft is up and loud is down. That is, the top curve shown is gain for soft inputs.

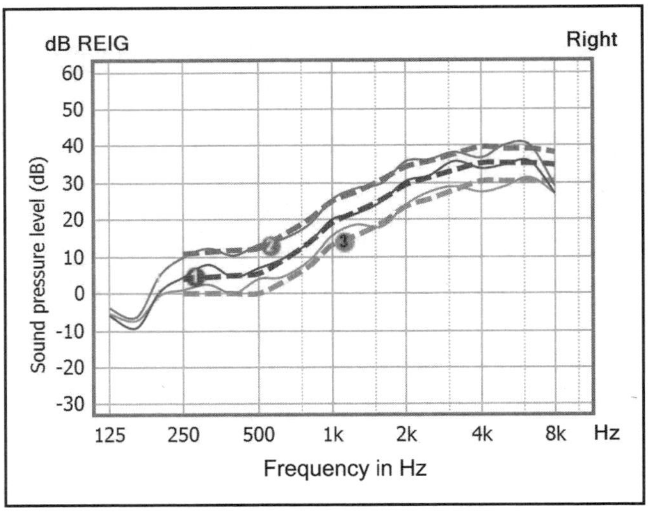

Figure 5–3. Example of REIG measures obtained with ISTS stimulus, with match to NAL-NL2 fitting targets, shown for three input levels (50, 65, 80 dB inputs).

Overall, we would consider this a good fitting—a very nice match for all input levels. Note that for this hearing loss, the NAL-NL2 calls for a fair amount of gain in the high frequencies—around 30 dB. What happens on occasion is that you will see a dip in the gain in the highs for the loud input. When this does happen, the first

TIPS AND TRICKS: Using REIGs to Construct Aided Audiogram

Those of you in clinical practice know that every now and then you will be asked to provide an aided audiogram. In some cases, this is to facilitate counseling for parents and teachers. In other cases, it may be because of a government form left over from the 1950s, or constructed by someone who thinks that this is something that we routinely do. Given that research has shown that insertion gain is the same as functional gain, and functional gain does indeed provide an aided audiogram, it seems reasonably okay to us to use the REIG findings (for soft inputs) to construct an estimated aided audiogram. That is, you simply take the REIG findings and improve the earphone thresholds by that amount (e.g., if earphone thresholds are 60 dB at 2000 Hz and the REIG for soft inputs are 35 dB, then the predicted aided threshold will be 25 dB). Yes, there are some concerns with expansion and compression, but these same issues will exist when the patient uses the hearing aids in the real world. At least one manufacturer of probe microphone equipment has simplified this process for you—it automatically adjusts the earphone thresholds by the REIG and provides the data on a handy audiogram. Figure 5–4 shows an example of this for the right and left ears.

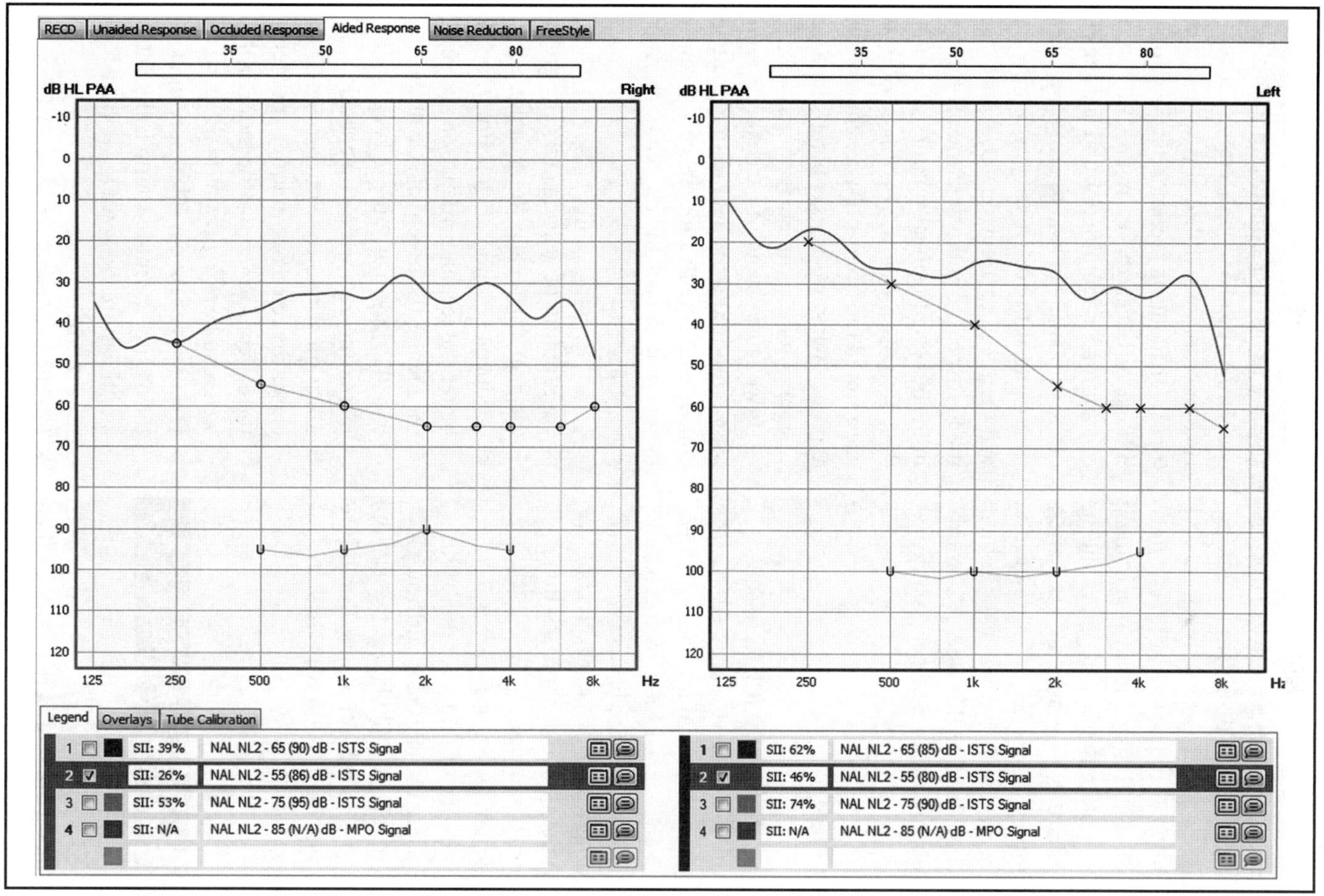

Figure 5–4. Example of one manufacturer's use of correcting the earphone thresholds using the REIG to obtain predicted aided thresholds on the same graphic, which can be used in counseling and cases where an "aided audiogram" is requested.

thing to check out is whether we've reached the MPO kneepoints, which would then be what is limiting gain. We wouldn't expect WDRC to create a gain pattern like this, and we know from our 55 dB SPL input findings that adequate gain has been programmed, so a low MPO would be likely the case. Raising the MPO in this frequency range might allow us to obtain the desired gain. But the MPO is where it is because we set it there based on the patient's LDLs. So we need to make sure we don't create a new problem while trying to solve this one. A compromise would maybe then be necessary.

Fitting Tips

- We used the average REUG for our measurement. As we discussed in Chapter 4, you could use the measured REUG, and some experts recommend this. There is no simple answer regarding what is "best" and it could be that there is not one approach that is best for all patients.
- The display shown in Figure 5–3 illustrates one of things we don't like about using the REIG for verification. Observe that, at 4000 Hz, we have about 40 dB of gain for soft inputs. But did we make soft sounds audible? How do we know?

Open-Ear Canal Fittings

Open fittings are very common, with some clinics fitting more than 50% of their patients with this earmold configuration. For the most part, probe microphone verification is the same whether the fitting is open or closed, but there is one significant difference—the on-ear calibration process for the input signal. As we discuss in Chapter 3, there is a reference microphone at the ear for all probe systems. Traditionally, we've used a concurrent modified-pressure method of equalization: The reference microphone continually monitors the input signal during presentation. With open fittings, however, there can be issues using this approach. Amplified sound leaking out of the ear canal can lead to erroneous measurements at the reference position, which will then lead to an erroneous signal from the loudspeaker and a subsequent mistake in the observed real-ear output (less output than actually present). For this reason, we use a stored modified-pressure equalization approach when we assess open fittings (see Chapter 3 for a complete explanation).

If we fail to switch to the stored equalization mode and conduct testing using the concurrent equalization method, several factors will impact the degree of the measurement error:

- Gain/output of hearing aid: The greater the gain, the greater the mistake.
- Feedback reduction algorithm: The better the feedback reduction system, the greater the potential size of the mistake, as you are able to keep increasing gain without feedback.
- Location of reference microphone: The closer the reference microphone is to the ear canal opening, the more likely we are to have a measurement error.
- Openness of the fit: The more open the fitting, the more sound leaks out, and the more likely we are to have a measurement error.
- Residual ear canal resonance of the patient: The measurement error usually occurs at the point of ear canal resonance; the mistake will be greater if the patient has a large resonance and the ear is left mostly open.

Test Protocol

- Change equalization method from modified pressure to stored equalization (*Note:* On most systems, this simply requires selecting "open" or similar descriptor of the hearing aid style).
- Enter patient's audiogram and measured LDLs. If conductive loss is present, enter bone conduction thresholds (conductive losses impact calculated targets). The LDLs will impact targets for DSL, not NAL.
- Select your choice of validated prescriptive method in probe microphone fitting software, and also select appropriate variables that could influence target calculation (e.g., adult versus child, gender, experience, tightness of fitting, and unilateral versus bilateral fitting—not all choices are available with all manufacturers, or all fitting methods).
- Program hearing aid to desired fitting algorithm using manufacturer's software control process (again, select appropriate patient and fitting factors).
- Place the probe tube in the ear at an appropriate depth, mute the hearing aid, and fit it to the patient's ear.
- Conduct stored-equalization, free-field calibration, then unmute the hearing aid. (*Note:* Probe microphone system manufacturers refer to this process using several different terms, including open calibration, equalization, and leveling.)
- From this point forward, all speech mapping testing is the same as for the traditional modified-pressure approach, *except* the patient must keep his head in the calibration position and cannot move it during test signal presentation.
- If the patient moves, it is important to mute the hearing aid, repeat the equalization procedure, unmute the hearing aid, and continue! Failure to complete this step can lead to fitting errors as great as 10 dB or more.

Sample Findings

To illustrate the potential mistake that can be made in real-ear output, we conducted speech mapping for an open fitting using both types of equalization. In Figure 5–5A, observe the bottom LTASS output tracing (dark line), which is a close match to NAL-NL2 targets, although it falls slightly below in the 3000 Hz region. This output was recorded using the concurrent equalization approach. The LTASS that is slightly higher at 3000 Hz was recorded using stored equalization—this is the "correct" output. In this case, you would think you were about 3 to 4 dB below target at 3000 Hz, when in fact you're 3 to 4 dB *above* target at this frequency. Not a huge problem, but significant nonetheless—a net difference of 6 to 8 dB.

Let's assume, however, that the audiologist doing this fitting failed to use the stored equalization approach, and wasn't happy with falling 3 to 4 dB below target at 3000 Hz, so she or he, raises gain at this frequency until target is reached. After this change, we repeated our testing using the concurrent equalization approach—see the bottom LTASS line in Figure 5–5B. Observe that, indeed, there is now a perfect match to target at 3000 Hz. But what *real output* is being delivered to the ear for this frequency range? That is shown in the upper LTASS line, obtained using the stored equalization procedure (but the same input signal). What had been a measurement mistake of around 6 dB is now nearly a 20 dB error. Why? Because as the audiologist turned up gain, leakage increased (essentially at a 1 to 1 rate), and the fitting error increased

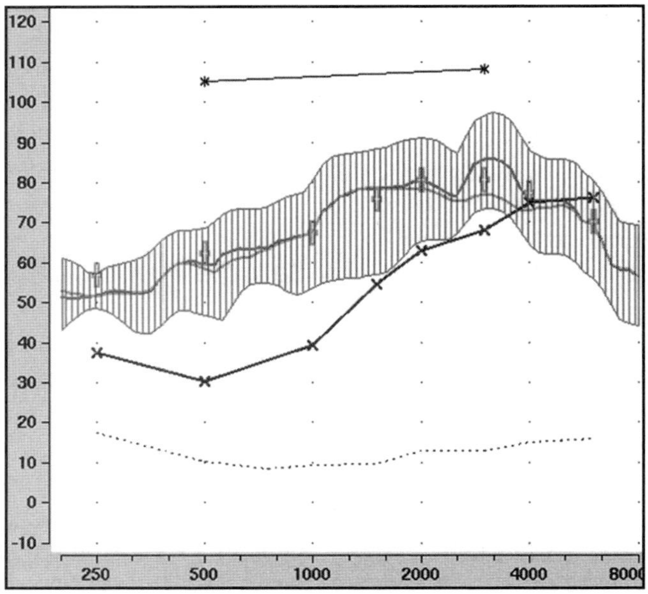

A

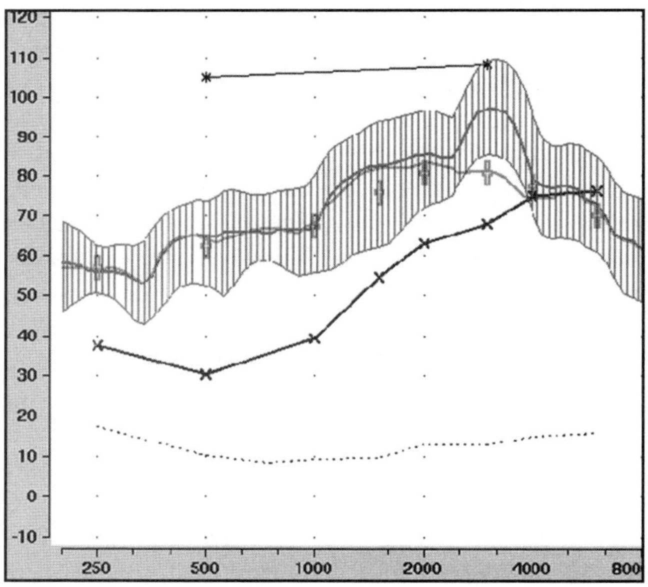

B

Figure 5–5. Repeat testing for an open fitting for the same patient using both modified pressure and stored equalization at-ear calibration procedures. In panel **A**, note that the output for the two measurement procedures is essentially the same except for a 5 dB or so increase around 3000 Hz for stored equalization (this is the true ear canal output). In panel **B**, gain has now been increased in the 3000 Hz region, and the output for the stored equalization is now nearly 20 dB greater (this is the true output) than what was obtained using the modified-pressure approach

accordingly. Imagine that an audiologist is using the wrong equalization process in a real fitting (and it *does* happen), the patient is saying, "That is really harsh sounding," and the audiologist is thinking, "I'm right at targets; I don't understand why he has a problem with that."

Fitting Tips

- Probe microphone manufacturers have made it very easy to access the stored equalization mode. There may be a software setting for "Open" or something similar.
- Remember, when using the stored equalization approach, the patient must keep her/his head in the same position as when the equalization is conducted, and not move her/his head during the testing (usually not a problem with adults).
- The measurement error is usually present only when the fitting is considerably open and gain is at least 18 to 20 dB or so, but given the simplicity of using stored equalization, we see no reason not to simply use it routinely whenever an open or even partially open fitting is assessed.
- While we recommend using concurrent equalization for closed fittings, there is no harm in using stored equalization with closed fittings as long as the patient's head and body movements aren't an issue.

TIPS AND TRICKS: One Limitation of REAR for Open Fittings

As we have indicated a few times, we prefer to use REAR over REIG verification procedures for a number of good reasons. Sometimes a REAR limitation is related to not having an obvious picture of hearing aid gain. When completing an open fitting, we sometimes see a good match to targets at 500 Hz and below and at 2000 Hz and above, but no matter how much we increase mid-frequency gain, we just can't reach targets. Sometimes, this problem is evident as a relatively narrow notch around 1500 Hz that results from a phase cancelation interaction between the amplified and direct signal pathways. This notch artifact is not easily remedied, but is often narrow enough that it does not affect sound quality (see Mueller & Ricketts, 2006). A different problem is that because the fitting is so open, we have little or no gain below 2000 Hz. So you ask—why then are we matching our REAR targets in the 500 Hz region? Because this is not "gain." The patient had normal-hearing thresholds at 500 Hz and lower, so we were able to match REAR targets because no gain was required (i.e., what we are observing in the REAR is the delivered speech input passing directly to the tip of the probe tube—we would have matched REAR targets with the hearing aid turned off!). While we would eventually come to this conclusion clinically without the REIG, it's an example of how not having a simple picture of gain can lead to a misinterpretation. Of course, we probably could glean this same information from the REAR if we also measure the REOR on the same screen. An example of this is shown ahead in Figure 7–7 (p. 261).

Verification of MPO

As we discussed earlier in Chapter 4, getting the maximum output right is an important aspect of fitting hearing aids. You certainly don't want the output too high, but you don't want it too low either, as that reduces headroom and possibly the quality of speech, and especially music. Verification to ensure that the aided output is correct is a three-pronged process (see Chapter 6): aided loudness ratings using speech material, aided loudness measures using obnoxious noises, and real-ear measures of the hearing aid's MPO—the topic of focus here. As noted earlier in the chapter, the new probe microphone standard refers to this as REAR85 or REAR90, and previously it was referred to as the real-ear saturation response (RESR; although not in the standard). For simplicity, we use the REAR85 for our discussion and sample findings here.

Some audiologists have expressed concern that driving the hearing aid to an output this high is risky business because of the potential for loudness discomfort, acoustic trauma, or even inducing tinnitus. We do not consider this procedure to be a significant risk for the following reasons:

- You already have the hearing aid programmed to a level below the patient's LDL, so discomfort caused by loudness will not be an issue (this assumes you conducted frequency-specific LDLs and adjusted to MPO accordingly—see Chapter 6).
- The signal is very brief.
- The hearing aid will likely be driven to this level in the real world, so if a problem exists, it is best to fix it now.
- The level will be no louder than what the patient will experience when feedback occurs.

Test Protocol

- This procedure is completed using the REAR approach described in Chapter 4. It is completed on the individual patient after verification of a validated prescriptive method.
- Adjust the overall gain of the instrument to just below feedback or to max user gain if no feedback is present. If the patient does not have control of gain with either a VC or remote device, conduct testing at the programmed use gain.
- Even if you use REIG for verification, go to the REAR screen. The measured LDLs that were entered earlier should be displayed and referenced to ear canal SPL.
- Provide the patient with the Cox loudness anchors chart (see Appendix B), and read appropriate instructions (see Appendix C).
- Deliver a frequency-swept tone or tone pips (may vary among manufacturers) at 85 dB SPL; observe the output relative to LDL targets, and have the patient rate the signal on the loudness chart (the objective and subjective findings should agree).
- If the output is either too high or too low, make appropriate changes and retest until REAR85 output falls to desired levels. (Note: the patient can also note exact frequency ranges where fine-tuning of the response may be required.)

Sample Findings

Figure 5–6A shows the test results for the REAR85. The measured LDLs are represented by the horizontal line going from 105 dB at 500 Hz to 110 dB at 3000 Hz. In

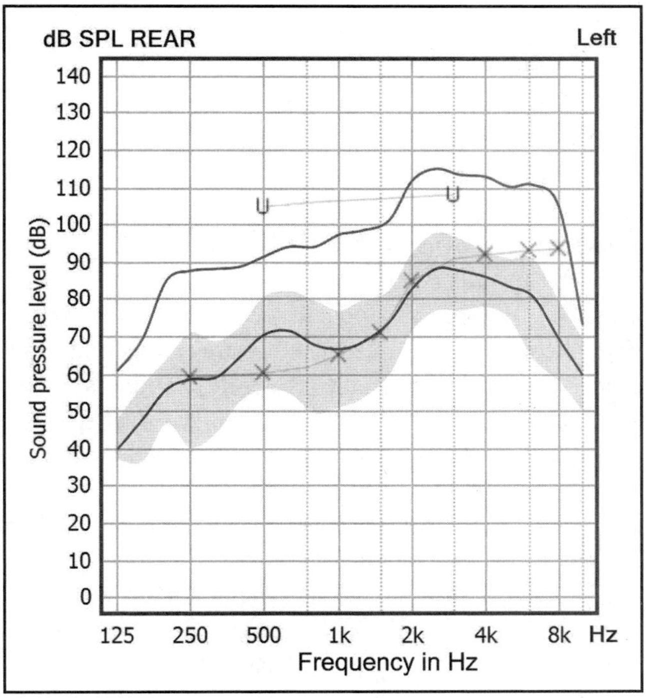

A

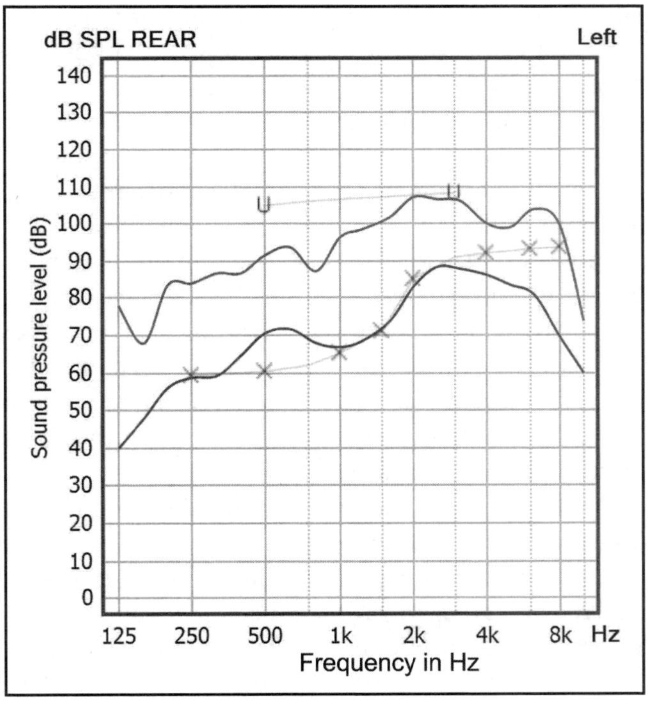

B

Figure 5–6. A. Example of maximum output set too high. The measured LDLs are represented by the horizontal line around going from 105 dB at 500 Hz to 110 dB at 3000 Hz. The top curve is the initial REAR85 measure. **B.** After adjustment, the maximum output falls below the LDLs.

this instance, the audiologist did not go into the software and set the MPO kneepoints to correspond with the LDLs but used the manufacturer's default settings instead. The initial REAR85 measure is shown in the top curve, which peaks around 3000 Hz. It exceeds the patient's LDL by 5 dB, and to no one's surprise, the patient also rated this as uncomfortably loud (some patients will actually point to screen to show where it was uncomfortably loud—it was quite obvious in this case). The REAR85 curve in Figure 5–6B shows the final setting that was achieved after some adjustments of the MPO (lowering AGCo kneepoints in the corresponding channels). Note the advantage of multichannel AGCo, as we were able to lower the problem frequencies while having minimal effect on the MPO for other frequencies. In the not-too-distant past, with a single channel AGCo, we would have had to lower all frequencies by the same amount just to achieve the desired outcome where the peak existed, which then would have resulted in too little headroom for much of the fitting range.

There also are instances when you will find that the REAR85 is much too low—15 dB or so below the LDL—unnecessarily reducing the patient's headroom. In some of these cases, you will find that after you raise the MPO (AGCo kneepoint in most cases) the REAR85 doesn't change. What does this tell us? That output is being limited by the WDRC, which we adjusted aggressively to meet targets for the 75-dB input. So, if we make the WDRC less aggressive to raise the MPO and increase headroom, we will have too much gain for 75 dB SPL (unless the hearing aid had a second or third AGCi kneepoint at 75 dB SPL) The solution? We would probably try a compromise and involve the patient in helping us decide whether loud speech is becoming too loud as we increase the MPO by making the WDRC less aggressive. A point to remember: Do not assume that the MPO setting in the software is necessarily controlling the MPO.

Fitting Tips

- It is useful to explain to the patient why we are conducting this test, "We want to create a loudness situation that is as bad as you will ever encounter in the real world, so if there is a problem, we can fix it now."
- Even after appropriate instructions, what sometimes happens is that when the first REAR85 run is conducted, even when the output falls below the patient's LDLs, the patient will indicate that the signal was uncomfortably loud on the loudness chart. We suggest repeating the testing once or maybe even twice to see if this is a constant rating, before you start changing the MPO. Sometimes the initial run startles the patient a bit, and he/she reacts to this sound, rather than process whether the output is truly uncomfortable.
- It is tempting to think that when fitting a relatively mild gain mini-BTE instrument with an open fitting, MPO issues will never be a problem. This is not true, though, as it is very possible that with some hearing aids, the MPO will be higher with an open fitting than with a closed fitting (Mueller, 2012). This is because the open-ear resonance (REUG) often is maintained, which boosts the ear canal hearing aid output by that amount. (With a closed mold this resonance is no longer a factor.)
- Another concern with open fittings, the ones that are truly open, is that the maximum output that you see on the fitting screen might not represent the MPO of the hearing aid, but rather the signal going directly to the TM. This can be even more of a problem for

higher level test signals (e.g., REAR90). We know of audiologists who have worked diligently lowering the MPO in the software, only to discover later that no hearing aid adjustment changed the output. If a person has a large REUG—note from Figure 4–2 that a 20 dB peak is not that uncommon—then an ear canal SPL of 105 dB or so certainly is possible, which could exceed the person's LDLs, if they were somewhat lower than average (See Figure 7–8 for an example of this).

- We have often recommended conducting an obnoxious noise test as part of the MPO verification (see Chapter 6 for details). We find it helpful to conduct ear canal SPL measures while we're doing this testing because it helps to determine if there is a peak and what channel of MPO might need to be reduced. This real-ear testing is conducted in the "live speech" or spectral analysis mode of probe microphone systems. Figure 5–7 is an example. This is the output for rattling marbles in a glass jar, indeed an obnoxious noise, written about by Robyn Cox (2009). In this case, the noise was rated as uncomfortably loud by the patient, so we will lower the MPO. By observing the real-ear output, we clearly see that the peak is around 2000 Hz, and we'll lower the MPO for this region. If these data were not available, we would have to guess about what MPO channel was causing the problem, or perhaps unnecessarily lower MPO across all frequencies. Granted, the patient may never hear rattling marbles in a glass jar again, but there are other intense environmental sounds that can create the same real-ear aided output.

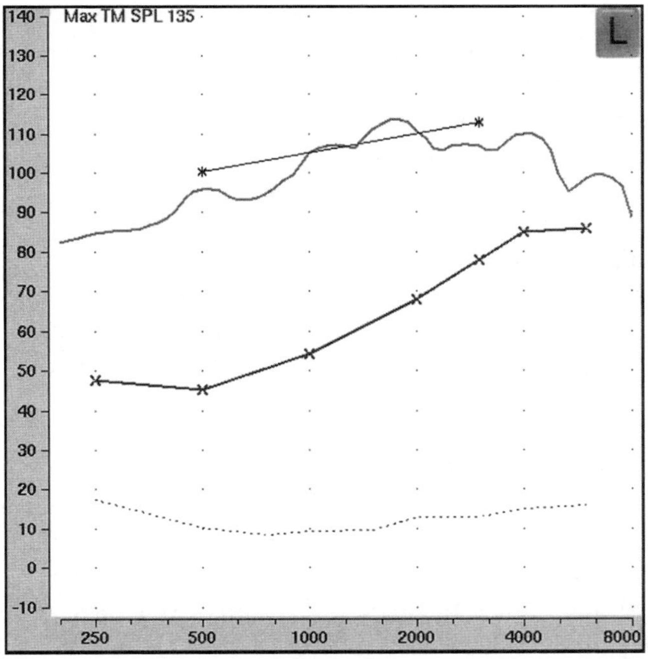

Figure 5–7. Example of REAR obtained by shaking a jar full of marbles. Note that the output of the hearing aid exceeds the LDL values in the mid-frequencies.

Directional Microphone Technology

Many different special features can and should be assessed with probe microphone measures, and directional microphone technology is among the most commonly examined ones. Several 2cc-coupler test box systems allow for the measurement of directionality, so you might ask, "Why do the testing in the real ear rather than the coupler?" A reasonable question. First, it isn't really an either/or thing. We recommend conducting the coupler measures when the hearing aid arrives for quality control purposes. But, even if the hearing aid passes this testing, as most will, there are still several reasons to also consider testing in the real ear:

- The selection of the directional setting may influence gain (e.g., output, particularly in the low frequencies, might not be the same for directional compared to omnidirectional).
- The positioning of the hearing aid on the ear will influence directivity.
- The tightness of the fitting (magnitude of venting) will influence directivity, particularly in the lower frequencies.
- The process of doing the testing and having the patient present to view the results provides an opportunity to counsel the patient about the use and potential benefit of directional technology.

When this testing is conducted, it is important to remember that the purpose is to determine whether the hearing aid is functioning appropriately and to help with counseling, not to compare one product to another. Different products have different polar patterns, and real-ear measures from a single specific azimuth do not reliably predict the overall directional effectiveness when a typical diffuse noise is present (e.g., Ricketts, Lindley, & Henry, 2001). As we describe later in this section, compression can also affect the clinically measured directivity, while not actually affecting the patient's directional benefit.

Here's how you might use directional probe microphone measures clinically. Let's say that you usually fit one of two models of directional instruments, either a Sonotone or a Radioear. After testing four or five different models of the Sonotone, which default to a cardioid directional pattern, you find that the typical real-ear front-to-back difference (REAR @ 180° subtracted from the REAR @ 0°) for the 1000 to 4000 Hz range is around 12 dB with typical compression settings. The Radioear defaults to a supercardioid pattern, and the typical front-to-back difference for this product is 6 dB with typical compression settings. This gives you some clinical norms to work with. Now, if you're testing a patient with his new directional Sonotones and you see only a 5 dB front-to-back difference, you know something is wrong.

Test Protocol

- This procedure is completed by following the verification of prescriptive targets using either the REAR or REIG approach.
- Program the hearing aid to the "fixed directional" setting.
- Disable digital noise reduction if you want to use a noise test signal. (Note: If the attack time on the DNR is slow enough, you might be able to use noise and take the measure quickly before DNR begins to reduce gain.)

CLINICAL CONCEPT: Compression and Directionality Measures

When conducting probe microphone measures with directional technology, it's quite probable that the input levels will exceed the kneepoint of the instrument's multichannel WDRC. Because of this, the directional effect assessed in the clinic will be less than that observed by the patient in the real world. The reason for this was explained by Mueller (2001c), and we'll summarize here. We all know that when WDRC is employed, greater gain is applied as the signal becomes softer. So consider this example: Your patient's WDRC hearing aid (2:1 compression ratio) is programmed to apply 20 dB of gain for a 70 dB input. He is in a room where there is a 70 dB input originating from in front of him (the person he's talking to), and there is also 70 dB originating from behind him (party noise). With an omnidirectional setting, in theory, the amplified SNR will be 0 dB. But you wisely fit him with a directional instrument, and we'll say that it reduces the input from the back by 12 dB. You might think that the front-to-back ratio (FBR) will be +12 dB (70 + 20 = 90; 58 + 20 = 78; 90 minus 78 = 12 dB), and this would be true for linear processing. Remember, however, that as the input goes down, gain goes up for a WDRC instrument. Therefore, for a 2:1 compression ratio, the 58 dB input will receive 6 dB more gain than the original 70 dB input; hence the gain will be 26 dB, not 20 dB. In other words, the WDRC is adding back in one-half of the gain that the directional microphone so diligently took away, and the measured FBR will be only 6 dB. This doesn't sound like a good thing.

This effect, however, is present only when the different test signals from different azimuths occur in isolation, with no other sounds present, an unlikely event in the real world, and a situation when directional amplification isn't needed. In all real-world situations of interest, the signals from the front and back are occurring at the same time; therefore, the same hearing aid gain is applied to both after directional processing. Based on this reality, it's perhaps not surprising that Ricketts et al. (2001) clearly showed that, for real-world use, directional processing coupled with WDRC will be just as effective as when it's used with a linear fitting.

It's possible to obtain a fairly accurate estimate of true FBR in the test box using a method that produces and analyzes two signals simultaneously from the front and back location. A speech signal can also be introduced during testing so that DNR processing doesn't also affect the results. This type of testing is also available with some probe systems for real-ear evaluation. When this method is used, the FBR is the same for both the WDRC and linear settings of the hearing aid. The bottom line of this Clinical Concept is that the probe microphone assessment of directionality isn't to predict the degree of directionality in the real world, but to determine whether the instrument is working as expected and to help with counseling patients.

- With the patient sitting in the usual test position (0 degree horizontal and vertical azimuth), conduct REAR measure using standard real speech (e.g., ISTS), a shaped speech signal, or a speech-shaped noise at an input of 75 dB SPL.
- Swing the patient around 180 degrees (carefully; hopefully he is in a swivel chair) and conduct a second REAR at the same input level from the back.
- By comparing these two outputs on the fitting screen, you will have a good estimate of the directional function—that is, are the results about what you would expect for that instrument? Some machines will automatically display a difference curve.

Rather than eyeball the differences in the REAR curves, you might want to have the probe microphone equipment plot the frequency-specific front-to-back difference. If so, then try out this test protocol:

- Program the hearing aid to the "fixed directional" setting.
- Set your probe microphone equipment for REIG calculations. Hopefully, you can do these measures using real speech. If not, disable DNR in the hearing aid if you want to use a noise test signal. (Note: If the attack time on the DNR is slow enough, you might be able to use noise and take the measure quickly before DNR begins to reduce gain.)
- Turn your patient around 180 degrees so that you conduct the first measure with the loudspeaker of the probe system located behind the patient using a 75-dB input signal. Tell your probe system that this run is the REUR.
- Turn the patient back so that he or she is in the normal test position and conduct a second measure. Tell your probe system that this run is the REAR.
- Because the probe system thinks you are doing an REIG, it will automatically subtract the first run from the second. What is then presented on the monitor is the frequency-specific front-to-back ratio (FBR) of the directional hearing aid.
- This approach will work with any probe microphone system. With some equipment, it may even be easier to display a difference curve for two REARs. And, as stated earlier, some systems have a special mode for directional testing, and will automatically display a difference curve. You don't have to "trick" the equipment.

Sample Findings

Figure 5–8 shows front-to-back directional testing for a mini-BTE RIC product. Figure 5–8A is for a standard eartip (moderate tightness) and Figure 5–8B is for a more open fitting; the hearing aid is programmed the same for both measures. First, we consider this a product with good directivity, and it likely is programmed with very little compression. With the partially closed eartip (A), note that we have a front-to-back difference of 25 dB or so for much of the frequency range. Directivity begins to disappear around 500 Hz because we have leakage from the eartip, and we do not have much gain programmed for this lower frequency range. Notice that, when we move to an open fitting (B), directivity for the higher frequencies stays about the same, but from around 1500 Hz and moving downward, directivity is reduced because of increased leakage from the open fitting, and the direct path of the input signal to the tympanic membrane.

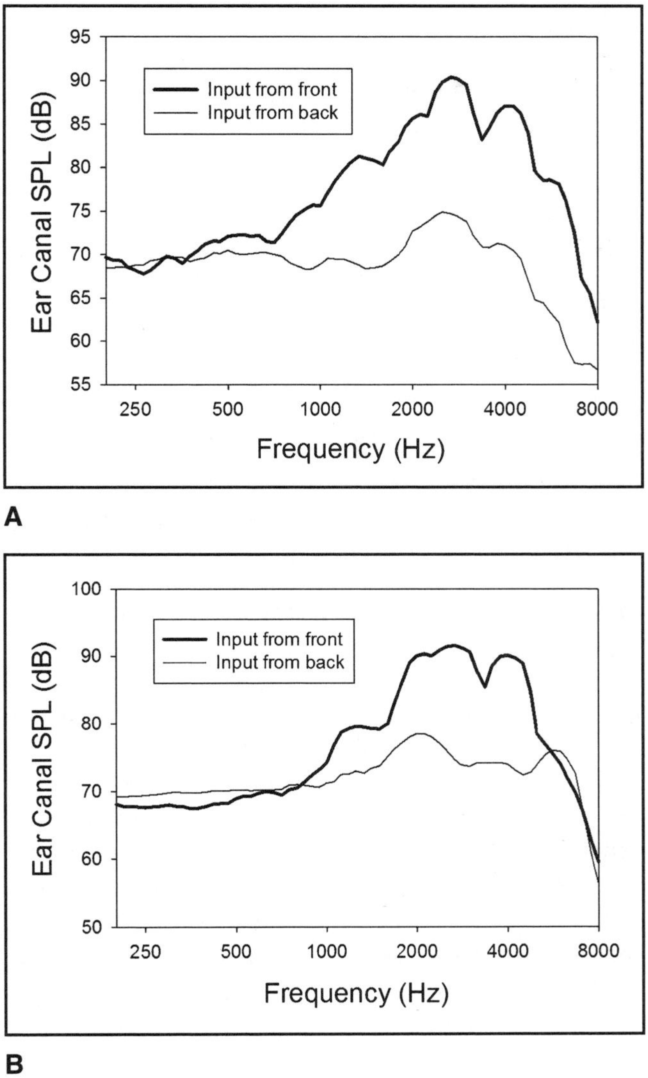

Figure 5–8. Examples of front and back curves measured for mini-BTE product. **A.** Results for a standard eartip (moderate tightness). **B.** Results for a more open fitting. The hearing aid is programmed the same for both measures.

Results are not always as impressive as shown in Figure 5–8. We conducted the same testing for a mini-BTE RIC, fitted with an open eartip, from a different manufacturer. Those findings are shown in Figure 5–9. Except for a 10 dB effect around 4000 Hz, this product is functioning like an omnidirectional product, although set to "directional." The difference between this hearing aid and its mini-BTE competitor shown in Figure 5–8B is quite significant, certainly significant enough to be noticed by a patient in some listening environments—an obvious reason why this type of testing is important.

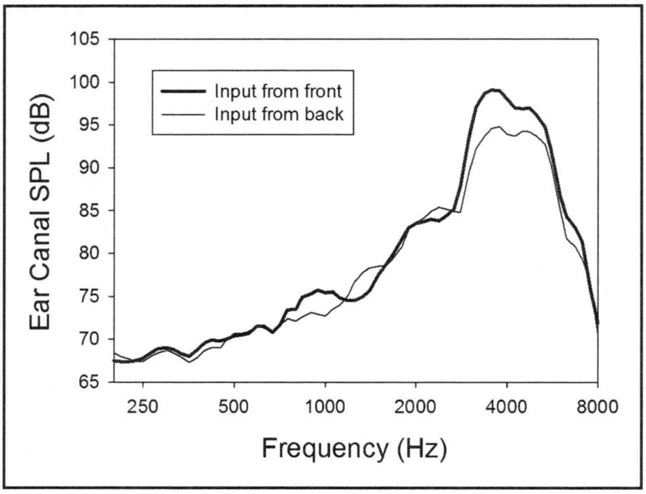

Figure 5–9. Examples of front and back curves measured for mini-BTE product with an open eartip. Except for the separation in tracings at 4000 Hz, the hearing aid, in the directional setting, is functioning as an omnidirectional instrument.

It is tempting to simply think it's a poor directional technology design, but it could be related to the positioning of the hearing aid on the ear (e.g., microphone ports not parallel to horizontal plane). It is possible, that in a test box, the directivity of this product would be more impressive—one of the reasons we mentioned for doing a quick on-ear test.

Fitting Tips

- The primary cause of poor directional function is dirt and debris in the inlet ports of the microphones. Therefore it is as important to evaluate directional processing on repeat visits, as on the day of the fitting. It is important, however, to also have a measurement on the day of fitting or during the initial electroacoustic evaluation to provide a baseline.
- It is very common to fit mini-BTEs that are designed to be cosmetically appealing and to fit comfortably behind the ear. Those two factors may work in opposition to good directional processing. When doing real-ear directional testing with these instruments, you will find that the directionality can vary significantly relative to how they are positioned on the ear. It is hard to say how you should base your final decision, but we can say that the best directionality often will not be the position that is the most comfortable, or the prettiest. Because we certainly can't have a hearing aid that is uncomfortable, this matter may turn into a counseling issue regarding the limitations of benefit.
- We recommend conducting your probe microphone assessment of directionality with the hearing aid programmed to "fixed directional." However, if you are curious (and who isn't, really), you can easily determine the "trigger" for directionality for a given product by setting directional

processing to "automatic" and then testing at input levels of increasing intensity, starting at 50 to 55 dB or so. When you first see a separation between the 0-degree and 180-degree signals, you know you've exceeded the activation point.

- Related to the preceding Fitting Tip, when you have directionality set to automatic directional, it is then controlled by the signal classification system. The hearing aid will not switch to directional unless certain parameters are met, which include an intensity of a certain level (probably around 60 to 70 dB SPL, but varies among manufacturers) and detection of some type of background noise. Hence, whenever conducting directional testing with the instrument in the automatic setting, be sure that you are using a fairly intense input (70 dB SPL or so should work) and a signal that *will not* be classified as speech-in-quiet. Some probe systems allow you to present speech and noise simultaneously.
- Because you often will be using a non-speech signal, it is probable that noise reduction will be activated. Hence, unless your goal is to observe the combined effects of directionality and noise reduction, we suggest that you disable noise reduction when the directional effects are assessed.
- Some probe systems allow you to present speech and noise simultaneously. If you are the curious type, this a great way to examine the directional effects for different SNRs. You could look at this for both fixed directional and automatic—the results will give you some insight regarding a given product's classification system.

Digital Noise Reduction

Most of today's hearing aids have two or three different types of noise reduction, working simultaneously and independently in each channel. The most common of these is modulation-based, effective in reducing noise when it is steady state, and the dominant signal is in a given channel. Another type is fast-acting spectral subtraction, or *Wiener filtering*, designed to clean the signal by subtracting noise in gaps between words or syllables and, like the modulation-based noise reduction, also reduces steady-state noise in the absence of speech (ambient room noise, for example). Finally, some hearing aids also have a fast-acting impulse noise reduction algorithm that reduces the amplitude peaks of impulse noises (e.g., the clinking of dishes in a busy restaurant). While the latter two are very fast-acting, modulation-based noise reduction may have a relatively slow onset and/or offset (a few up to several seconds), which does vary among manufacturers. Manufacturers' software typically allows for changing the magnitude of the noise reduction for a given patient (e.g., min-medium-max), although, among different manufacturers and different products from the same manufacturer, the range from min to max may vary from as low as 5 to 6 dB to as much as 12 to 20+ dB.

In the previous section, we talked about how with directional technology, the positioning on the ear can have a very significant effect, and the processing easily can be affected by other issues regarding the sound reaching the two microphones (e.g., dirt and debris in microphone inlet ports). These are not concerns with DNR. If you know how a given manufacturer's product XYZ worked for Mary, you can pretty much be assured it will work the same way for Bob—except, the tightness of the fitting will have an impact (see our following sample findings). If you are unfamiliar with a product, it is helpful to evaluate the DNR at least once to better understand the workings, but is it really worthwhile to conduct real-ear DNR measures with all patients? Maybe not, but there are a couple reasons why you might want to consider it with some patients:

- As we mentioned, the tightness of the fitting will impact DNR significantly in the low frequencies, to the extent that there may be no effect at all. This will help determine situations when increasing DNR will not solve a patient's complaint of a given noise.
- Ever had a patient ask why hearing aids are so expensive? Conducting this testing with the patient watching the screen can be quite impressive and leads to many counseling opportunities. Moreover, both you and the patient will be able to observe the time constants of the effect firsthand.
- For some manufacturers, the amount of gain reduction for noise inputs increases with increasing input signal levels. In such cases, a demonstration of this effect to a patient can help with expectations relative to function in their everyday environments.

Test Protocol

- This procedure is completed after the verification of prescriptive targets using either the REAR or REIG approach has been completed.
- Although for most testing we want to use real speech, in this case, select a signal that is truly noise. This could be speech noise, white or pink noise, or different noises that might be available on your probe microphone equipment for this purpose (e.g., air conditioner, bus, vacuum, etc.). See examples in Figure 3–6.
- Conduct an REAR with the DNR turned off using a 75-dB input to establish a baseline.
- Program hearing aid to the DNR planned for the patient's everyday use and conduct REAR—leave noise on for 10 seconds or so to ensure maximum reduction has occurred. (Note: For at least one manufacturer, maximum reduction may take up to 20 to 30 seconds!) Observe difference from baseline REAR and note time required to reach maximum reduction. (Note: Rather than requiring a baseline, some systems require only a single measure that compares the level very soon after the presentation begins to the level after the signal has been presented for a period of time.)
- Check DNR effects for different programs if DNR is programmed differently, or check the effect of different settings of DNR for future reference.

Sample Findings

Shown in Figure 5–10A are the effects of DNR set to "max" for a closed fitting. The upper two curves are the REARs for noise reduction off versus on, and the lower chart is a difference curve (amount of noise reduction). Note that we have nearly 20 dB of reduction for the lows, and considerable reduction for all frequencies. Figure 5–10B is the same fitting, but we now have re-progammed the hearing aid, and set noise reduction to "mid." Note that this had a substantial effect above 1000 Hz, but not too much for the low frequencies. Figure 5–11 illustrates the DNR effects for the

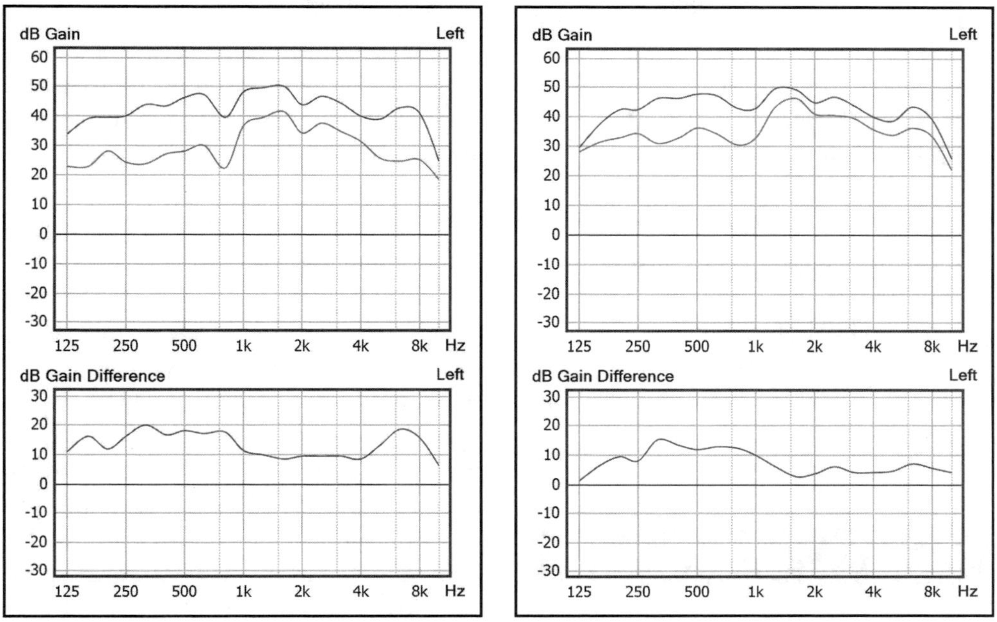

A B

Figure 5–10. Example of DNR testing for different levels of DNR. The top output is DNR set to off. **A.** DNR set to maximum. **B.** DNR set to medium.

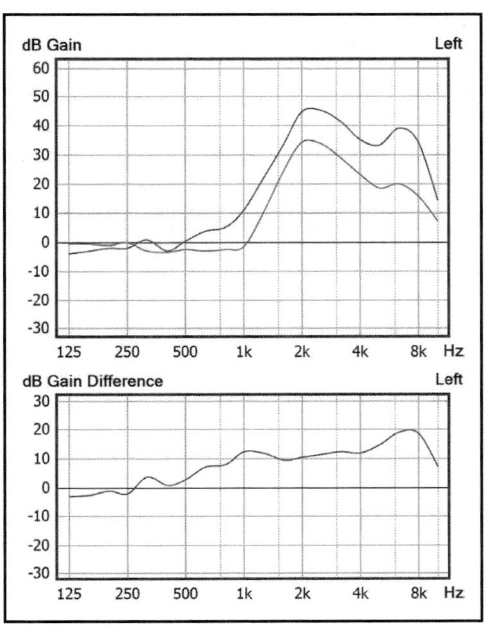

Figure 5–11. Example of DNR testing with an open-fit hearing aid. The top output is the reference "DNR-off" condition. Note the minimal DNR effect in the lower frequencies.

same hearing aid, with the same "medium" setting, except now with an open fitting. Note that the effects in the high frequencies haven't changed much from Figure 5–10B. But, because the ear canal is open and little gain is present, the low-frequency effects are minimal, even at the medium DNR setting.

Fitting Tips

- Some products have DNR that increases with increasing intensity—that is, the effect may be only 5 dB for a 60-dB input but 10 dB for an 80-dB input. Although we suggest routinely using a 75-dB input, it may be useful to check softer inputs for different products on occasion just to gain information regarding how different algorithms work.
- To observe the release time of the DNR, you can try talking while the noise is

present (raise your voice well above the noise). You should observe the release of the DNR on the screen (the time for this to happen will vary among instruments, but it usually is quite fast—one second or less).

- DNR should have no effect when the patient is listening to speech. To confirm this, you may want to check products by simply conducting an REAR using real speech with the DNR turned on versus off at a relatively high input level (e.g., 75 dB SPL).

Frequency Lowering

With downward sloping hearing loss, there are times when the loss in the high frequencies reaches a level of severity at which it is not realistic to make speech audible with conventional amplification. For these patients, we sometimes simply choose to roll off gain, to help prevent feedback. A second option is to use frequency lowering to make speech in this area audible, albeit at a different frequency. Frequency lowering can be accomplished by using frequency compression, linear frequency transposition, or frequency duplication (for review, see Alexander, 2013, 2016; Mueller, Alexander, & Scollie 2013; Scollie, 2013).

Regardless of the approach used to lower the frequencies, the fitting application remains the same—move high-frequency speech (and environmental sounds) from a frequency range where they are inaudible to a frequency range where they are audible. As we show in our sample findings, it is fairly easy, using probe microphone measures, to determine whether the algorithm has been activated, as you will observe frequencies missing from the usual aided speech spectrum when speech mapping is conducted. Determining whether the high-frequency sounds have been made audible at a lower frequency, however, is a more difficult task because the lowered signal will blend in with the amplified signals that originate at this frequency.

Some probe microphone systems provide calibrated speech signals, such as the Ling 6–Sound Test, that can be used to more directly observe the effects of the higher frequencies (e.g., /s/ and /sh/ sounds). In some cases the level of these sounds represents the actual peak level we would expect in running speech based on analysis of the ISTS or other speech samples, such as we show in Figure 3–8. Signals such as this have been developed by the research group at the University of Western Ontario (Scollie et al., 2016).

One system has filtered the standard speech passage so that only higher segments of speech are present (options include speech segments centered at 3150, 4000, 5000, or 6300 Hz), which then allows for observation of each signal when it is lowered. As we review in Chapter 3, there is some concern that these signals are not as representative of real speech as the excised /s/ and /sh/.

In the absence of recorded speech, live voice presentation of the /s/ and /sh/ sounds will provide a rough idea of the effects of the lowering. However, we recommend using a calibrated speech signal whenever possible if you are interested in not only the amount of frequency lowering but also the audibility of the lowered signal in the individual patient (see review of frequency-lowering verification procedures by Scollie et al., 2016).

Test Protocol

- This procedure usually is completed after the routine verification of prescriptive targets has been conducted using either the REAR or REIG approach.

- Conduct speech mapping for 65-dB input for reference; display the full amplitude spectrum of the amplified signal.
- If your system has an excised /s/ stimulus, present it at 65 dB SPL. If the stimulus does not fall above the patient's threshold, frequency lowering may be warranted to improve audibility and should be activated. (*Note:* Deactivate noise reduction for all testing using excised /s/ and /sh/ stimuli.)
- Activate frequency lowering and present the speech signal; observe change in speech spectrum, showing that frequency lowering indeed has been activated.
- Deliver one or more high-frequency signals to observe the placement and level of the lowered signal.
- If the signal does not appear to be audible, adjustment may be needed regarding either the target location frequency or the gain at the lowered region, or both. For example, if your system has the excised /s/, fine tune until the signal falls just above threshold using the weakest frequency lowering setting possible. In some cases, the signal may still be audible even though it does not appear to be so—more on that later in this chapter.
- Optional: Play a slightly lower frequency stimulus (e.g., /sh/) that is band-limited around 5000 Hz and make sure there is frequency separation. If the output from the two signals overlap too much, the listener may have difficulty perceiving them as two different speech sounds.
- After activating noise reduction, have the listener listen to ensure they can distinguish between /s/ and /sh/.

Sample Findings

It is initially of interest to observe whether the frequency compression has indeed been activated but our real interest is its effect on the test signal. Figure 5–12A (from Mueller et al., 2013) shows the output for a 65 dB SPL speech input with frequency lowering deactivated and with two nonlinear frequency compression settings: one starting at 2000 Hz with a 2.2:1 frequency compression ratio and another starting at 1500 Hz with a 3.2:1 frequency compression ratio, for the same hearing aid programming. No gain adjustments were made as the settings were changed. As shown, the output for the frequency-compressed regions (between the start frequency and response roll-off) is essentially the same as it is without frequency lowering, which suggests that the lowered signals are being treated as though they originated at their new frequencies. It is also possible to observe the presence of frequency lowering by viewing the REAR85. Illustrated in Figure 5–12B is the real-ear MPO of this same hearing aid for the same two different frequency compression settings. As we noted previously, REAR85 and REAR90 measurements using swept pure tones are invalid when frequency lowering is activated. In fact, it is not unusual to see an REAR85 for a swept pure tone that appears to be lower than the REAR observed in response to a 65 dB SPL-shaped real-speech signal! This artifact occurs because, during signal acquisition, a filter is used by many probe microphone systems that surround the test frequency and "sweeps" along with it. Because the output frequency is not the same as the input frequency after frequency compression, this filter does not correspond to the test frequency, and the REAR is artificially lowered. This really does not affect operation of the hearing aid in the real world. It just means we need to disable

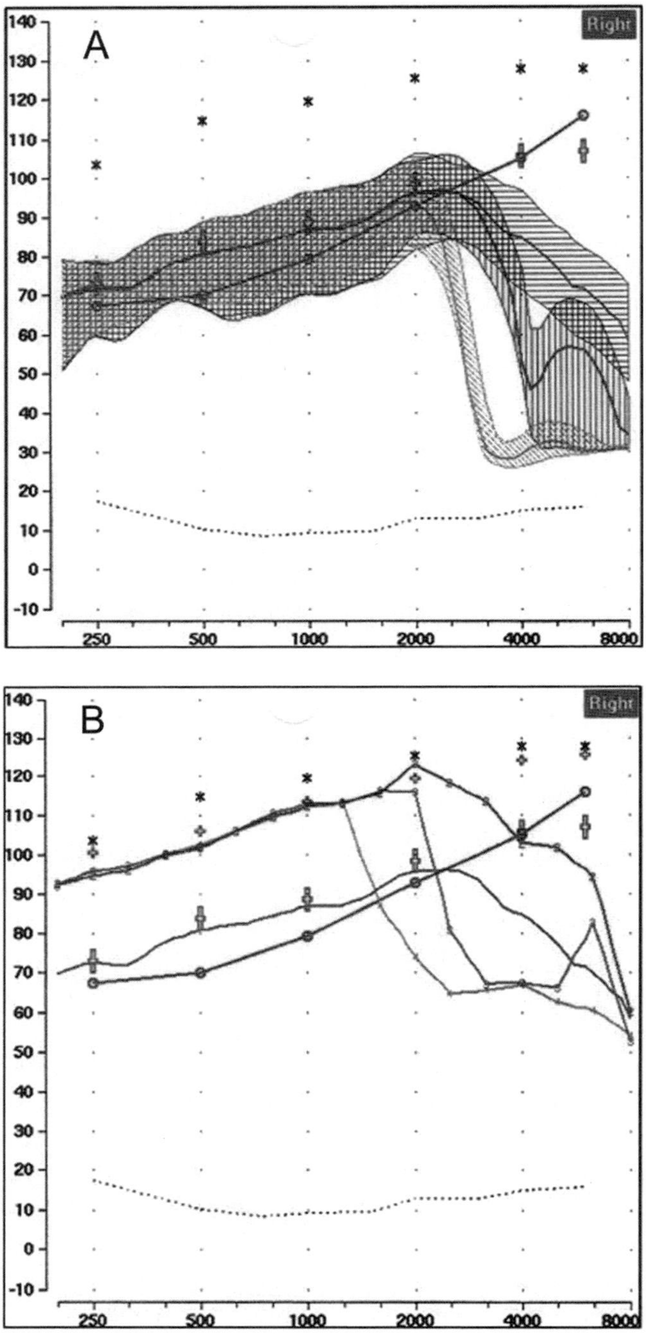

Figure 5–12. A. The output for a 65 dB SPL speech input with frequency lowering deactivated, and with two nonlinear frequency compression settings: one starting at 2000 Hz with a 2.2:1 frequency compression ratio, and another starting at 1500 Hz with a 3.2:1. **B.** The real-ear MPO of this same hearing aid for the same two different frequency compression settings. Adapted from Mueller et al., 2013.

frequency lowering in order to measure REAR 85/90 accurately.

In Figure 5–13, we show the findings for a patient whose hearing loss drops to 80 to 90 dB at 4000 to 6000 Hz, and we decided to apply frequency lowering for these frequencies. Although the use of the real-speech /s/ and /sh/ might have been the best choice, in this case we used the equipment's calibrated speech signal for the /s/ and /sh/ segments of speech. In Figure 5–13A, you see the output for these two signals following activation of frequency lowering in the default mode. From this figure, it appears that the signals are *inaudible*. Actually, they probably are not *totally* inaudible. Previously, we described how speech peaks could be audible even when the LTASS is below the threshold and the signal appears to be inaudible. The same issue is present here. Specifically, because the LTASS averages over time (and energy is not present at all frequencies all of the time) and speech segments vary in level, the speech peaks are not captured by this average. Instead, the speech peaks fall approximately 10 to 15 dB above the signal shown in this figure. As mentioned, this example is the manufacturer's default setting, with the hearing aid programmed to the manufacturer's proprietary algorithm. We show you this to point out that most, if not all, manufacturers take a very conservative approach to frequency lowering, and rarely will you find that their default settings accomplish the desired goal (of course, if you did not conduct this type of probe microphone testing, how would you know?).

In Figure 5–13B, you see these same two signals after adjustments are made. Observe that we changed the target destination to the 2000 to 2700 Hz range and increased gain slightly to obtain increased signal audibility. We do want to maintain separation of the signals after lowering, as shown here. We, of course, involve the perceptions of the patient during this testing to confirm that the signals are audible, but not to the extent of distorting the overall speech signal. In this case, we were probably too aggressive, in that the LTASS falls above threshold, even for speech energy centered at higher frequencies. This over-aggressiveness was confirmed by patient complaints of "too hissy sounding." Reducing frequency lowering so that the /s/ test signal fell a couple of dB below the patient's threshold led to peak energy that was still 8 to10 dB above threshold and a patient who was satisfied with the sound quality.

Fitting Tips

- It is important to remember that the gain applied to the lowered signal is the same as a signal originating at the frequency. Therefore, as we demonstrated in Figure 5–13A, if the hearing aid originally was not programmed appropriately (e.g., use of the manufacturer's proprietary fitting), then it is unlikely the lowered signals will be optimally audible.
- Related to the preceding fitting tip, when attempting to make the lowered signals audible, it is tempting to keep increasing gain for the lowered region. We cannot forget, however, that this is also affecting signals originating at the target frequency, and you may end up with a fitting that has strayed far from the NAL-NL2 targets. A compromise often is necessary.
- If your probe system does not have specific speech sounds for use with frequency lowering testing, you can download a Ling 6–Sound Test App that is compatible with iPhone, iPad, and iPod Touch and is optimized for

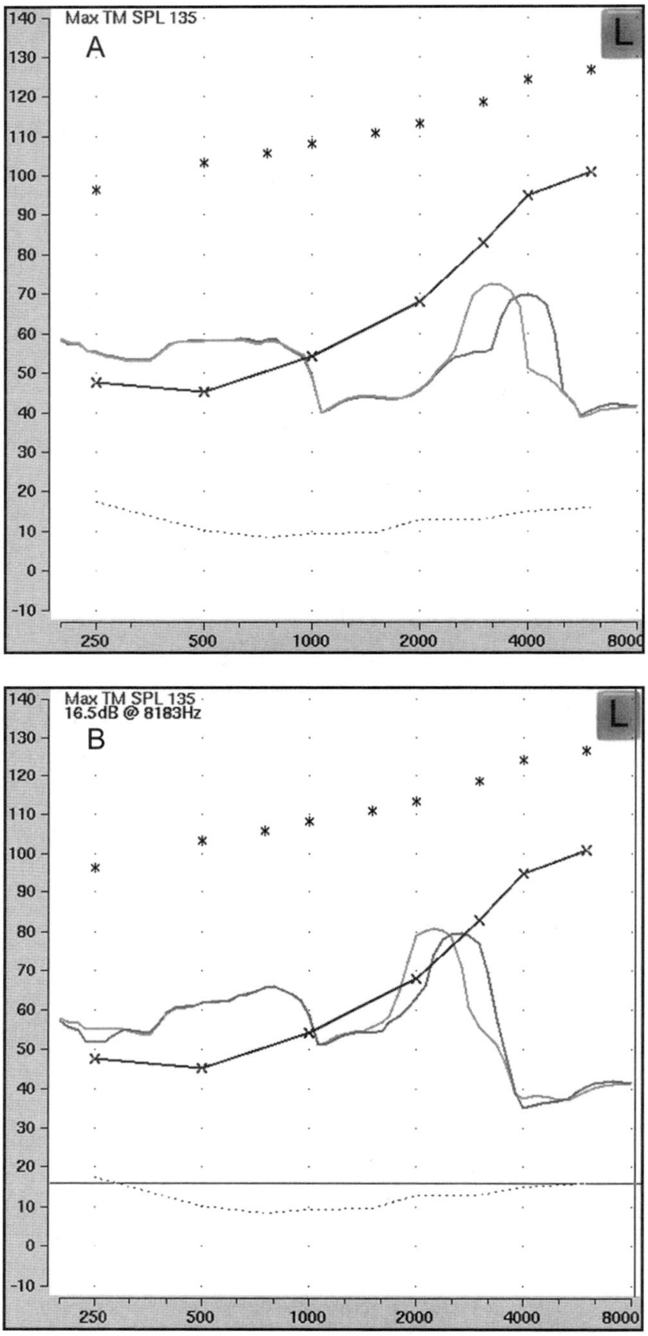

Figure 5–13. A. The output of this manufacturer's high-frequency speech bands, centered at 4000 Hz and 6300 Hz for the manufacturer's proprietary fitting and default frequency lowering settings. **B.** The same patient after adjustments have been made to gain and the frequency compression parameters. The 6300 Hz signal is now around 3000 Hz, and the 4000 Hz signal is lowered to the 2000 Hz region.

iPhone 5. This App allows for delivery of the sounds at a consistent SPL. Wave files are available from the University of Western Ontario. Guidelines for conducting these measures using the UWO ISTS excised /s/ and /sh/ can be found in Scollie et al. (2016).

Assessment of Feedback Suppression

For some hearing aid features, such as compression, there may be considerable similarities across at least some manufacturers in how the features work, as well as the expected outcome. For others, such as DNR, there are some differences across manufacturers in how the feature operates and how it affects the patient's listening experience. One feature with considerable published differences across manufacturers, however, is digital feedback suppression (DFS) (e.g., Ricketts, Johnson, & Federman, 2008).

Over the past decade or so, DFS has significantly affected how we select and fit hearing aids. Without feedback suppression, open fittings are restricted to listeners with no greater than mild-to-moderate high-frequency hearing loss. Therefore, the current popularity of mini-BTE hearing aids when used with open and other non-custom eartips has often been attributed in large part to effective DFS technology. The differences in how well the DFS technology works, however, greatly influence the hearing loss configurations and the degree of high-frequency hearing loss that can be fitted appropriately.

We assume that you will be completing probe microphone measures on each patient, so determining the effectiveness of DFS on every individual patient is not necessary (or even particularly informative). As we noted, however, there are large differences in the effectiveness of this technology across manufactures, and the effectiveness of this technology often changes with each new generation of hearing aids. These differences include how much gain is available before feedback, as well as any audible artifact that is introduced by the feedback suppression system—sometimes referred to as *entrainment.* The speed with which a feedback suppression system can adjust to eliminate feedback generated by the introduction of a cell phone, or other new surface, is also of interest. In addition, considerable differences (approximately +/− 10 dB) occur across individuals in the maximum stable gain before feedback within the same product. While we can't do a lot to control for individual differences across patients, having a general idea of the effectiveness of a DFS technology is tremendously useful for both selection of an appropriate hearing aid and effective counseling. Consider a patient who has normal hearing in the low frequencies, sloping to a moderately severe hearing loss in the highs. This patient is an excellent candidate for an open fitting because hearing thresholds are normal through 1000 Hz. With some models of mini-BTE hearing aids, you will not be able to reach high-frequency NAL-NL2 targets without significantly decreasing the amount of venting. With other products, we can match targets with a non-custom open eartip, but only with audible artifacts. With still other products, we easily can match targets with a non-custom open eartip without entrainment. If you do not previously evaluate the hearing aids with your probe microphone tests, how do you know which is which? So while you don't need to do this testing with each patient, information that is highly useful clinically can be gained from testing each product.

Test Protocol

- This procedure can be completed by using either an REAR or REIG approach. Select a speech or speech-like test signal (e.g., shaped speech, ISTS).
- Select a patient for testing; it might be useful to have access to the same individual multiple times for assessment of multiple new instruments as they are introduced over time. The magnitude of hearing loss does not matter that much as long as the individual is willing to listen to feedback for a short period of time; even a coworker with normal hearing will work.
- Change the equalization method from concurrent to stored equalization. (*Note*: On most systems this simply requires selecting "open" or similar descriptor as the hearing aid style.) Select an average patient's audiogram and LDLs that reflect a good candidacy for open fitting (e.g., normal hearing in the low frequencies sloping to moderate hearing loss in the high frequencies).
- Select the verified prescriptive method in the probe microphone fitting software that you use for a typical patient and usual fitting factors.
- Program the hearing aids to the desired fitting algorithm using manufacturer's software control process (select the same patient and fitting factors entered into the probe microphone software).
- Place the probe tube in the ear at an appropriate depth and measure the REUR.
- Fit the hearing aid to the patient's ear with a fully open, non-custom eartip.
  - Activate feedback suppression and calibrate the feedback suppression system if recommended by the manufacturer.
  - If there is more than one DFS setting, consider repeating this entire protocol for all available DFS settings.
- Mute the hearing aid and conduct stored-equalization, free-field calibration.
- Unmute the instrument and begin testing and making gain adjustments using a 55 dB input level. A lower signal level is used, as compression processing will provide increased gain with decreased input, increasing the likelihood of feedback.
- Adjust frequency-specific gain to achieve a reasonable match to target. It may be the case that you are unable to match the gain targets because of feedback or gain limiting resulting from the hearing aid's feedback calibration routine, or because you reach the gain limits of the hearing aid. If so, either (1) attempt to match the same gain shape as the targets, or (2) consider using better thresholds for the hearing loss that you enter into the probe microphone system.
- Once you match the shape, increase overall gain across all frequencies until (1) you or the patient hear feedback, (2) you reach the hearing aid gain limits, or (3) you reach the gain limit imposed by the feedback calibration routine.
- If you reach audible feedback, decrease and increase overall gain slightly, talk, whistle, and have the patient open and close her mouth until you determine the gain setting that is just below the presence of feedback for typical listening conditions.
- Remeasure the REAR to display the maximum REAR before feedback. If you are interested, compare these values to the REUR; this difference is the maximum real-ear gain before feedback.

- Turn gain down a couple of dB, and if they are available, plug monitor headphones into your probe microphone system in order to "listen in" to the sounds in the patient's ear. Have the patient sit quietly while you talk, whistle, and make other sounds. Listen for any artifacts or problems with the sound quality.
- If the maximum additional gain before feedback is of interest, for quick comparisons to other products and manufacturers, repeat the maximum REAR procedure with the feedback suppression system disabled. In this way, you can calculate the difference between DFS-on and DFS-off REARs.
- Repeating the sound quality procedure we just described with DFS disabled is also useful as a benchmark for comparing possible degradation in sound quality related to DFS processing.
- It may also be informative to increase the thresholds entered into the probe microphone software until the prescriptive targets are similar to the maximum REAR you measured. This procedure provides an indication of the maximum hearing loss you're able to fit before feedback.

Sample Findings

We selected a new hearing aid from Bob's-Pretty-Good Hearing Aids to test its new DFS processing. This is a mini-BTE instrument, and we fitted it to a patient's ear using an open eartip. This manufacturer recommends completing the DFS calibration routine in its software, so we did. Two separate DFS settings, "normal" and "turbo," were available, and we tested turbo first. A sloping hearing loss (normal in the low frequencies sloping to 65 dB HL thresholds in the high frequencies) was entered into the probe microphone system and we adjusted gain to match NAL-NL2 targets. Gain was then increased. Rather than reaching feedback, we stopped seeing gain increases in the high frequencies after increasing overall gain a few steps. This gain limit, the maximum REAR before feedback, is shown in the upper curve in Figure 5–14. Given that this curve falls 5 to 10 dB above our original targets, we estimated we could successfully match targets even for a patient with high-frequency hearing thresholds of 70 to 75 dB, or perhaps greater at some frequencies. We then lowered gain, disabled the DFS, and searched for feedback. We found it quickly! Just to make Figure 5–14 interesting, we captured the response with the aid in feedback (this is also a reminder that feedback is loud—about 115 dB in this case). To reach a stable REAR with DFS deactivated, we had to lower the gain by several dB.

By comparing the final adjusted curve to the first REAR, we found that approximately 15 to 20 dB of additional high-frequency gain was available before feedback after activating the DFS system—clearly, this is a DFS system that works, and works well!

We then turned gain down two clicks (about 2 dB in this instrument) and plugged headphones into the probe microphone system. Right away we heard a soft but audible roughness that sounded a bit like a distant motorboat. We then repeated the entire procedure on the normal setting, which resulted in a decrease in maximum REAR of about 4 dB and the elimination of roughness in the sound quality. From this information, we know we can fit a wide range of high-frequency hearing loss with this product. We further know that we probably want to activate the turbo setting only if we cannot reach targets with the normal feedback reduction setting. Finally, we know that if the patient has a range of normal hearing, counseling

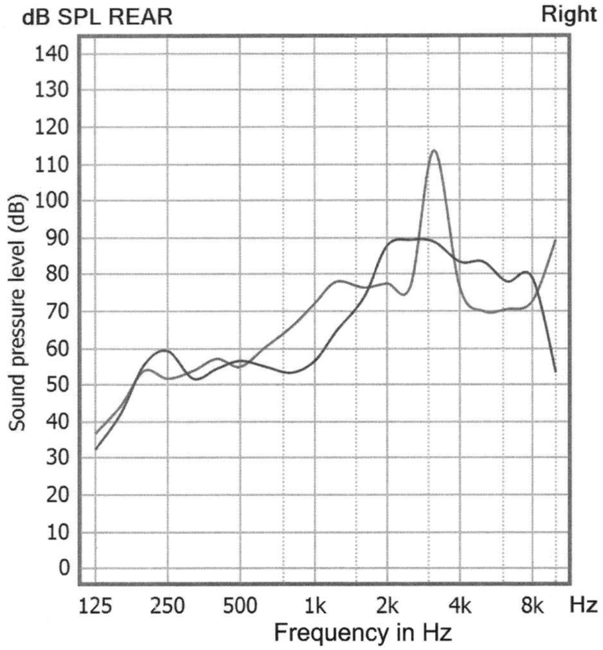

Figure 5–14. An example of the maximum output available before feedback with the feedback cancelation turned "on" (*upper curve*) and "off" (*lower curve*). Also shown is the peak caused by feedback.

may be necessary for acceptance of the turbo setting, or there may be a trade-off involving decreasing venting and using the normal setting to achieve desired target gain.

Fitting Tips

- It is often useful to examine not only the limits of high-frequency gain and REAR corresponding to the DFS function but also the gain in the middle and low frequencies. A lower power receiver can greatly limit low-frequency gain in open fittings. Therefore, consider using a power receiver to really test the maximum limits of additional gain before feedback in a product.
- Plugging in headphones to the probe microphone system to search for audible artifacts will add another potential path for feedback. Therefore, consider not plugging the headphones in until you reach this testing phase. Furthermore, it may be necessary to limit headphone gain and/or reduce hearing aid gain to ensure there is no feedback during the sound quality assessment.

Contralateral Routing of Offside Signal (CROS) Fittings

When a patient has an unaidable ear, head shadow can reduce speech recognition in specific listening situations (speech from the bad side). One way to improve performance is to place a microphone on the ear that is unaidable (usually housed in a hearing aid), which wirelessly transfers signals from this side to a hearing aid on the good ear. This is referred to as a *CROS* (Contralateral Routing of Offside Signal) *fitting*. If the better hearing ear has a hearing loss, then a microphone is activated for this side, too, and the fitting is termed a *bi*lateral CROS, or BiCROS.

Fitting the on-side hearing aid when a BiCROS is employed is no different than fitting any other unilateral hearing aid. Fitting the signal from the off-side microphone, however, requires some adaptation to the usual probe microphone test approach, particularly when the patient has normal hearing in the better ear, which often is the case. When normal hearing is present, the goal of the fitting is simply to eliminate the head shadow effect. So, we want to place the signal originating from the side of the bad ear into the good ear, but apply 0-dB insertion gain (no gain, but no loss). In other words, the REAR should equal the REUR; therefore, the REUR is our fitting target. For BiCROS fittings, the REAR targets for the better ear are also the targets for the signal delivered from the poorer ear. Some probe systems have a dedicated method for conducting CROS/BiCROS fittings on their systems using two probe modules.

Test Protocol (CROS)

- Initially, position the patient as you do for conventional probe microphone testing. Properly position the probe tube in the better ear.
- Use stored equalization to calibrate the system (as you do for an open fitting).
- Measure the REUR using a standard real-speech signal (e.g., shaped speech or ISTS). This now becomes the fitting target. For a BiCROS fitting, you can skip measuring the REUR and instead simply use the targets for the better ear.
- Fit the CROS system to both ears and with it muted, measure the REOR to confirm that it is similar to the REUR. Remember the goal is that there is an open fitting on the good ear and the eartip does not serve as an earplug. Unmute the system. For a BiCROS system, begin by fitting the better ear to targets using the standard REAR fitting we described previously.
- Carefully swivel patient in chair so that loudspeaker is directly facing the bad ear (i.e., 90 or 270 degrees). The patient's head should be the same distance from the loudspeaker. In the case of a CROS, conduct the REAR using a speech signal at 65 dB SPL (the probe tube remains in the good ear). Adjust programming until the aided output matches the previously measured REUR. In a true CROS fitting, this typically involves increasing gain only in the high frequencies. In the case of a BiCROS, adjust programming until the aided output matches the better ear REAR targets.

Sample Findings

Our CROS fitting is for a patient with an unaidable left ear and essentially normal hearing for the good (right) ear (thresholds around 15 dB HL). For conducting the fitting, with the hearing aid turned off, we first obtained the REUR for the right ear (with the patient at 0-degree azimuth). We then positioned him/her so that the loudspeaker was directly facing the left ear (270-degree azimuth relative to the patient). For counseling purposes, we conducted an REOR measurement (hearing aid turned off) to illustrate the head shadow effect—this is shown in Figure 5–15A. All testing was

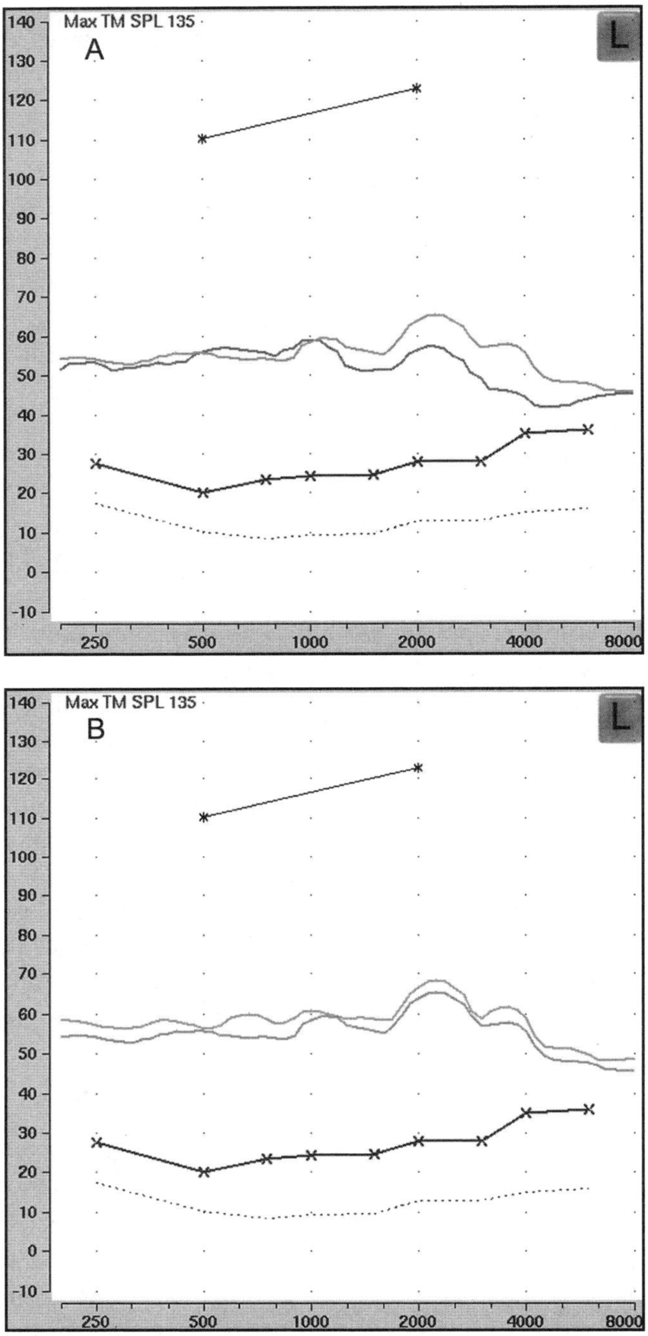

Figure 5–15. Example of CROS fitting. The hearing aid is turned off and the patient positioned so that the loudspeaker is directly facing his good/left ear (270-degree azimuth relative to the patient). **A.** The head shadow present with the hearing aid off. **B.** After the hearing aid is turned on, the head shadow is gone, indicating the functionality of the CROS.

conducted in the stored equalization mode, as in this case, we do not want the monitor microphone to control the input signal. The upper response is the patient's REUR, and the lower response is the signal presented from the off-side. This finding is fairly typical if the fitting is truly open, showing a 10- to 12-dB head-shadow effect for the higher frequencies. We then turned the off-side microphone on and conducted an REAR. As shown in Figure 5–15B, we programmed the hearing aid to mirror the REUR, falling just a few dB higher for most frequencies.

Fitting Tips

- Hearing aids generally do not provide much amplification for frequencies above 5 to 6 kHz. Consequently, for a true CROS fitting, some patients will prefer a fitting that is a few dB higher than the REUR, similar to what we provided in the example above.
- There has been some work with fittings termed *transcranial CROS,* which is when a power instrument is placed in the unaidable ear, and the desired signal is transferred to the good ear via bone conduction vibrations generated in the ear canal. If you want to try this interesting fitting approach, you'll find your probe microphone measures will come in handy to determine specific crossover levels for the fitting (Valente, Potts, Valente, & Goebel, 1995).

Telephone and Streaming Devices

Wireless streaming from telephones, personal music systems, wireless microphones, television, and a variety of other devices has gained considerable traction in the past few years as a convenient way to bring aided signals to a patient's ears and, in some cases, provide considerable benefits when compared to traditional routing methods (e.g., Picou & Ricketts, 2011, 2013). The testing and programming of wireless streaming is typically completed in the test box by matching the frequency response from the streaming to the hearing aid's frequency response after fitting to a validated prescriptive target using the techniques we described earlier in this chapter. However, there are at least two reasons we may want to complete probe microphone measures for demonstration and counseling purposes. First, we may want to demonstrate wireless streaming from a telephone while completing probe microphone measures to allow the patient to visualize the audibility of the streamed signal using speech-mapping techniques. Both electromagnetic handsets and bilateral measurements available from some probe microphone systems can be useful to demonstrate specific conditions such as streaming telephone signals from one ear to the other and streaming all types of signals to both ears. Having the patient call a telephone number with a recorded standard message like the weather number can also be useful for this demonstration—the output of this call easily then can be displayed on the screen.

Another more important reason to complete probe microphone assessment relates to the bandwidth of streamed signals. Modern hearing aids differ considerably in audible bandwidth, with the high-frequency limit ranging from as low as 3 to 4 kHz to as high as perhaps 8 to 10 kHz. The effect that these audible high frequencies have on sound quality depends on the listener. That is, extended high-frequency audibility could be either negative or positive (Ricketts et al., 2008) so it is useful to know how high into the high frequencies audibility extend here. Venting can contribute to an even greater extent to a reduction in the sound quality of wireless streamed signals, particularly music. Specifically, a large vent as is typical in open-fit hearing aids can preclude delivery of the low-frequency energy from a streamed source and result in music that sounds tinny and unacceptable. This problem is not observed for sounds in the listener's environment because the low frequencies reach the listeners' ears through the vent. Therefore, this potential problem is unique to wireless streaming.

Test Protocol

- This protocol should occur after the hearing aid is already fitted to a validated prescriptive target using the REAR or REIG techniques previously described, so we are assuming that you have already entered the patient's audiogram and measured LDLs, placed the probe tube and hearing aid, and calibrated the probe system appropriately.
- Set equipment to spectral analysis mode, which may be the same as "live speech" mapping for some equipment.
- Activate wireless streaming in the hearing aid from a smartphone or personal music player. Some audiologists we know keep a Bluetooth-capable wireless music player on hand for this specific testing purpose—this can be a great use for that old smartphone you replaced last year.
- Select and play music of the patient's choosing.
- View the audible bandwidth and discuss the sound quality in consultation with the patient.

Sample Findings

Our patient came to us as a typical open fitting and had relatively normal hearing in the low frequencies. He indicated no real difficulties on the telephone but was interested in streaming music, text to speech, and other signals from his smartphone. We activated his music program and streaming and had him play one of his favorite songs. The resulting REAR is marked "Open" in Figure 5–16. The patient indicated that it sounded "tinny" and "very shrill." Just to see the difference, we tried replacing the open eartip with closed tips. The patient indicated that things sounded much better but were still shrill and that the high pitches sounded like mechanical noise. We then reprogrammed the hearing aid master program so that there was again a match to NAL-NL2 targets with his new closed domes. Based on this complaint of shrillness, we then turned down gain above 5000 Hz in his music program until the patient indicated he was happy with the sound quality. The resulting output is labeled "Closed" in Figure 5–16. As you can see, even though the same low-frequency REAR targets were matched for the open and closed fittings, the open fitting resulted in a reduction in the low frequencies for the streamed signal of about 30 dB—no wonder it sounded tinny!

But have we just created other problems? Somewhat surprisingly, the patient indicated he liked the sound of the hearing aids in general with the closed domes and felt satisfied with the sound of his own voice. A quick measure of the occlusion effect with the closed fitting (as we describe in the next section) indicated it was much greater than with the open tip, but not terribly high (about 12 dB). After trying the closed domes for a couple of weeks, the patient indicated he was very satisfied overall with how the hearing aids worked—so this fitting worked out pretty

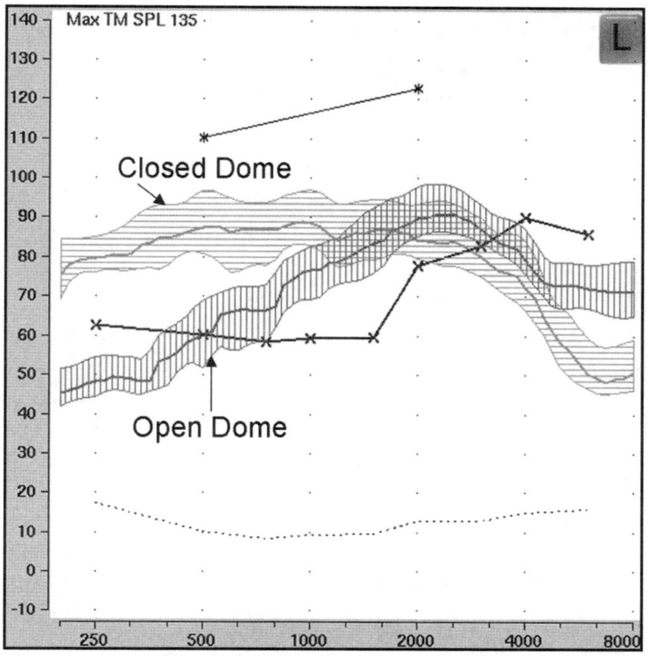

Figure 5–16. Example of verification of a wireless accessory. The two curves represent the output measured for the same music signal with an open eartip (Open) and a closed eartip (Closed). In both cases, the REAR was matched to the patients NAL-NL2 targets through 4000 Hz, but gain was reduced in the higher frequencies for the closed fitting per the patient's request.

well. We would not have been surprised, however, if he had returned and asked for some middle ground, with a little more venting.

Fitting Tips

- For some patients, it may be necessary to select a more closed eartip to obtain desirable sound quality from streamed media. If so, it will be necessary to refit the hearing aid to targets and ensure that the sound quality for external sounds and the patient's own voice are still acceptable. Finding the right balance in this trading relationship for patients can take a bit of effort. With some patients who prefer a completely open hearing aid fitting, the best solution will be to remove the hearing aids and listen to music through headphones or insert earphones.
- When you are attempting to maximize sound quality for extended high frequencies, probe microphone testing may be less useful because standing wave issues make accurate assessment of the higher frequencies challenging and, in some cases, impossible (see Vaisberg, Macpherson, & Scollie, 2016). In these cases, it's sometimes best to just rely on patient feedback and/or move the audibility assessment in the coupler using simulated REAR and average RECDs. Some newer systems use a variety of techniques to provide a visual representation of hearing aid output through 10 kHz or even higher.

Assessing the Hearing Aid Occlusion Effect

There seem to be several misconceptions surrounding the occlusion effect and its treatment, so before we go through our probe microphone test protocol, we'll provide a little background regarding this common nemesis to a successful hearing aid fitting. The occlusion effect is best described as an echo, "boomy" (as in an overabundance of low-frequency energy) or hollow sensation occurring when the patient is speaking or chewing. Older patients may describe it as sounding like they are "talking in a barrel" (young people don't talk in barrels so much). This sensation can be highly annoying, and it is more likely to be annoying for patients having better than 30 to 40 dB HL thresholds in the low frequencies. Addressing the possibility of the occlusion effect is part of the verification process, and fortunately, as we will show here, it's relatively easy to measure with your probe microphone equipment at the time of the fitting. Nevertheless, there will always be situations where a patient was not bothered by the occlusion effect initially but, after using the hearing aids for a while, finds it distracting. Some patients report using only one hearing aid rather than two to minimize the annoyance, which of course is not the preferred solution. Hopefully, this issue can be resolved during follow-up visits.

Why the Occlusion Effect Happens

So what causes the occlusion effect? As reviewed by Mueller, 2003b, the process goes like this:

- When we talk, certain sounds, especially vowels, reach 120 to 130 dB SPL, or more in the back of the throat.
- The high intensity sounds travel via the mandible (bone conduction) to the condyle, which is adjacent to the ear canal.
- This bone-conducted signal (typically below 750 Hz) then becomes an air-conducted signal by vibrating the cartilaginous portion of the ear canal (in general, the lateral two-thirds).
- In normal situations, this low-frequency energy escapes out the open ear canal and doesn't contribute significantly to our perception of our own voice.
- If the lateral portion of the ear canal is plugged with a hearing aid or earmold, this signal cannot escape, and the resulting trapped energy in the residual ear canal volume is reflected back to the eardrum and transmitted to the cochlea in the typical air conducted manner.
- These sounds will then change the perception of our own voice and can also increase the sounds of chewing (particularly crunchy foods), and even vascular noise and breathing.
- Importantly, the occlusion effect process is not related to the signal going through the hearing aid or to amplification provided by the hearing aid. In fact, the occlusion effect will be the same whether the hearing aid is turned on or off!

There are basically two ways to treat the occlusion effect. One is to make an earmold or hearing aid shell that fits deeply into the ear canal. By sealing the earmold or shell beyond the second bend of the ear canal, the vibration of the cartilaginous portion of the canal is held to a minimum, and the occlusion effect is mostly prevented from occurring. Figure 5–17 shows the occlusion effect findings for two different CIC instruments, fitted to the same individual. Displayed is the ear canal SPL generated for the /ee/ vocalization by the patient at 80 dBA

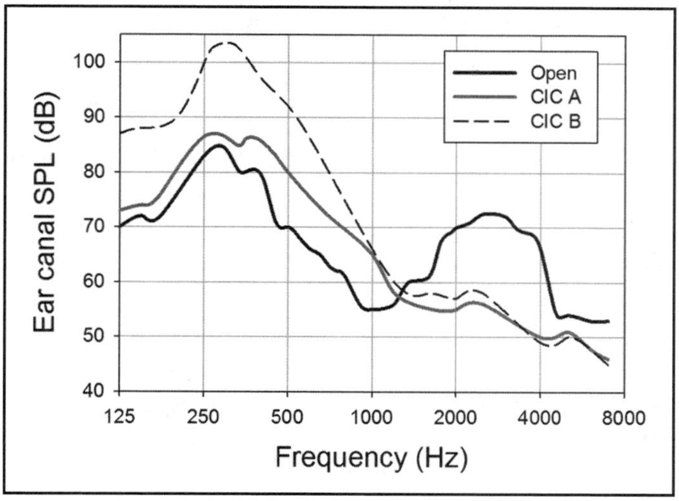

Figure 5–17. Example of the occlusion effect for two different CIC hearing aids. CIC **A** was fit deeply in the ear, whereas CIC **B** was a more shallow fit.

SPL (12 inches from mouth). The measures were taken with the hearing aids turned off. Observe the output for the open ear and for when the two different CICs were placed in the ear. One CIC terminated about 12 mm from the eardrum, a fairly common depth. The other was fitted deeply and terminated 3 to 4 mm from the eardrum. The occlusion effect, with a peak around 300 Hz, was about 20 dB for the CIC that was fitted shallowly (102-dB output versus 82 dB for open ear). Note that the deep fitting reduced the occlusion effect by 15 dB or more, to a point where it likely would not be noticeable for this hearing aid user.

Although tackling the problem in this manner is an earnest goal, the side effect of a deep-fitting earmold or shell is that it can cause significant discomfort and even pain for some patients. The hearing aid also can be difficult to insert. Therefore, this solution, although theoretically sound, is not very practical for many patients. Also, this treatment cannot be applied immediately because it involves making a new ear impression (unless the first one was scanned), ordering a new earmold or ear shell, and then waiting for it to arrive. This process may also decrease a patient's confidence in the overall fitting process or the use of hearing aids in general.

The second, and by far more popular, way to fix the occlusion-effect problem is through venting. When a vent of 2 mm or more is created, sound energy can readily escape. The larger you make the vent, the more likely you are to solve the occlusion problem. If you are using the manufacturer's eartips or domes for the fitting, the same general application applies; switch to a more open or looser fitting style.

Not all occlusion-effect problems have the same peak frequency, which is exactly why the probe microphone measurements can be your best friend. If the peak of the effect is around 200 Hz, the problem is much easier to solve with venting than if the occlusion peak is around 750 Hz or higher. Once the vent reaches 3 mm or so (equivalent of an open fitting tip), most subjective occlusion effects are eliminated. Increasing venting will not provide a solution for more severe losses, where the low-frequency gain is needed for audibility. That is, gain before feedback limits will eventually be reached in listeners needing the most amplification, even in the presence of effective, modern feedback-suppression processing. Increasing venting often will not work with many custom hearing aid fittings either, where it often isn't possible to create a vent this large.

In many cases today, the patient is fitted with a mini-BTE and an open mold, often a stock open-fitting dome or tip. These couplings don't have a vent per se, but their "openness" (using the most open dome) commonly results in the venting equivalent of a large traditional vent. In some cases, however, what is labeled an "open" fitting tip may be occluding for someone with a small ear canal. Probe microphone measures of the REOG will quickly determine whether the ear canal is open or not (see Chapter 4).

The general treatment process for the post-fitting complaint of the occlusion effect goes something like this:

- Determine that indeed the patient is reporting the occlusion effect, and not a general dissatisfaction of too much low-frequency amplification (see our Tips and Tricks).
- For fittings not expected to be open, measure the magnitude of the occlusion effect using probe microphone techniques.
- If the occlusion effect is less than 5 dB or so, the complaint may be related to low-frequency gain, not the occlusion effect. Many patients do not find the occlusion effect to be particularly bothersome until it reaches 10 to 15 dB.

CLINICAL CONCEPT: Ampclusion—What Is It and Should I Measure It?

You might have seen the term "ampclusion" used in articles about the hearing aid occlusion effect. And unfortunately, the term has led to some misunderstanding regarding the treatment of the occlusion effect. The term was coined by Steve Painton in a 1993 article. According to Painton (1993, p. 152), ampclusion is "the combination of occlusion and low-frequency amplification that results in the 'hollowness' or 'head in the barrel' complaints." So, if we are understanding this correctly, if you know that the patient's problem is caused by the occlusion effect, then the patient would not have ampclusion, as there is no combined effect.

We do not use the term ampclusion because usually, the combined effects are not the major clinical issue. First, consider that if the occlusion effect and the hearing aid output were at the same frequency range and the same intensity, the combined effect would be no more than 3 dB (and that is only if the two signals were equal). True, it is possible that there could be an occlusion effect problem at 200 Hz, and too much gain at 500 Hz, but usually the problem is one or the other. For effective treatment and management, you really need to determine which of the two factors is the prime contributor to the problem. So, while you *could* measure "ampclusion" with your probe microphone equipment—use the procedure we recommended but have the hearing aid turned on rather than off—we see no reason to do so, and its unlikely the results will help you in your treatment of the problem.

- For fittings using an open eartip, determine whether the fitting is open through the use of REOG measures or by measuring the occlusion effect. If the REOG shows the fitting is open (or nearly open) or that the occlusion effect is near zero, reconsider whether the complaint is truly the occlusion effect.
- If the fitting is not open, use increased venting or a different fitting tip to allow for a more open ear canal (again, you can monitor this with REOG measures).
- If the fitting was made more open, before the patient leaves the clinic ensure that you have not created a feedback problem.
- Ensure that increased venting did not remove necessary low-frequency information needed for speech understanding (i.e., you still have adequately matched your desired low-frequency gain targets).

Test Protocol

- Set equipment to spectral analysis or live monitoring mode. This may be termed "live speech" mapping in some equipment. Other equipment may have special software for assessing the occlusion effect.
- Place the probe tube in the ear at an appropriate depth.
- Without the hearing aid in place, have patient vocalize /ee/ at 75 dBA and hold for 5 to 8 seconds. Some equipment will have a monitoring microphone to show the SPL of the vocalization. If not, an inexpensive sound level meter or smartphone app can be used. (*Note:* Some probe microphone equipment will monitor the level at the probe microphone, not the reference microphone—this level cannot be used for this purpose.) Some older patients may have difficulty holding this level. If so, 70 dBA will also work.
- Place earmold/hearing aid in ear, but keep hearing aid muted.
- Again have patient vocalize /ee/. This vocalization needs to be at the same input level as open-ear measure.
- Compare the two outputs. The degree that the occluded output is greater than the open-ear output is the occlusion effect. Some equipment might automatically subtract these two curves and provide an on-screen difference curve.

TAKE FIVE: Occlusion Effect—Greater for Males?

We often hear clinicians say that they find more occlusion effect problems with male patients. Is this because males have a lower fundamental frequency and, therefore, more hearing aid-induced occlusion? Probably not. Mueller et al. (1996) compared the occlusion effect for males and females, all fitted with similar custom instruments. There was no significant difference between genders for either the peak or the magnitude of the occlusion effect. It could be that the perception of a larger occlusion effect for males is because males fitted with hearing aids are more likely than females to have normal or near-normal hearing in the low frequencies. Because of occupational and recreational activities, more males have noise-induced hearing loss, which leads to more complaints of the occlusion effect, not necessarily larger occlusion effects.

Sample Findings

To illustrate how we might handle occlusion effect problems in the clinic, we have a case study of a 55-year-old woman with a unilateral hearing loss (sudden onset at age 52) who was fitted with a mini-BTE RIC instrument using a double-dome eartip (reasonably tight fitting). She had a relatively flat hearing loss (40 dB in the lows, sloping slightly to 65 to 70 dB in the highs). The degree of hearing loss in the lows is what prompted the audiologist to select a relatively tight fitting dome. The patient returned to the clinic after one week of using her hearing aid, reporting that the hollowness of her own voice was very annoying, to the point that she was not using the hearing aid. Here is the step-by-step procedure an audiologist might use to address this patient's issue:

- Step 1: We ask the patient to read a passage that contains vowels that trigger the occlusion effect with the hearing aid on, and also turned off. We suggest the following passage (see related Tips and Tricks): "Through three cheese trees three free fleas flew." If the problem is truly an occlusion effect, it should be present with the hearing aid turned off.
- Step 2: For this patient, we want to determine whether using a dome that is not as tight fitting can solve the problem—without creating a new one. Our probe microphone equipment will provide the data to ensure that we are approaching things correctly. We first measure the REOG for the dome she is using and for a second dome that does not fit as tightly. We also measure her REUG just to have a reference

TIPS AND TRICKS: What Doesn't Work Very Well

It is important to talk about treatments that do not reduce the occlusion effect. Recall that the effect is produced by a signal traveling along the mandible to the ear canal, not a signal traveling though the hearing aid. So it is only logical that changing the programming of the hearing aid (reducing low frequencies, for example) will not reduce the occlusion effect. Let's say that again: "Reducing low frequency gain does not reduce the occlusion effect." In fact, this approach could have a negative effect if a person needs the low-frequency amplification in order to understand soft speech. If you have a follow-up patient with the complaint of the occlusion effect, and if turning down low-frequency gain made the occlusion effect go away, then the problem probably wasn't the occlusion effect in the first place—it probably was too much gain for the low frequencies, which is a different problem.

Some have suggested that you add low-frequency gain to fix the occlusion effect. The rationale is that the gain of the hearing aid will sound more natural than that produced by the occlusion effect (and this may be true because the occlusion effect is different for different vowels). The extra-low frequencies from the occlusion will still be there, but the effect might be masked. However, the added low frequencies from the hearing aid might work against understanding speech in background noise, so again, this isn't the preferred solution.

regarding the degree of openness. These results are shown in Figure 5–18A. Observe that, indeed, the REOG for the replacement dome (Dome B) is more similar to the REUG than the original dome (Dome A), suggesting that the fit is more open. So we know we're going in the right direction.

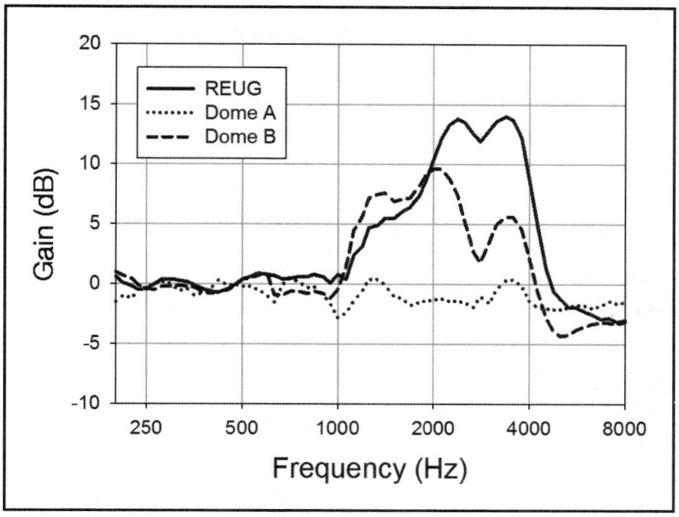

A

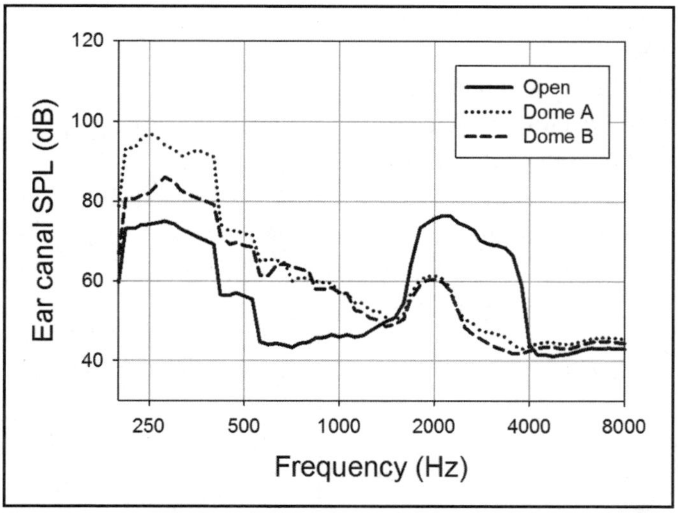

B

Figure 5–18. A. Observe the REOG for the replacement dome (Dome B) is more similar to the unaided curve (REUG) than the original dome (Dome A), suggesting that the fit is more open. **B.** Observe that the occlusion effect for the open ear (for reference), the original tighter fitting dome (Dome A) and the new dome (Dome B), which is more open, are shown. Notice that with the original dome, our patient had over 20-dB occlusion effect, with a peak around 250 Hz. With the new dome, we reduced this occlusion effect by approximately 15 dB.

- Step 3: The REOG, of course, is not a direct measure of the occlusion effect, so our next step is to assess the occlusion effect directly. In the clinic, we may skip Step 2 and jump straight to Step 3 to save time, if we planned to measure the occlusion effect all along. Figure 5–18B shows the occlusion effect for the open ear (for reference), the original tighter fitting dome (Dome A), and the new dome (Dome B), which is more open. Notice that with the original dome, this patient had more than 20-dB occlusion effect, with a peak around 250 Hz. With the new dome, we reduced this occlusion effect by approximately 15 dB. The patient also reports a very noticeable improvement.
- Step 4: Now that we have successfully reduced the occlusion effect, we must determine what effect this looser fitting dome has on the hearing aid output. We expect some reduction in the low frequencies because the increased venting caused the reduction in the occlusion effect. We now go back and complete speech mapping, as we described earlier.
- Step 5: After the hearing aid is reprogrammed, we ensure that this "more open" fitting does not create a feedback issue.

Fitting Tips

- If open fittings are truly open (e.g., the REOG is very similar to the REUG), the occlusion effect will nearly always be no more than a few dB—see research by MacKenzie (2006) comparing eartips/earmolds of different sizes and tightness.
- Annoyance from occlusion is rated slightly higher for a bilateral fitting than a unilateral one (Jespersen, Groth, Kiessling, Brenner, & Jensen, 2006). Some patients report using only one of their two hearing aids for this reason.
- We are not aware of convincing data to support this, but our general notion is that, if you can reduce the occlusion effect to no more than 8 to 10 dB, it will no longer be bothersome for most patients.
- Some probe microphone equipment provides an average occlusion effect—a single value for a range of low frequencies. This is handy, but we have found it underestimates the effect (there may be only one peak that is annoying) and we prefer doing a complete frequency analysis.
- For patients who simply cannot sustain an /ee/ vocalization, it is possible to conduct these measures using bone-conducted signals from an audiometer (for review, see Stender & Appleby, 2009).

TIPS AND TRICKS: Occlusion Effect, or Not?

When patients say that their voice sounds "hollow" or "booming," we usually assume it is the occlusion effect, but the complaint could be related to too much low-frequency gain. A quick test is to have the patient read a passage with the hearing aid turned on and then again with it off. If the hollow sound goes away with the hearing aid turned off, it's not the occlusion effect. As we mentioned earlier, we suggest a sentence using words with vowels that trigger the occlusion effect such as, "Through three cheese trees three free fleas flew."

In Closing

For those of us who use probe microphone measures routinely, it is difficult to imagine how hearing aids could be fitted without this testing. Certainly, using either the REAR or the REIG is essential for verification of prescriptive targets and determining appropriate audibility of the amplified signals—there is no alternative choice. And, it's important we follow appropriate test protocols when we conduct this testing. As Thomas Edison said: "A good intention, with a bad approach, often leads to a poor result."

Along with being the most important clinical measure, as we have described in this chapter, this procedure is also helpful in assessing and adjusting several hearing aid features and in troubleshooting post-fitting problems. Moreover, conducting these measures can be fascinating and educational, and sharing the results with the patient is a very effective counseling procedure. Clearly, the routine use of probe microphone assessment and making reasoned decisions based on the findings in combination with other important information is one of the most important components in the overall fitting of hearing aids. Without this information we are forced to make choices based on hunches, guesses, or clinical intuition instead of data. This is certainly not something we want to do if we are truly interested in providing evidence-based services.

6 Putting It All Together

Great things are done by a series of small things brought together.
—Vincent Van Gogh

This book is dedicated to the clinical applications of probe microphone measures, with an emphasis on the verification of gain and output using modern speech mapping techniques. While this, in fact, might be the most important component of the hearing aid fitting process, it is not used in isolation. There are many other steps needed in the protocol to assure that the end result is a satisfied patient who is obtaining optimal benefit from his or her hearing aids. As succinctly stated above by Van Gogh, if you bring all these small things together, great things will happen (well, at least most of the time)!

There are tests and patient questionnaires to be administered prior to the fitting, verification procedures that can be used during the fitting, (which complement the real-ear findings), and there are outcome measures and follow-up procedures needed following the fitting. We have detailed these tests and procedures in two other separate books (Mueller, Ricketts, & Bentler, 2014; Bentler, Mueller, & Ricketts, 2016). In this chapter, we provide some highlights from the different areas; in particular, the relationship between the overall protocol and your probe-microphone test procedures.

Before the Hearing Aid Fitting

Pre-fitting tools are used to assess the patient, the patient's hearing handicap, and his or her communication needs in order to begin making decisions regarding hearing aid candidacy and selection. Given the time limitations in a typical clinic setting, it is necessary that an appropriately small number of measures are selected that provide the most important information for each specific patient in an efficient manner. Because every patient is different and there is not time to gather exhaustive clinical data, this handful of assessment tools must be selected individually for each patient's situation out of the large group of possible assessment measures available. This is often an iterative process, during which the clinician uses information gathered earlier (e.g., general case history, type and degree of hearing loss, general patient goals, and problems) to determine what additional information is most critical to gather for the individual patient via additional assessments.

Using the Audiogram for Counseling and Predicting Audibility

A big part of the success of the overall fitting relates to making speech audible, with the caveat that it also must have the appropriate loudness, minimal distortion, and a reasonable sound quality. This is why we include a soft speech input when we conduct our real-ear verification—to verify that, indeed, soft speech is appropriately audible. It is helpful during the pre-fitting appointment to ensure that the patient understands this fitting goal. For the new hearing aid user, who still might be questioning the need for hearing aids, it might be necessary to illustrate how much of the average speech signal is *not* audible. For the experienced hearing aid user obtaining a new pair of hearing aids, it might be helpful to explain why the new hearing aids will sound different from the old ones. For example, if more high frequency gain is being added, an explanation of the importance of these speech cues might encourage the user to be more accepting to this new amplification strategy. These visual demonstrations can also be very helpful for family members, who might be wondering why Mom can "hear but not understand."

There are several methods of using the patient's pure-tone audiogram for pre-fitting counseling. Some are more detailed than others, and the method selected often relates to the sophistication of the patient, the level of interest in learning about hearing loss, and how the loss might impact speech understanding. As we discussed in previous chapters, when we plot the LTASS of average speech on the HL scale, it more or less resembles a banana—so much so, that even many lay people know what the *speech banana* is. This is commonly used for counseling patients regarding their hearing loss. Some audiologists have only the banana shaded on the audiogram, other forms have symbols for common environmental sounds, or have the various speech consonants or vowels printed on the audiogram—this is a common option in the software of computer-based audiometers. Usually this is not the audiogram placed in the patient's records or sent out to referral sources, but rather simply something unofficial that can be used for counseling, and that the patient can take home for review.

Using the Speech Banana with Dots

In previous chapters, we discussed how we can use the SII to roughly assess the "goodness" of the amplified signal—something that is calculated automatically on most probe microphone systems. These calculations also can be used during the pre-fitting process. One handy procedure is the count-the-dots audiogram, originally introduced by Mueller and Killion in 1990. In 2010, Mueller and Killion modified their 1990 count-the-dot procedure (Killion & Mueller, 2010); the change provided a new SII importance function that gives more weight to higher frequencies. The new version, therefore, slightly redistributed the 100 dots and includes weightings for 6000 and 8000 Hz.

The revised 2010 audiogram is shown in Figure 6–1 (a template can be found in Appendix A). Note that the density of the dots varies by frequency, related to the importance of that specific frequency for understanding speech. We have plotted a typical hearing aid candidate's thresholds on the audiogram. Observe that this person has only about 20 dots audible—an estimated SII of .20 (20%).

We have found the count-the-dot audiogram to be particularly helpful when counseling patients who are in denial regarding the degree of handicap that they might have. Using a percentage to make the point

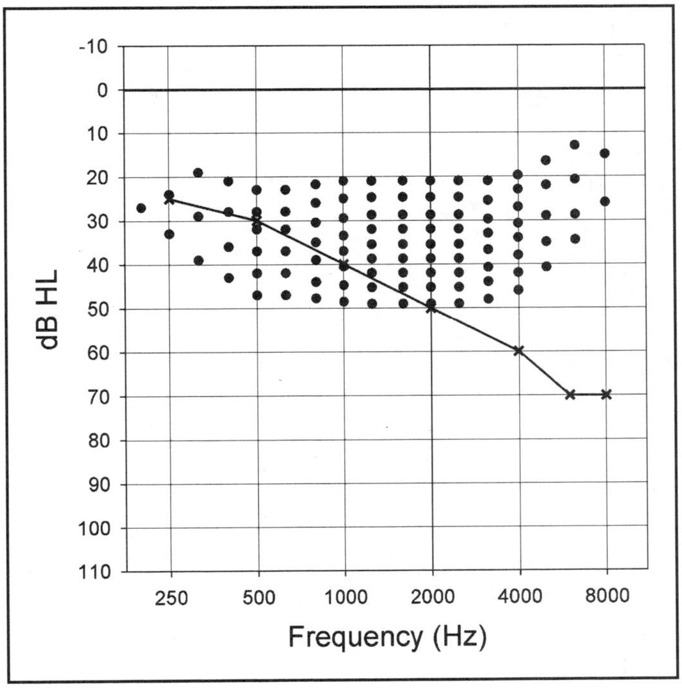

Figure 6–1. Typical downward sloping hearing loss plotted on an audiogram displaying the 2010 Killion and Mueller count-the-dots SII speech spectrum.

is something that everyone can relate to. Graphically showing someone that they are missing 80% of average speech, when they have just said they hear everything, can be a convincing message. Patients often forget much of what we tell them during the prefitting counseling process, but they usually remember the percentage of dots they could hear!

Although the audibility calculations that we have been discussing can easily be computerized (and they have been), there is something to be said about using the paper-and-pencil version. Sitting at a desk with a patient, plotting the audiogram, having the patient help you count the audible dots, showing what happens when the low-frequency dots are covered up because they are masked by noise, all tends to have a memorable counseling impact. The patient takes the sheets home with them, and in general, they seem to get it. But, computer automation is a good thing too, so we discuss how the illustration of audibility also

> **CLINICAL CONCEPT: Hearing, Not Understanding**
>
> Although we believe that using *percent audibility* of average speech can be effective for patient counseling, we do need to mention a fine point that often needs to be clarified. It is important to clearly state that this is the percentage of speech that the patient *hears,* not the percentage of speech that he or she *understands.* Patients sometimes want to think of it as percentage understanding, or even percentage hearing loss.

TAKE FIVE: Pick Your Banana Carefully!

As we have mentioned, it is common to place the speech banana (average LTASS with percentiles) on the audiogram and use this for counseling. There have been several studies of defining average speech over the years, and LTASS findings do vary somewhat from study to study, but they are more or less in fairly good general agreement. So why is it then, that if we would do a Google image search on *Speech Banana* today, we find audiograms (apparently used in offices and clinics somewhere) with the 1000 to 2000 Hz frequency region of the LTASS ranging anywhere from 15 to 45 dB for the upper boundary and 40 to 70 dB for the lower boundary, with everything in between also used? A 25 dB difference! Since this is a fundamental concept of audiology, wouldn't it be nice if we all could get it right? We recently saw a speech banana in the software of a major hearing aid manufacturer that was plotted 10 to 15 dB too low on the audiogram.

Imagine if you took your three-year-old son in for testing, and the audiometric results revealed that he had a 35 dB loss (or is it really a loss?). If he were tested at Clinic A, where they use the 15 to 45 dB banana, you would be told that your son was missing about two-thirds of the important sounds of average speech. On the other hand, if he were tested at Clinic B, where the audiologists use the 40 to 70 dB speech banana, you would be told that all is well—he is hearing 100% of average speech! In our opinion, this borders on malpractice, as a child suffering from middle ear effusion, which often results in a hearing loss of 30 to 35 dB, might go untreated for months or years, simply because the parents were given the wrong counseling based on the wrong banana.

In general, we recommend using a spectrum that has the soft components for the mid-frequencies around 20 to 25 dB HL, with the loud components of the LTASS at 50 to 55 dB HL, similar to what is shown in Figure 6–1.

can be used with your fitting software and probe microphone equipment.

Using Fitting Software or Probe Microphone Equipment

Most hearing aid fitting software also provides a counseling module, which often includes a method to relate the hearing loss to average speech. As previously stated, we have observed that some of these do not use the correct level for the banana, so proceed with caution if you choose to use this approach.

Another way to illustrate how the patient's hearing loss relates to the average speech signal is to use your probe microphone equipment. The advantage of this is that we now have converted everything to ear canal SPL, and we are using an SPL-O-Gram, a display method where loud sounds actually fall appropriately above soft sounds, unlike the standard audiogram. One way to use this display is to plot the patient's hearing threshold, and conduct an REUR for a 65 dB SPL speech signal. In general, this is more intuitive for patient counseling than the standard audiogram, as we see that what is *not audible* falls below the patient's thresholds, and what is audible falls above (Figure 6–2). What you see here are the same hearing thresholds as before (see Figure 6–1), converted to ear canal SPL, compared with the measured real-ear output of the calibrated real-speech signal. Most probe microphone systems will calculate an SII for this measure. The Killion-Mueller spectrum was based on a 60 dB SPL overall level, so if that is also used with the probe equipment, the findings should be similar. The patient's free-field-to-eardrum transfer function will also impact these measures—large REUGs will show more audibility and a higher SII. In fact, the patient used for the measure shown in Figure 6–2 had an REUR slightly larger than average. The probe microphone system calculated an SII of 28%, slightly better than what was obtained using the count-the-dots method. Depending on the time that is available, this counseling and demonstration can be expanded by presenting speech of different input levels (soft, average, loud), or even using the live speech of family members to illustrate to the patient what he or she is missing.

Loudness Discomfort Level Testing

The most critical aspect of the hearing aid verification process is ensuring that the gain and the maximum output are adjusted

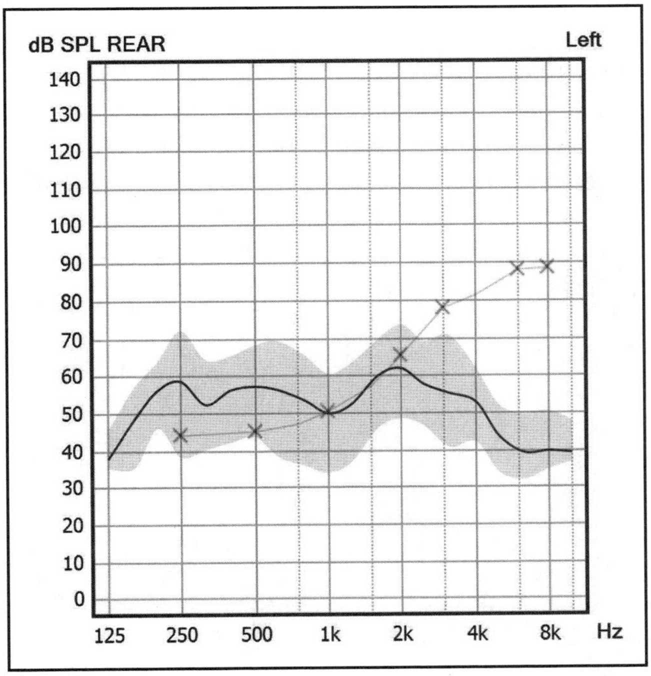

Figure 6–2. Typical downward sloping hearing loss plotted in the SPL-O-Gram format (reference = ear canal SPL). Rather than displaying the average speech spectrum, the spectrum shown was obtained from a real-speech signal (65 dB SPL) delivered to the patient's open ear with the probe microphone tip at the patient's eardrum.

correctly for a given patient. Although these two adjustments are not totally independent (one could not achieve high gain levels for average inputs without a moderately high output setting), for the average patient, it is usually possible to vary the gain by 40 to 50 dB, and the MPO (for maximum power output) by at least 20 dB. Gain prescriptions are typically based on audiometric thresholds, but how do we determine the best MPO setting? The logical approach, which also has been specified in best practice guidelines for the past 25 years, is to conduct frequency-specific loudness discomfort level (LDL) measures, and use these values to set the hearing aid MPO (often by manipulating the output compression limiting kneepoint) so that loud sounds are loud, but not too loud.

These frequency-specific LDL measures are a routine part of the pre-fitting hearing aid battery. As we discussed in Chapters 4 and 5, the REAR85/90 is used to verify that the hearing aid's MPO falls below the patient's LDL. But if you don't know the patient's LDLs, how will you establish the targets for these measures? As we'll soon discuss, taking a guess based on the patient's hearing thresholds can be risky business.

Although intuitively, it seems likely that the maximum output of the hearing aid could influence use, benefit, and satisfaction, one might question if there are data to suggest that this is a problem? There are. In 2003, in a large survey of audiologists, Jenstad, Van Tasell, and Ewert (2003) reported that "aids too loud" was the most common complaint audiologists received from patients fitted with hearing aids. "Satisfaction with loudness" also has been a common question on the MarkeTrak surveys. Although overall satisfaction with hearing aids has gone from a low of 53% (1994) to a high of 81% (2015), as recently as 2008, the MarkeTrak VIII survey revealed that satisfaction for "comfort with loud sounds" was only 67%, which had a .60 correlation with overall satisfaction (Kochkin, 2010).

So what happens if we fit a hearing aid and the MPO is not right? Perhaps the biggest problem would be to select an output that is too high, exceeding the patient's LDL.

CLINICAL CONCEPT: Does the Terminology Really Matter?

There are many terms used to denote the point at which loud sounds become uncomfortable—UL, UCL, ULL, TD, LDL, and so on. Does it matter what term we use? For reasons unknown, many clinicians prefer "UCL." We review many of the terms that have been used relative to loudness and hearing aid output in Table 6–1. It has been suggested by some (including Dr. Ruth Bentler) that TD is the most appropriate term, as dimensions other than the *loudness* of a perceptually abusive sound play a part in what is considered uncomfortable—it is not determined by the RMS level of the signal alone. Factors that tend to cause LDLs to be rated lower include annoyance, peakiness, high-frequency content, and the subjective perception of tinniness. These factors are particularly important during the aided verification process, which we'll discuss later in this chapter. Despite some fondness for the TD descriptor, we will use the more common LDL term to describe this loudness perception.

Table 6–1. Terminology Associated with the Measurement of Loudness Discomfort

- Uncomfortable Loudness (UCL): This is perhaps the most commonly used term among clinicians to describe the point at which loud sounds become uncomfortable. The common use of the letter "C" in the abbreviation is somewhat puzzling and, indeed, some simply use the abbreviation UL. The abbreviation ULL is also used, with the final "L" referring to *level.*
- Loudness Discomfort Level (LDL): This is the term that we prefer and what we will use throughout this chapter. It is used interchangeably with UCL/ULL.
- Threshold of Discomfort (TD). This is another term for the same measure. For the most part (see Clinical Concept on this topic), it can be used interchangeably with LDL, UCL, and ULL.
- Upper Level of Comfort (ULC): This is the category of loudness falling just below the LDL. When using the 7-point Cox Contour Anchors we discuss later, this is the #6 Loud, but an Okay rating. In general, we want the output of the hearing aid to fall at this level; the DSL prescriptive software has used ULC values for this purpose.
- Highest Comfortable Level (HCL): This is the same as the ULC.
- OSPL90: This is the broadest, most powerful output of a hearing aid with the gain control "full on" measured in a 2-cc coupler using 90 dB swept pure tones. This is a component of ANSI standard S3.22 and used for hearing aid specification, documentation, and quality control.
- Maximum Power Output (MPO): In some cases, the term MPO is used synonymously with OSPL90. More commonly, however, in the clinic, MPO refers to the maximum output of the hearing aid when specific settings have been made (e.g., settings of gain, input and output compression), and not the *potential* maximum output of the instrument (the OSPL90). The MPO, therefore, cannot be higher than the OSPL90, and it is often significantly lower. For example, lowering the AGCo compression kneepoint for a given patient would lower the hearing aid's MPO.
- Real-Ear Saturation Response (RESR; REAR 85/90): This is an MPO measure obtained with the hearing aid fitted to the patient's ear, rather than in a 2-cc coupler. Typically, this measure is made with the hearing aid's gain and compression parameters set to approximate use conditions using an 85–90 dB swept pure tone.
- Real-Ear Coupler Difference (RECD): This is a measure that compares the output of a hearing aid in the real ear to the output in a 2-cc coupler with identical settings. If the RECD is known, it can be added to the hearing aid coupler MPO (*not* the OSPL90) to predict the maximum output in the ear canal.
- Reference Equivalent Thresholds in SPL (RETSPL): This is the difference between HL dial setting and output in a 2-cc or 6-cc coupler. Because insert earphones (which are calibrated in a 2-cc coupler), are typically used for HL LDL testing, RETSPL values can be used to convert HL LDLs to 2-cc coupler values (so you can speak the same language as your fitting software).
- Real-Ear Dial Difference (REDD): This is the addition of the RETSPL and the RECD (or it can be measured directly); using this you can convert from HL LDL to ear canal SPL. This provides the RESR output targets you see on the probe-mic fitting screen.
- Automatic Gain Control-input (AGCi): This is input compression, typically having a low activation kneepoint, (in which case it is referred to as WDRC). It can be used to control the hearing aid's MPO if kneepoints are low enough and the ratios are big enough.
- Automatic Gain Control-output (AGCo): This is output compression, typically having a high activation kneepoint and high compression ratios, (in which case it is referred to as compression limiting)—the most common method to control the MPO.

Some probable adverse outcomes are as follows:

- Because there is no control for MPO, the patient will turn down gain (and will then not have appropriate audibility for soft and average inputs).
- The patient will only use the hearing aids when knowing that no loud sounds will be present (missing out on appropriate amplification for the majority of listening situations).
- The patient will have some initial negative experiences and will simply stop using the hearing aids.

So what if the MPO is set unnecessarily lower than it needs to be? Unlike setting the output too high, this probably will not result in rejection of amplification, but there are several potential negative consequences.

- Speech may sound somewhat distorted, as the peaks often will be limited by the MPO of the hearing aid (typically an AGCo algorithm).
- Speech may not have the necessary amplitude dynamics, as the peaks will be limited or clipped. Music may sound dull.
- The range of loudness perceptions will be limited—average and loud inputs may only differ by a few decibels following processing.
- For some speech-in-noise listening situations (those with a slightly positive SNR), unnecessary MPO limiting could make the SNR more adverse.

Can We Predict LDLs from the Audiogram?

A busy clinician might be tempted to simply use the "average" LDL based on the patient's hearing loss. This can be very risky, as shown in the finding from the most extensive study of LDLs that was reported by Bentler and Cooley (2001). They determined LDLs for a total of 433 subjects (710 ears), with presumed cochlear pathologies, using an ascending method of limits similar to our recommendations in the next section. Their data (averaged for five test frequencies) is displayed in Figure 6–3. Several important teaching points are evident:

1. From 20 to 60 dB hearing loss, there is no average change in LDLs.
2. Above 60 dB, average LDLs go up roughly 5 dB for each 10 dB increase in hearing loss.
3. The range of LDLs for different individuals with the same hearing loss is 40 to 50 dB or greater for most hearing loss levels.

Other findings from the Bentler and Cooley (2001) study that have clinical importance (multiple regression analysis using almost 2,000 LDLs; subjects ranging in age from 11 to 97 years):

1. LDLs did not vary as a function of the frequency tested (when hearing loss was matched).
2. There were no gender differences.
3. There were no age differences.

As mentioned above and readily observed in Figure 6–3, the variability of LDLs for individuals with the same degree of hearing loss is very large. For example, if we take a common 50 dB hearing loss, we see that values ranged from the mid-70s to over 130 dB —nearly a 60 dB range. Perhaps more important than the range per se, is that there were not just one or two outliers, but a fairly even distribution between the lower and upper values. If we were to use average values to predict the correct MPO setting

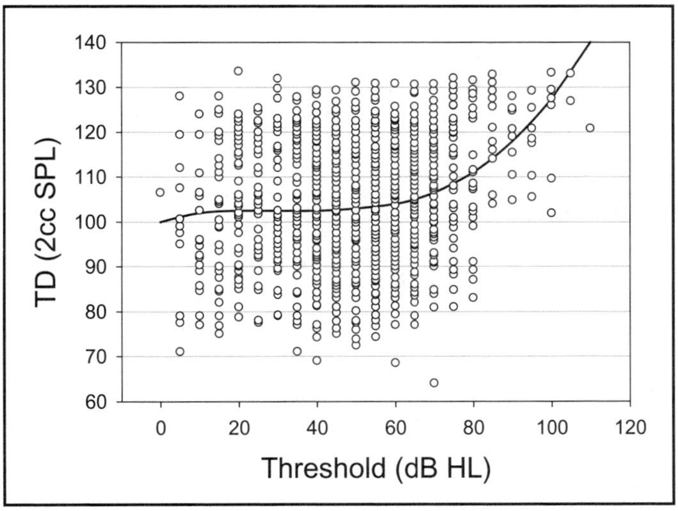

Figure 6–3. Display of LDLs (TDs) referenced to a 2-cc coupler as a function of hearing loss obtained from 710 individual ears. Data points averaged for frequencies 500 to 4000 Hz. Adapted from Bentler and Cooley, 2001.

in this example, the value would be around 102 dB (re: 2-cc coupler; see regression line). Bentler and Cooley (2001), however, report that only 32% of measured LDLs fell within ±5 dB of this average. Assuming that we would not want an MPO mistake of greater than 5 dB, this clearly points out the problems that can exist when average values are used.

Conducting the Testing

Although measuring LDLs is usually considered a fairly simple task and can be conducted effectively by a technician, there are two important procedural conditions that, if not followed correctly, will significantly reduce the validity and reliability of the task: the use of loudness anchors and appropriate instructions. In fact, we suspect that when audiologists state, "I don't do LDL testing because the results are just too unreliable," it is probably because these two critical components have not been implemented into the test protocol.

Loudness Anchors

Loudness anchors are used to give the patient a reference for the loudness perceptions that he or she will be experiencing. It indicates boundaries and intermediate steps, which facilitates the understanding of the task and improves reliability; the patient has words to attach to a perception. The loudness anchors that we recommend, shown in Figure 6–4 (and also Appendix B), are from Robyn Cox (1995) and were used in the development of the Cox Contour Test, which became part of the hearing aid fitting protocol of the IHAFF (Independent Hearing Aid Fitting Forum; Cox, 1995; Mueller, 1994b).

Prior to the testing, the patients are familiarized with the loudness anchors, and they are provided the chart to use during testing. They can respond either by stating

Loudness Anchors

#7. Uncomfortably Loud
#6. Loud, But Okay
#5. Comfortable, But Slightly Loud
#4. Comfortable
#3. Comfortable, But Slightly Soft
#2. Soft
#1. Very Soft

Figure 6–4. Loudness anchors used for LDL testing. Anchors adapted from those used for the Cox Contour Test. Adapted from Cox, 1995.

the loudness category or by simply giving the number. We prefer to have the chart quite large (e.g., 2′ × 3′), mounted on cardboard, which patients can hold in their lap during testing. They then have the option of pointing to the category rather than calling out the term or the number. (Savvy clinicians have learned to associate the certainty of the judgment with different pointing techniques—a true #7 hits the board with a little more force than an uncertain one!) The pointing technique of course only works if you have the patient positioned in the booth so that you can observe the response. Many audiologists simply have the chart printed on standard size paper and hand it to the patient, or have the chart mounted on the test booth wall. However you do it, our main point—*use the anchors!*

Instructions

Going hand-in-hand with the anchors, are the instructions. The measured LDL can vary by 15 to 20 dB simply based on the instructions that are used. Given that we are using the loudness anchors of Cox (1995), it is appropriate to also use the instructions that were developed in association with these anchors. They are provided in Figure 6–5 (and also Appendix C). We have modified Cox's instructions slightly, by adding the sentence, "It is okay to repeat a loudness category, and it is okay to skip a category," as we've found that patients sometimes have problems regarding these issues. For example, they give a #6 rating when it really is a #7 because they think they have to say #6 at least once, or they immediately go from #4 to #5 because the tone got louder, and they already had said #4 once. Perhaps the most important statement of the instructions is at the end, " . . . louder than you would ever choose on your radio no matter what mood you are in." What we are looking for is when the sound is *first* uncomfortable. Audiologists who are somewhat haphazard in delivering LDL instructions often say something

AUDIOID: I See the Twitch!

As we mentioned, it is critical to use the correct instructions when conducting LDLs. The loudness level we are looking for is when the signal first becomes uncomfortable. Over the years, there have been instructions used that obviously were looking for a loudness level much higher. Some instructions used phrases such as, "what you can tolerate for ten minutes." One of the most intriguing set of instructions comes from a hearing aid fitting protocol published by Wallenfels in 1967. It states, "As soon as you see the muscles around his eyes start twitching, you have your measurement."

LDL Instructions

THE PURPOSE OF THIS TEST IS TO FIND YOUR JUDGMENTS OF THE LOUDNESS OF DIFFERENT SOUNDS.

YOU WILL HEAR SOUNDS THAT INCREASE AND DECREASE IN VOLUME. YOU MUST MAKE A JUDGMENT ABOUT HOW LOUD THE SOUNDS ARE. PRETEND YOU ARE LISTENING TO THE RADIO AT THAT VOLUME. HOW LOUD WOULD IT BE?

AFTER EACH SOUND, TELL ME WHICH OF THESE CATEGORIES BEST DESCRIBES THE LOUDNESS. IT IS OKAY TO REPEAT A LOUDNESS CATEGORY, AND IT IS OKAY TO SKIP A CATEGORY.

KEEP IN MIND THAT AN UNCOMFORTABLY LOUD SOUND IS LOUDER THAN YOU WOULD EVER CHOOSE ON YOUR RADIO NO MATTER WHAT MOOD YOU ARE IN.

Figure 6–5. Instructions that are read to the patient prior to administering LDL measures. Adapted from Cox, 1995.

like, "we want to see what you can tolerate." The difference between *uncomfortable* and *tolerate* can be 10 to 20 dB for some patients. We can assure you that when new hearing aid users experience an environmental noise that exceeds their LDL, they do not sit back and say, "Gee, I wonder if I could tolerate that?" Rather, they turn down gain as quickly as possible, which often makes soft speech inaudible. Alternatively, in cases where there is no volume control, the patient may reject the hearing aids completely.

We find it convenient to paste the written instructions on the back of the board that has the loudness anchors on the front. This way you can be reading (yes, *reading)* the instructions while the patient is looking at the anchors. We cannot overstate the importance of using precise and consistent instructions when the goal is a reliable and valid measure.

Test Procedures

Typically, LDL testing is conducted in the test booth, as that is where the equipment is located, and the patient is already seated and hooked up to earphones for the diagnostic testing. If the equipment is available in a hearing aid fitting room, there is no reason that earphone LDL testing could not be conducted there instead, as ambient room noise is not an issue. Once the patient is seated, the earphones have been inserted properly (deep fit of foam tip), the patient has the loudness anchors and the instructions have been given, we recommend the following protocol:

- Use pulsed pure tones as test signal and select frequency.
- First, conduct a practice run.
- Begin testing at or near the patient's MCL (e.g., 60 to 70 dB HL).
- Present a signal and obtain a rating (will probably be #4).
- Use an ascending approach in 5 dB steps and obtain loudness rating for each subsequent level.
- Stop the run at the level that results in the first #7 rating.
- Following the practice run, repeat the procedure.

- After again establishing the #7 rating, conduct a second run.
- If the #7 rating of the second run is within 5 dB of the first, average the two and record this as the patient's LDL. If the difference is larger than 5 dB, conduct a third run and average the last two.
- Repeat the procedure for other selected frequencies. (A practice run is no longer necessary.)
- Repeat the procedure for the other ear.

We recommend testing at two frequencies for each ear; usually one lower (500 or 1000 Hz) and one higher (3000 or 4000 Hz) frequency is selected to roughly map the loudness function. The frequencies tested are based on the degree of hearing loss—the loss must be great enough that you are planning on providing gain, yet not so great that providing useful gain is not possible. For example, if a person has normal hearing through 500 Hz, and then a hearing loss that drops to 90 dB at 3000 Hz, you would probably conduct LDL testing at 1000 and 2000 Hz, certainly not 500 and 3000 Hz.

So, now that the LDLs are measured and recorded, what happens next? How do you use these numbers to program the hearing aids? Will this extra effort and time (five minutes or so) result in a better fitting?

Clinical Applications

As we discussed earlier, when programming the hearing aids, one option is to enter the measured LDLs into the fitting software. The impact this has on the setting of the hearing aid MPO varies considerably among manufacturers. If you fit most of your patients with hearing aids from a single manufacturer (as 85% of audiologists do), then it might be worth taking some time and entering different LDLs into the software (e.g., all 80s, all 90s, all 100s, etc.) and observe how this influences the MPO settings. Do they change? Do the settings agree with your beliefs? It is possible that the manufacturer(s) that you use will do these calculations correctly. If not, we recommend the procedure outlined below.

A continual disconnect in the fitting of hearing aids is that we conduct testing in HL; manufacturers commonly provide hearing aid software referenced to 2-cc-coupler levels in SPL, and we verify hearing aids in ear canal SPL. As a result, we are continually converting between the three references. If that makes you feel like you are going in a circle, you might want to go back and review the Larry Revit figure at the end of Chapter 4. So, for our task at hand, we have LDLs in HL, but we want to program hearing aid MPO for specific frequencies, which are defined in the fitting software in 2-cc coupler SPL. How do we get from HL to the 2-cc coupler levels? Fortunately, this is more of a common correction than you might think, and we have an ANSI standard (S3.6-2004) for making these corrections. These values are referred to as *RETSPLs*. This is an acronym for the Reference Equivalent Threshold in SPL and is pronounced *Rhet-Spull*, which we reviewed in Chapter 3. For our discussion here, things work out conveniently, as insert earphones, which you used for conducting the LDL measures, are calibrated in a 2-cc coupler, just like hearing aids. If we convert HL values using the RETSPL, it makes it easy to talk to the fitting software, which also is in the language of 2-cc SPL, when adjustments are needed.

The RETSPL values for insert earphones are contained in ANSI Standard S3.6-2010, and should be easy to locate with a quick Google search. These are mostly positive numbers, which means that they are *added* to the HL values to convert to 2-cc. Let's say our patient's LDLs were 95 dB at 500 Hz and 105 dB for 3000 Hz. The RETSPLs for these two frequencies are 6.0 and 2.5 dB, respectively. We then do the following calculations:

For 500 Hz:

100 + 6.0 = 106 dB (re: 2-cc coupler)

For 3000 Hz:

105 + 2.5 = 107.5 (108) dB (re: 2-cc coupler)

This little bit of simple math gives us the values that we need to go into the fitting software and make the necessary adjustments for this patient. Be sure to go to the MPO tab, which is often different from "Gain for loud sounds." We want to adjust the AGCo, not the WDRC. (See Mueller et al., 2014 for a complete description of related hearing aid adjustments.) These frequency-specific HL values will also be carried into the probe microphone equipment, converted to ear canal SPL, and will provide targets for your REAR85/90 verification. If the MPO is initially set based on the earphone values, it's very unlikely you'll experience any surprises during the real-ear verification.

Speech-In-Noise Testing

It is common in best practice guidelines related to the fitting of hearing aids to recommend speech recognition in noise as a routine measure prior to the hearing aid fitting, and we certainly agree. There are several reasons why these tests are important, besides the fact that the speech recognition score in quiet is a poor predictor of a patient's speech-in-noise performance, including:

- To address the patient's complaints: It is very likely that problems understanding speech in background noise are the primary reason why the patient is seeking assistance. Conducting this testing conveys to the patient that you understand, and are interested in learning about his or her problem.
- To select the best technology: The results of these tests can impact your selection of the fitting arrangement (e.g., unilateral versus bilateral), the hearing aid style, and/or the need for special features such as remote microphones.
- To establish a baseline: The information collected during this testing can be used as a baseline for measuring aided benefit.
- To monitor performance over time: A patient's ability to understand in background noise may become significantly poorer without an associated change in hearing thresholds or speech understanding in quiet.
- To assist with counseling: How does the patient's score compare with individuals with normal hearing, or other individuals with the same degree of hearing loss? Part of the fitting process is to maintain realistic expectations for the patient. The results of speech-in-noise testing will assist in identifying real-world situations where the patient may or may not do well.
- To help a patient make a decision: Many times, a patient may be on the fence regarding the use of hearing aids and maybe has heard that hearing aids do not work. An aided versus unaided speech test during the initial visit provides an example of potential benefit (see example later in this chapter), and often provides that shot in the arm to encourage the patient to move forward.

CLINICAL CONCEPT: RIP Monosyllables in Quiet

You will notice that we are *not* recommending or even discussing the use of monosyllables in quiet. There are good reasons for this. This test is a very poor predictor of hearing aid candidacy, use, benefit, or satisfaction. Your time will be much better spent conducting speech-in-noise tests. If you *must* conduct speech testing in quiet, however, remember these four rules (from Mueller et al., 2014):

1. Always use presentation levels that optimize audibility (see the 2000 Hz threshold + SL approach reviewed by Mueller et al., 2014).
2. Always use a 50-word list, unless the patient passes the Auditec NU#6 ordered-by-difficulty 10-word or 25-word screening.
3. Always use critical differences for decision making when comparing scores between ears or test sessions (Thornton-Raffin critical differences provided in Appendix D).
4. Never use live-voice presentation. Repeat after us: "The words are not the test. The words are not the test. The standardized recording of the words is the test!"

Factors to Consider When Selecting a Clinical Test

There are several good speech-in-noise tests available that could be used to accomplish the goals we stated above. As a busy clinician, however, you'll probably simply select one or two favorites for routine use. When picking a test, there are several factors to consider, some of which might impact the clinical effectiveness of the test.

Words or Sentences? When conducting speech-in-noise tests, we have the option of using tools that require the recognition of single words, key words embedded in sentences, or entire sentences. There does not seem to be a consensus of what is best, as there are pros and cons of using either words or sentences. As reviewed by Wilson and McArdle (2008), advantages of sentence materials are:

- Better face validity similar to what the patient experiences in everyday listening;
- Perhaps better approximation of how a person understands conversational speech; monosyllables have a lack of lexical, semantic, and syntactic redundancies and dynamic phonotactic cues.

On the other hand, monosyllables have the following advantages (Wilson & McArdle, 2008):

- With sentence material, context contributes heavily to intelligibility and makes basic auditory function difficult to determine.
- The syntactic and semantic structures of sentence-length stimuli can influence performance.
- Sentences involve more complex cognitive skills; more working memory

AUDIOID: Olive, Twist, or Cherry?

For most speech-in-noise testing, it is common to use a multi-talker babble, sometimes referred to as *cocktail party noise*. You probably also have used the phrase *the cocktail party effect*, which if you didn't know, is a scientific term! In the early 1950s, much of the early work in this area was related to the problems faced by air traffic controllers. At that time, controllers received messages from pilots over loudspeakers in the control tower. Hearing the intermixed voices of many pilots over a single loudspeaker made the controller's task very difficult. The effect was first defined in a Journal of Acoustical Society paper in 1953, where is was named the "*cocktail party problem*" by Colin Cherry.

effort is required. These demands could differentially affect older versus younger patients.

Competing Noises. There are several different types of competing noises used with popular speech tests. The different noises have different characteristics, which can impact the performance for a given test. Most importantly, using the wrong noise can affect list equivalency, resulting in a clinician drawing the wrong conclusion about measured differences between test conditions (e.g., performance for the right versus left ear). It is important, therefore, to use the type of competing noise with each speech test that was used in its development, when normative data were collected.

Adaptive Versus Fixed SNR. In the clinic, speech-in-noise testing can be conducted by using an adaptive or a fixed SNR method. With adaptive testing, either the speech or the noise level is fixed, and the other signal level is then varied. The variance of the adaptive signal can be at predetermined intervals, with a wide range of SNRs tested (e.g., WIN, BKB-SIN, QuickSIN). Alternatively, the adaptive signal can be varied as a function of the individual's performance on the previous item. Examples of this are the HINT and the Matrix Test (English modification of the German OLSA), where the target sentence material is raised or lowered for each sentence and the background noise is fixed. In all cases, the purpose of the testing typically is to determine the SNR where the patient is obtaining a score at or near 50% correct. This is often referred to as the speech reception threshold (SRT) in noise (often denoted as SNR-50 or SRT50).

An alternative method of conducting speech-in-noise testing would be to use a test that has a fixed SNR. That is, the SNR is not adjusted for the individual patient but is presented at the same level for all. Speech tests that use a fixed SNR are the R-SPIN (+8 dB) and the Speech Recognition In Noise Test (SPRINT; +9 dB). The Connected Speech Test (CST) also is a fixed-level test, although the background multitalker babble can be adjusted to different SNRs.

There are clinical advantages to both the adaptive and fixed SNR methods of measuring speech recognition in background noise. First, some advantages of the adaptive model:

- It eliminates floor and ceiling effects (i.e., scoring nearly all correct or all incorrect), a common problem when a fixed SNR is used.

- The 50% correct point for most patients can be obtained more reliably and efficiently than a lengthy word list. With the adaptive model, we can more readily determine significant differences between patients or between the right and left ears of the same patient.

But, there are also some disadvantages of measuring the reception threshold for speech compared with using a fixed SNR approach:

- It makes it difficult to explain test results to the patient—telling a patient his or her speech reception threshold (SRT) in noise is 10 dB is not very meaningful.
- It makes it difficult for patients to relate their performance to the real world. Because of the way the test is designed, two individuals with very different speech recognition ability would both report that they got about one-half of the words correct.
- It makes it difficult to relate findings to third parties and referral sources. Even audiologists themselves are not always certain if an SNR-50 score of +4 dB is good or bad. And, the SNR-50 score that is good for one speech test might just be okay for another (e.g., see norms for BKB-SIN versus WIN).
- The administration and scoring may be somewhat more cumbersome.

Presentation Level. An important consideration when conducting speech-in-noise testing is the selection of an appropriate presentation signal. The level selected is directly related to the question being asked, and the overall purpose of the testing. Here are some examples:

- Choice #1: Conduct testing at the level at which the norms were collected. This is the most reasonable choice, as it allows for comparison with the norms and should ensure the best interlist reliability.
- Choice #2: Conduct testing at the level at which the best performance is predicted. This should provide the best indication of true recognition ability and best predict potential performance with amplification.
- Choice #3: Conduct testing at the average real-world levels, which should provide the best prediction of how the patient performs in the real world. (*Note:* We say best not accurate—clinical testing is not too good at predicting real-world performance.)
- Choice #4: Conduct testing at the specific level that relates to a patient complaint; a patient with a mild hearing loss whose primary complaint is understanding soft speech might be tested at the level of soft speech.

Earphones or Sound Field?

As with presentation level, the use of earphones versus sound field testing depends somewhat on the purpose of the test and how the test was normed. In general, there are compelling reasons to conduct the testing using earphones, including:

- Calibration/standardization is much easier.
- Individual ear information can be obtained.
- Masking of the non-test ear is easier, when necessary.

- Testing is not constrained by upper output limits of sound field speakers.
- Many audiologists fitting hearing aids do not have appropriate sound-field systems.

We have given you several considerations in this section to think about. We encourage you to keep these in mind as you select one or two tests for use with your patients. At this point, it is reasonable to ask, what test is best? Mueller et al. (2014) review in detail 12 different speech tests that could be used in the pre-fitting process. For one reason or another, an argument could be made for using any one of these. For this chapter, however, we'll just provide one example, the QuickSIN. We're not saying it's necessarily *the best*, but it is the most popular, and it meets most of the criteria that we believe is important.

Quick Speech in Noise (QuickSIN) Test

The QuickSIN was designed to be short enough for routine clinical use, and provides a reliable way to measure a listener's speech understanding ability in noise. The test certainly is quick, as a single list only requires about a minute to administer after instructions. The QuickSIN consists of 12 standard lists and three practice lists. Each list contains six sentences, with five key words per sentence. Sentences are spoken by a female talker who is reading sentences from the speech corpus of the IEEE (1969).

The QuickSIN sentences are presented in a multi-talker background at six predetermined SNRs, which become progressively more difficult with each sentence in 5-dB steps. That is, the first sentence is presented at a +25 dB SNR, and the second sentence is presented at a +20 dB SNR. The final sentence is the most difficult and is presented at a 0 dB SNR. The presentation level of the speech is fixed, and the level of the multitalker background varies when SNR is adjusted. The competing signal is somewhat unique, as it is not a true babble as used with some of the other tests commonly used. It is only four talkers, and one of the talkers, a female, is the same talker who is reading the target sentences. At the adverse SNRs (when the multitalkers become louder) many patients report that they have a tendency to try to follow the woman in the competing noise, rather than the target speaker. You might say that this makes the test "unfair," but this type of background noise is not unlike what many of our hearing aid patients frequently experience in their daily life.

The most common method of administering the QuickSIN is using the commercially available CD in a CD player routed to a clinical audiometer. Most of today's computer-based audiometers, however, have the test available as a wave file, with an automated scoring procedure. The QuickSIN manual describes specific calibration and scoring methods.

- For standard measurement of the SNR-50, the presentation level should be 70 dB HL (83 dB SPL) for patients with pure-tone averages 45 dB or less and should be set to "loud but okay" (just below the patient's LDL) for patients with more hearing loss.
- The test can be administered under headphones (bilaterally or unilaterally) or in the sound field, depending on the desired use. For pre-fitting testing, we are interested in ear-specific headphone results.
- The patient's task is to repeat the sentence spoken by the female talker.

Each sentence consists of five key words, and patients receive credit for each key word correctly repeated.

- The test is easily scored (with minor math applications) using the standard score sheet, copies of which are available online. The clinician simply marks the number of key words correctly repeated for each sentence and then sums these numbers to calculate a total score, shown in Figure 6–6.

The QuickSIN is scored as SNR loss, rather than SRT-50 because the score is adjusted based on average performance for normal hearing individuals. That is, the number of correctly repeated key words is subtracted from 25.5 (SNR loss = 25.5 – Correct Key Words). This number reflects the SNR at which a patient correctly repeats approximately 50% of the key words, with the normal hearing correction (Killion et al., 2004). For example, let's say a patient repeated all the words correctly for the first four sentences (a total of 20 words; 5 key words/sentence), and was not able to get any of the words correct for the last two more difficult sentence presentations (presented at an SNR of +5 dB and 0 dB). We would then subtract 20 (words correct) from 25.5, and this patient would have an SNR loss of 5.5 dB.

Critical difference values for the QuickSIN are shown in Figure 6–7. You can see that these values drop fairly rapidly as the number of lists per condition increases from one to three. Given the quick test time of giving one list, we believe it is worthwhile to always present at least two lists/ear for pre-fitting testing. The time investment is still less than five minutes and the critical differences approach 2 dB with 90% confidence.

The most obvious clinical uses for the QuickSIN may be as a pre-fitting measure to aid in hearing aid selection and counseling decisions. Once a clinician has determined the SNR loss, this information can be combined with knowledge of the patient's communication needs to provide evidenced-based recommendations to the patient regarding hearing aid features, in particular microphone technology. For example, let's

TRACK 21

Practice List A		**Score**
1. The lake sparkled in the red hot sun.	S/N 25	_______
2. Tend the sheep while the dog wanders.	S/N 20	_______
3. Take two shares as a fair profit.	S/N 15	_______
4. North winds bring colds and fevers.	S/N 10	_______
5. A sash of gold silk will trim her dress.	S/N 5	_______
6. Fake stones shine but cost little.	S/N 0	_______
	TOTAL	_______

Figure 6–6. Sample list from the QuickSIN. Adapted from the QuickSIN manual, Etymotic, Inc.

Lists per Condition	1	2	3	4	5	6	7	8	9
95% C.D. +/-, in dB	3.9	2.7	2.2	1.9	1.7	1.6	1.5	1.4	1.3
90% C.D. +/-, in dB	3.2	2.2	1.8	1.6	1.4	1.3	1.2	1.1	1.1
80% C.D. +/-, in dB	2.5	1.8	1.5	1.3	1.1	1.0	1.0	0.9	0.8

Figure 6–7. Critical differences for the QuickSIN for different number of lists used. Adapted from the QuickSIN manual, Etymotic, Inc.

TIPS AND TRICKS: Do Not Use These QuickSIN Lists

For a standard administration, the QuickSIN is a quick and reliable method of estimating a patient's ability to understand speech in noise. As we have mentioned, you will want to use two or three lists per ear when conducting your testing. It is important, therefore, that all lists are equivalent. Research by McArdle and Wilson (2006) suggests that all 12 may not be. In studying individuals with hearing loss, they found that the range among lists was 10.0 to 14.3 dB SNR. The data from their study indicated that for purposes of homogeneity of test results, *for individuals with hearing loss*, lists 4, 5, 13, and 16 *should not* be used.

assume a patient has the communication goal of better speech understanding in a noisy mall, which you estimate the SNR to be around +5 dB. If the patient has a QuickSIN score indicating the SNR at which they can repeat 50% of words in sentences (SNR-50) of +7 or so, they might expect to obtain important benefits from directional technology for the shopping mall setting (e.g., the SNR improvement might be just enough to allow them to follow the conversation). Conversely, if the patient has a goal of communicating in a noisy club, in which you estimate the SNR to be +1 dB and their QuickSIN SNR-50 is +15 dB, we would predict that he or she would not obtain any benefit from directional technology, and an FM system or remote microphone may need to be considered, and you may have some counseling about realistic expectations to do as well! Mueller (2016) reviews eight illustrative cases where the QuickSIN can be used for fitting decisions and patient counseling.

The QuickSIN CD is available from Etymotic Research, and from Auditec of St. Louis, MO. (https://auditecincorporated.wordpress.com/)

Pre-Fitting Self-Assessment Scales

We have all heard the old saying, "You can't judge a book by its cover." A saying that is maybe not as well known, but even more true is, "You can't judge a hearing aid candidate by his audiogram." Patients differ in so many ways that are not displayed in Xs and Os or word recognitions scores. There is an excellent battery of validated preselection self-assessment inventories available. They are easy to administer and score. The results of these scales will shape the fitting process, assist in technology decisions, and become invaluable for developing counseling strategies and a relationship with the patient along the way. The routine use of these scales is not only a good thing to do, it is the right thing to do.

In some ways, these scales are not much more than an extended case history, but they allow the clinician to collect information in an organized manner, and in most cases, the patient's responses can be compared with average data from large samples. The information collected using these inventories can significantly influence pre-fitting counseling and in some instances alter fitting decisions. In some cases, the scores collected before the fitting serve as a baseline, as they may be compared with results measured after a patient wears hearing aids for a period of time to directly quantify subjective hearing aid benefit, reduction in hearing handicap, or other outcomes of interest.

In case you don't routinely conduct these tests, here are a few areas where self-assessment pre-fitting measures might be helpful for the overall hearing aid fitting process:

- They assist in determining if a patient is a candidate for hearing aids. Is the patient's report of communication problems consistent with the audiogram? Do they even report that they have problems?
- They assist in determining if a patient is ready to be helped. If a person denies they have communication problems, will he or she accept the use of hearing aids? Is counseling needed before even attempting to move forward?
- They assist in establishing realistic expectations. A patient is obtaining hearing aids because of problems understanding speech in background noise. His or her expectations show that he or she believes that the use of hearing aids will resolve 100% of these communication problems. It is probably best to readjust the patient's expectations before he or she begins to use hearing aids.
- They assist in establishing a baseline. Many of the same inventories used in the pre-fitting process also are used as outcome measures following the fitting. Obtaining pre-fitting unaided data will then be helpful in determining aided benefit.

There have been a large number of inventories that have been introduced over the years. We have selected a subset that we believe are useful, and each of which provides unique information. More specific, we have selected seven different self-assessment inventories that can be used in the pre-fitting process—these tests are all explained in detail in Mueller et al. 2014, complete with guidelines for administration and scoring, and related seminal references. Here is a brief summary:

- Hearing Handicap Inventory for the Elderly/ Adult (HHIE/A). Measures the degree of handicap for emotional and social issues related to hearing loss (see examples in Appendix E and F).
- Abbreviated Profile of Hearing Aid Benefit (APHAB). Provides the percent of problems the patient has for three different listening conditions involving speech understanding (in

quiet, in background noise, and in reverberation) and problems related to annoyance of environmental sounds (aversiveness scale). (Appendix G)

- Expected Consequences of Hearing Aid Ownership (ECHO). Measures the patient's expectations for four different areas: positive effect, service and cost, negative features, and personal image. (Appendix H)
- Client Oriented Scale of Improvement (COSI). Requires patients to identify three to five very specific listening goals/communication needs for amplification. Can then be used to measure patients' expectations related to these specific goals. (Appendix I)
- Hearing Aid Selection Profile (HASP). Assesses eight patient factors related to the use of hearing aids: motivation, expectations, appearance, cost, technology, physical needs, communication needs, and lifestyle.
- Characteristics of Amplification Tool (COAT). Determines the patient's communication needs, motivation, expectations, cosmetics, and cost concerns.
- Profile of Aided Loudness (PAL). Assesses the patient's loudness perceptions and satisfaction with these perceptions for 12 different everyday environmental sounds. (See Appendix J and K.)

During the Hearing Aid Fitting

In the previous section, we discussed various tests and procedures that can be conducted prior to the actual fitting. Now that you are prepared—the day of the fitting is here. As hopefully apparent from the title of this book, we believe that the most important aspect of the fitting itself is the real-ear verification of gain and output. We do recognize, however, that this verification procedure is not conducted in isolation. To some extent, the measures that are taken on the day of the fitting reflect the audiologist's gold standard regarding what is a "good" fitting, or, at the least, what is an "acceptable" fitting. For example, if the audiologist truly believes that the most important aspect of the fitting is the patient's opinion of sound quality, then some type of formal sound quality judgments would be implemented. This might, however, compromise the fit-to-target that we have been discussing throughout this book. Hence, we view the measures reviewed here as supplemental, not a replacement for the careful adjustment of gain and output using real-ear verification.

Aided Speech Recognition

The pros and cons of using aided speech testing to quantify the success of a hearing aid fitting has been debated since about as long as hearing aids have been fitted by someone with the professional title of audiologist. Consider that many, if not most, individuals purchase hearing aids because they have problems understanding speech, most commonly speech in background noise. As professionals, we sell them a device (usually two) designed to solve their problems and hopefully meet their expectations. Isn't it reasonable then, for a new hearing aid user to expect that during the fitting process a test would be conducted that assesses the improvement the hearing aids provide for understanding speech, the primary problem that triggered their purchase decision? To state the obvious corollary, a nearsighted person fitted with contact

TAKE FIVE: Verification Versus Validation?

If you look up dictionary definitions of verification and validation, you may be hard pressed to discriminate between the two words, which mean essentially the same thing. However, in the world of quality control, there has been a great deal of discussion on the topic, and several industries have provided definitions for these two words that are specific to their work. In most cases, verification is used when discussing if specific goals, often that design or manufacturing goals were met. In contrast, validation is used to describe whether the end user/target audience obtains what they wanted or needed. Stated simply:

- Verification: Are we building the system right?
- Validation: Are we building the right system?

Applied to the selection and fitting of hearing aids, hearing aid verification is often used to refer to the process of ensuring that the hearing aid meets specific criteria (are we building the system right?). For example, we verify that we achieve our target prescriptive gain and output, we verify that aided loudness does not exceed threshold of discomfort, or we verify that aided thresholds meet expected levels. In contrast, hearing aid validation is the process of ensuring we meet the goals set forth in the communication needs assessment (are we building the right system?). It's hard, however, to pigeonhole some clinical tests. For example, is aided speech recognition verification or validation? This question has generated a lively discussion or two between the three of us. Whatever you call it, in this section we provide a few tools to supplement your probe microphone measures.

lenses would expect that part of the fitting would be a before and after reading of the Snellen chart to ensure that an appropriate improvement in vision had occurred.

Speech recognition, when used for hearing aid selection or verification, has been fraught with reliability issues, but there are several other issues that also limit the usefulness of this tool. Typical speech recognition in noise tests used in the clinic do not reflect real-world conditions. Specifically, for testing in the clinic, reverberation is more limited, visual cues are typically not present, talkers have clear speaking voices, speech is usually presented at conversational levels (even though softer levels would be more challenging), and conditions tend to represent one-on-one conversations with very small speaker-to-listener distance (typically ~1 meter). In fact, the test conditions are so easy for listeners with mild and moderate hearing loss that there is little or no room to demonstrate hearing aid benefit. That is, we do not expect the speech recognition to improve with amplification based on calculated changes in audibility. Moreover, even if all these factors could be overcome, if you were using speech testing on the day of the fitting to determine the appropriateness of the fitting, you would still be left with the following practical questions for a given patient:

- How good does this patient's speech recognition have to be to be "good enough"?
- How do you know when you've reached the patient's optimal level of speech recognition?
- How do you know when one more change of programming won't make recognition better?
- How do you know when a different pair of instruments, with slightly different signal processing won't make speech recognition better?

Despite these considerable limitations, we believe it is sometimes useful to measure speech recognition benefit as a supplemental measure. Because it's not possible to have a specific aim (X% improvement in speech recognition, or an aided score of X%) it is not really a verification procedure. In addition, because it is somewhat unreliable, and the listening conditions don't really reflect those commonly experienced in the real world, it is not really a validation procedure either. Instead, its clinical value (when there is one) most often relates to counseling, or simply a demonstration. We also can't forget that simply using this measure in the fitting process seems to increase patient loyalty to the provider, satisfaction with the fitting process, and ultimately, increased satisfaction with amplification over time (see Mueller et al., 2014).

As we already mentioned, it may not be necessary, in many cases, to perform aided speech recognition testing. However, if you have the clinical time available, and you have a patient for whom this testing will enhance the fitting procedure through changes in counseling, counseling reinforcement, or other reasons, we encourage you to obtain as much information, or as specific information, as possible. The general purposes for completing aided speech recognition testing include:

- Demonstrate that the hearing aids improve audibility leading to improved speech recognition;
- Demonstrate that a technology aimed at improving SNR (directional microphones, beam-formers, FM systems, remote microphones, etc.) can lead to improved speech recognition in noise;
- Demonstrate the limitations of performance in noise (even with SNR improving technologies) to aid in counseling related to realistic expectations.

Illustrative Case Study

Our patient is a 72-year-old male who is obtaining his first pair of hearing aids. He recognizes that he has problems, but is still somewhat apprehensive about the use of amplification. He has a typical downward sloping hearing loss bilaterally, going from 25 to 35 dB in the low frequencies, to 60 to 70 dB in the 3000 to 4000 Hz region. Our probe microphone testing showed that we were able to obtain a good match to NAL-NL2 targets bilaterally through 4000 Hz for soft, medium and loud inputs. At this point, we decided to conduct some supplementary speech testing as part of the verification process. As mentioned earlier, this will not be used to alter the fitting, but rather to gather useful information that can be used in counseling.

Our pre-fitting test results from a week earlier showed that his unaided QuickSIN performance (conducted under earphones at 70 dB HL) was 8 dB SNR Loss for the right ear, and 9 dB SNR Loss for the left. Our testing today in the sound field (conducted aided bilaterally with an input of 65 dB SPL) revealed an SNR Loss of only 4 dB. This is a very encouraging finding. It shows that he is performing better with hearing aids than his best-ear earphone performance, and the input used today is considerably softer (conversational speech). Moreover, for many "noisy" environments, the SNR is around +5 to +10 dB, and these aided results suggest that he now should be able to follow a conversation in these settings. So, from a verification standpoint, these findings are more or less a pat-on-the-back for the audiologist who selected the technology and programmed the hearing aids. But what about the patient? He probably doesn't realize that he is doing any better—he still is missing several words—and of course, he doesn't realize that today's testing was conducted ~20 dB softer than the testing of last week.

To demonstrate the aided benefit to the patient, we conduct a second QuickSIN measure. We now present the signal at a soft-speech level (50 dB SPL) and test unaided versus aided bilaterally. Additionally, to make things more meaningful for the patient, we score the test as percent correct for each of the six SNRs (two lists = 10 words/SNR level). The results of this testing are shown in Figure 6–8. Once these results are graphed, and placed in front of the patient, we can have a meaningful discussion. We would start by first pointing out than when there is very little background noise (e.g., SNR +20 and +25), he does okay without hearing aids (he probably already knew that). We then might mention, that even with hearing aids, he won't do very well in the very difficult listening situations—the 0 dB SNR condition—but we also need to mention that neither do people with normal hearing! We then focus on the center portion of the chart, the most commonly encountered SNRs in daily activity, where the use of hearing aids improved his under-

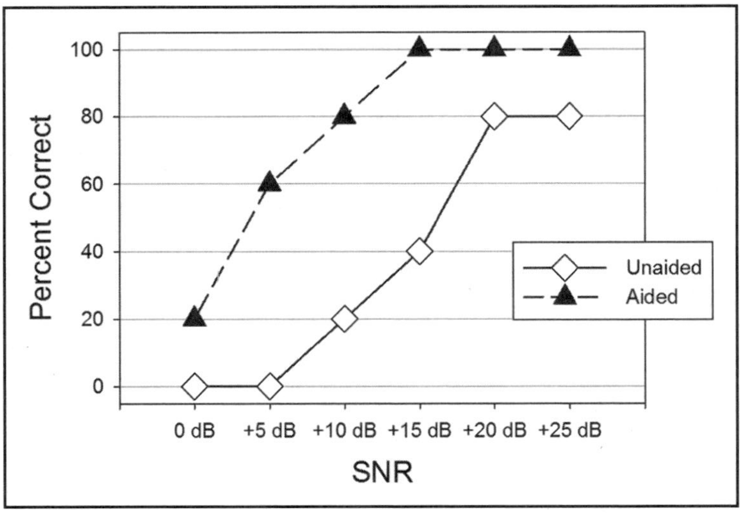

Figure 6–8. Worksheet to show patient scores as a function of the SNR for both the aided and the unaided conditions. Recall the testing was done with a soft speech level, so even if the scoring for the QuickSin is represented as SNR-loss, it is possible to see the percentage correct across the various SNRs to show the result of increased audibility.

standing by 60%. It's probable that he has already mentioned this to us on his own, as this degree of improvement is very noticeable to the patient during the procedure. The 5 to 10 minutes spent conducting this testing and explaining the results to patients can have a lasting impact on their attitude toward the use of hearing aids.

Verification of Loudness Comfort

A general goal of most all hearing aid fittings is to restore normal, or near-normal, loudness perceptions for the hearing-impaired patient. That is, when the patients are wearing their hearing aids, soft sounds should be audible, average sounds should be comfortable, and loud sounds should be loud, but not too loud (see Mueller 1999 for review). As we discussed in Chapter 2, to some extent, prescriptive fitting algorithms are geared toward loudness normalization, although a *true* loudness normalization approach tends to result in too much gain for most patients and too high of compression ratios. In general, our initial approach for providing appropriate loudness for speech is to measure hearing thresholds and then program the hearing aids based on these thresholds to a validated prescriptive method. As we reviewed in the previous chapters, verification is probe microphone measures—but these values are not directly related to the patient's loudness perceptions.

A related, and perhaps more important issue regarding loudness, is testing to assure that the frequency-specific hearing aid MPO is set correctly and that outputs do not exceed the individual patient's LDLs. In general, our approach to accomplish this is to first measure frequency-specific LDLs, and then use these values to set the MPO accordingly (via adjusting AGCo kneepoints) for the different frequency channels. As we describe in Chapters 4 and 5, verification is through probe microphone measures, comparing the REAR-85 for a swept tone to the patient's LDLs—but again, these values are not directly linked to loudness perceptions.

If prescriptive gain has been achieved and verified with probe microphone measures, and the MPO has been set correctly based on the patient's LDLs and REAR-85 testing, one might question why it is still necessary to include aided loudness testing as part of the hearing aid verification process? There are several reasons:

- Average values: Regarding soft and average inputs, prescriptive gain targets are for the "average" patient. While these values typically place the amplified speech signal at or near the patient's preferred loudness levels, adjustments are needed for some patients.
- Measurement errors: Regarding the MPO settings, errors in the earphone LDL assessment are possible, which would have influenced AGCo settings. If the manufacturer's default MPO settings were used, or if earphone LDLs were not obtained, then the need for behavioral aided LDL testing is even more critical.
- Monaural summation: Previous testing involved pure-tone stimuli. The monaural summing of broadband signals such as speech varies from individual to individual.
- Binaural (bilateral) summation: At this point in the overall fitting process, behavioral testing only has been conducted monaurally. Summation has been accounted for in the prescriptive method (see Chapter 2), but again, these are average values and summation

could vary by 5 dB or more among different individuals. The bilateral LDL may not be too different from the unilateral one, but it remains important to account for this.

- Channel summation: There is a summing of the signal when multiple channels are used in the processing, which occurs with all modern instruments. The exact degree varies depending on the number of channels, how much they overlap, and the settings of the instrument; therefore, this also is difficult to predict.

All of these factors have the potential to affect loudness perceptions with hearing aids, or to cause bilateral aided judgments for speech to differ from what would be predicted based on unilateral earphone testing with using pure tones. We know that nearly 50% of patients are not satisfied with the loudness of their hearing aids (Kochkin, 2010). This tells us that aided loudness testing and related MPO adjustment, is well worth the clinical time investment.

Clinical Testing

Before conducting the aided loudness testing you will need two tools discussed earlier in this chapter that were used for the unaided earphone LDL measures: the Cox Contour Anchors (see Figure 6–4; Appendix B) and the written instructions for the loudness rating task (see Figure 6–5 and Appendix C).

The next step is to ensure that your equipment is calibrated—consider that for this testing we will be focusing on SPL values, not HL values. Loudness verification can be conducted in an audiometric test booth via the sound-field speakers, or in the hearing aid fitting room using some other sound source like your probe microphone equipment. We will start with a protocol for conducting the testing in a test booth (adapted from Mueller & Hall, 1998):

- Obtain an SLM (inexpensive models will work just fine for this measure; a good smart phone App will work fine too).
- Set the audiometer dial to a fixed HL value (e.g., 50 dB HL) and present speech via the loudspeaker. Most any recorded, calibrated speech signal will likely work, but we recommend a continuous discourse passage—CD recordings are available from Auditec of St. Louis, MO.
- Place the SLM at the presumed location of the patient's head. Observe the average levels of the peaks of speech with the SLM set to "linear" weighting (e.g., for the 50 dB HL signal, the peaks of speech might be measured to be 66–68 SPL range).
- The correction values for "average speech" will be 2 to 3 dB below the noted peak level. If the peaks were 68 dB SPL, we would then predict the average speech signal to be around 65 dB SPL.
- Subtract the HL value from the sound field SPL value and you will have a correction factor for all presentation levels; 65 minus 50 = 15. Therefore, for this example, for loudness testing you know that you would use 30 dB HL (45 dB SPL; soft), 50 dB HL (65 dB SPL; average), and 70 dB HL (85 dB HL; loud). These corrections would be easy to remember, but usually the numbers don't work out quite as well—if you had measured peaks of 72 dB SPL, which would give you an overall level of 69 dB SPL, the correction factor would have been 19 dB, and the presentation levels would be 26, 46, and 66 dB HL.
- Fit the hearing aids to the patient, set at projected "use gain." Provide the

patient with the Loudness Anchors, and read the instructions from above. Most patients will remember the procedure from the previous unaided loudness testing

- Present the soft speech signal (45 dB SPL)
  - Desired rating: #2 (Soft)
  - Acceptable ratings: #1 (Very Soft) or #3 (Comfortable, But Slightly Soft)
- Present the average speech signal (65 dB SPL)
  - Desired rating: #4 (Average)
  - Acceptable ratings: #3 (Comfortable, But Slightly Soft) or #5 (Comfortable, But Slightly Loud).
- Present the loud speech signal (85 dB SPL)
  - Desired rating: #6 (Loud, But Okay)
  - Acceptable rating: #5 (Comfortable, But Slightly Loud).
- For any judgments that do not fall into the acceptable range, conduct intuitive tweaking and repeat judgment. Most manufacturers provide easy-to-use tabs in the fitting software for this purpose. Our experience has been that many patients, especially new users, tend to be a little startled by the 85 dB SPL input, which prompts them to assign it a #7 rating. We suggest that before making programming changes, repeat the testing for this level a couple times, after providing a little more instruction: Was it truly uncomfortable, or was it just startling, or annoying? Many times, once the patient is aware the signal will be produced and are prepared, the rating is a #6—Loud, But Okay.

In our previous example, we discussed how you would use an audiometer to conduct aided loudness testing in your audiometric test booth. This setting is efficient for producing the different signals at desired levels in a controlled setting, but it is not very practical. It's possible that the results of this testing will indicate that programming changes must be made, and this needs to be done efficiently. What works best, therefore, is to conduct this testing at the fitting site, with the patient's hearing aids attached to the programming cables, so that immediate changes and retesting can be conducted.

TIPS AND TRICKS: Unilateral or Bilateral Loudness Testing?

In a perfect world, we would first do aided behavioral loudness testing for each ear individually, make gain and output changes if necessary, and then conduct the testing again with the patient aided bilaterally. In this way we could first correct for any measurement errors, and address issues related to the patient being different than average for monaural summation, and preferred gain. The impact of binaural summation could then subsequently be assessed. While this approach is ideal, it does require more time, and therefore unilateral loudness testing is usually skipped, and only aided bilateral measures are conducted. This does have some face validity, as we assume the patient will most commonly be using both hearing aids. The downside is that if there is a problem, how do you know if it's being caused by the right hearing aid, the left hearing aid, or both? The patient can sometimes help with this, but not always.

CLINICAL CONCEPT: Open Fittings and Loudness Measures

We are reminded of an interesting case regarding aided loudness judgments for a patient fitted with open earmolds. The student clinician was dutifully conducting aided LDL testing using the Cox Contour Anchors (she had not conducted REAR-85 measures when she conducted the probe microphone prescriptive verification—more on that in a moment). When the 85 dB SPL "obnoxious noise" signal was presented, the patient indicated it was a #7 on the loudness chart (Uncomfortably Loud), meaning that an MPO programming change was warranted. We noticed a peak around 2000 to 3000 Hz. The student appropriately reduced the MPO (using multichannel AGCo kneepoints) for the peak frequency of the stimulus by 5 dB (this is why knowing the location of the peaks of different noise stimuli is important), and repeated the testing. The rating was still a #7. Another 5-dB reduction took the AGCo kneepoints to their lowest level. Again, a #7 rating from the patient. At this point, the fitting screen showed that the kneepoint was lower than the input signal, yet the patient's loudness perceptions were not changing? What's going on? This prompted a move back to the probe microphone equipment, to see what was happening regarding ear canal SPL. While the fitting screen was showing a lowering of the AGO kneepoints, maybe this wasn't really happening? The REAR-85 for this noise signal showed a peak around 103 dB SPL, which indeed exceeded this patient's lower-than-average LDL for this frequency. But the AGCo setting should have kept the output around 95 dB SPL. It was then that we had an "aha!" moment. We turned the hearing aid off and conducted another REAR-85. Exactly the same as the previous one with the hearing aid turned on. So what we were seeing was the patient's REUG (which was larger than average) added to the input signal. Lesson learned: When conducting behavioral loudness testing, don't forget about the signal going through the open ear canal.

This means that the patient must be sitting in the fitting area, not the test booth, and a different sound source must be used. The best source for this of course is your probe microphone equipment. Not only does it produce the desired signals, but the monitor microphone of the system can then be used to calibrate each signal at the ear to the desired presentation level. Some probe microphone systems also have environmental sounds that can be used, or if PC-based, allow for different wave files to be added. Figure 6–9 shows a pull-down menu of the

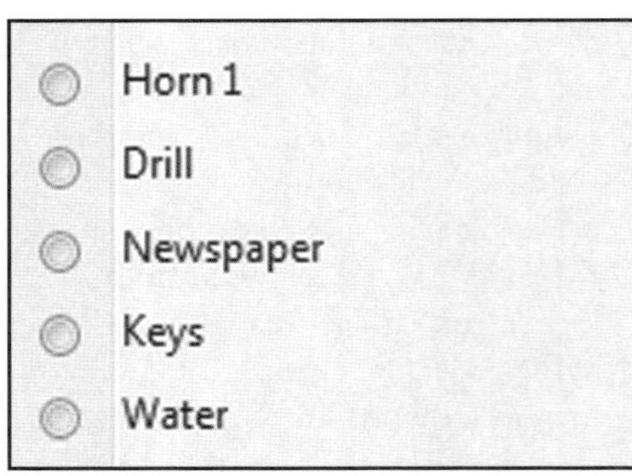

Figure 6–9. Example of the sound files available on a manufacturer's fitting software for use in the loudness judgment testing.

different sounds that are available, and this is only a partial listing.

Verification of MPO

We have discussed the aided verification procedures for assessing loudness perceptions for soft, average, and loud inputs. This is usually accomplished using speech or speech-like materials. For some patients, however, the primary interest simply is to ensure that loud sounds are not uncomfortably loud. For this testing, we suggest the use of loud obnoxious noises. By obnoxious noises, we mean everyday sounds such as door slam, toilet flushing, baby crying, dog yapping, dishes clattering, and so forth. There are two reasons for using these types of signals. First, some of the noises are composed of relatively narrow bands—this will drive the hearing aid to a higher MPO than a broadband signal such as speech. Secondly, the quality of the signal can impact the LDL; LDLs tend to be lower for noises that are not pleasant to listen to. In the clinic, on the day of the fitting and verification, we typically want to create a "worst case scenario" so that the patient has no unpleasant surprises when he starts using the hearing aids in his everyday environment.

The following is a step-by-step procedure for conducting this testing using your probe microphone equipment.

Step 1. Place the patient 1 m from the speaker while wearing the hearing aids (fitted bilaterally) with the gain adjusted a little higher than their "average use level"—we want to account for the possibility that the patient will tend to use slightly more gain as he or she becomes accustomed to the amplification.

Step 2. Provide the patient with the Cox Loudness Anchors, and read the patient the instructions. We typically emphasize the fact that the signals will be loud and annoying, but that he or she should decide when they are "okay" or if they indeed are "uncomfortable."

Step 3. One by one, present several obnoxious noises to the patient at a level of 80-85 dB SPL, and have them rate the loudness level on the Cox scale. Patients should rate the noise to be a #6 on the chart. If the patient rates a given noise as #7, (and this is verified on retest), the output (AGCo kneepoint) of the hearing aids (or at least one hearing aid) needs to be adjusted downward. If the peak of the noise signal is known, adjust only the AGCo for this frequency region (Note: You easily can conduct simultaneous REARs, which will show you the peak of the noise in the ear canal).

Step 4. Following the AGCo adjustment, repeat testing until a consistent #6 rating is obtained. If this cannot be obtained using the AGCo setting, it might be necessary to make the compression ratio larger for the WDRC—this is termed "gain for loud sounds" in most fitting software.

A few caveats:

- As discussed in the associated Clinical Concept for open fittings, when a #7 rating persists after lowering the MPO, it is important to ensure that the *unaided signal* is not uncomfortably loud—simply conduct testing with the hearing aid turned off to check for this.
- While we are normally concerned that loud sounds are too loud, you might also consider changing the programming for the patient who has a #5 rating for the 85 dB SPL input signals that should be perceived as #6.

While "loud sounds too soft" does not seem to lead to the same rate of hearing aid rejection as "loud sounds too loud," there is little reason not to use all of the patient's residual dynamic range. In our experience, when the patient has the lower-than-average ratings, it is usually because of an overly aggressive WDRC setting, and unrelated to the AGCo. A few mouse clicks and probe measures will quickly tell you if it is the input or output compression that is controlling the MPO.

After the Hearing Aid Fitting

We are now to the point of discussing what to do after the patient has been fitted with his or her new hearing aids and has left our clinic or office. There will likely be follow-up counseling required, and maybe a little troubleshooting for some problems that were discovered during real-world use—we talk about those in Bentler et al. (2016). In this section, however, we are going to focus on self-report validation measures. Recall that earlier in this chapter we encouraged the use of some type of formal questionnaire to be completed by the patients that relates to their hearing difficulty and communication needs. Many of these same pre-fitting tools are used as outcome measures in the validation stage. The results of these outcome measures are useful in and of themselves, and when compared to pre-fitting test results, they allow us to determine the benefit afforded by the intervention.

An outcome measure allows us to quantify the impact of the management or treatment scheme. They can be useful for answering the following important clinical questions:

- How did the intervention impact the individual?
- Did the management improve the communication abilities of the individual?
- Did our intervention improve the person's overall lifestyle?
- And most important clinically, did we meet our intervention goals that were identified during the hearing needs assessment?

You might ask why do we really need self-report measures of real-world outcomes? Why not just stick with probe microphone measures and speech perception scores as indicators of success? We can think of at least four reasons why self-report outcomes are a good idea:

- First, for largely economic reasons, health care is becoming more consumer-driven. In this evolving system, the consumer decides what treatment is selected and when it is complete. The major index of quality of service is self-reported outcome and satisfaction. Consumer-driven health care places an added emphasis on the patient's point of view. Therefore, it is critical to measure the real-world benefit and satisfaction of hearing aid use. Because today's patients are, on average, more savvy and better informed than our grandparents, they want to know how much benefit they are receiving in everyday listening situations. Using a self-report of hearing aid outcome allows us to measure and report to patients how they are doing compared to an average.
- Second, self-report measures of outcome are gaining importance, due in part to the fact that many real-world experiences simply cannot be measured effectively in laboratory conditions. The traditional hearing aid outcome measures (e.g., speech recognition in

quiet and in noise) do not capture the true experiences of hearing aid use in everyday listening situations. Consider hearing aids with automatic and adaptive beamforming and directional technology. The effectiveness of features such as these depends heavily on the lifestyle and listening environments of the individual patient. In order to quantify the true impact of hearing loss and its associated treatment on activity limitations, lifestyles, and so on, self-report measures need to be used.

- Third, even when laboratory conditions are used to simulate real-world listening situations, they do not always resemble the patient's impression of the actual real-life situation. Assessing speech perception in noise with a defensible signal-to-noise ratio is rarely perceived by patients as bearing any resemblance to their own experiences. Self-report outcome measures give us a scientifically defensible way to measure the real-life success of the hearing aid fitting.
- Finally, if you choose not to use outcome measures, it is likely that your patients will find other ways to report their satisfaction, or lack of satisfaction. There are several Internet sites devoted to rating doctors and other health care providers, and we suspect that these will become even more commonly used in upcoming years. Increasingly, hospitals and clinics are sending out provider satisfaction surveys following a clinic visit. Figure 6–10 shows an example of an audiologist's rating from

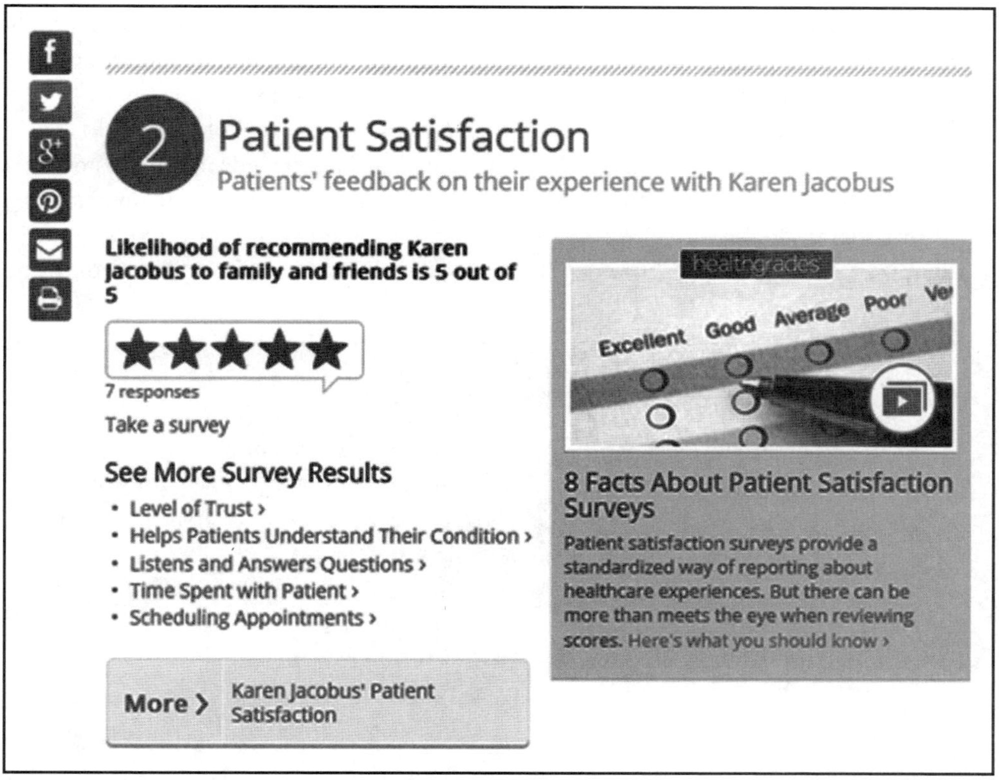

Figure 6–10. Sample rating of patient satisfaction for audiologist from the website http://www.healthgrades.com. Although not a direct measure of satisfaction with amplification, it is unlikely that dissatisfied hearing aid users will recommend a given audiologist to their family and friends.

the website http://www.healthgrades.com, showing the rating for "likelihood to recommend this audiologist to family and friends." Many prospective patients will likely view these ratings before making an appointment—just like your patients now use TripAdvisor or Yelp to decide where to have dinner. It makes good sense, therefore, to obtain these ratings yourself so that, if there are problems, you can take care of them before they are made public on the Internet.

To get started, we'll first list a few areas where self-assessment tests might be helpful for the overall process of fitting hearing aids. Here are some practical reasons for using standardized scales as part of the fitting and validation process:

- Assist in determining the success of the hearing aid fitting by comparing the patient's score to normative data. Example: A patient has a very mild hearing loss; normal hearing through 2000 Hz, dropping down to a 40-dB loss in the 3000 to 6000 Hz range. His unaided scores showed significant handicap and considerable communication problems. Following the fitting of new hearing aids and a reasonable adjustment period, the patient's aided scores suggest fewer communication problems. In fact, the patient's aided scores reveal that he is performing at the 40th percentile of people with normal hearing.
- Assist in determining if pre-fitting goals are met or if additional intervention is needed. Example: The patient identified "easier to understand my daughter on the phone" as a pre-fitting goal. After three weeks of wearing the hearing aids, the patient indicates continued difficulty and no benefit in this area. Additional hearing assistive technologies including amplified telephones, wireless streaming, and speakerphone solutions are explored.
- Assist in determining if pre-fitting goals are met or if additional counseling is needed. Example: The patient established the goal of wearing his or her new hearing aids in more listening environments. Because the inventory can be used to monitor progress, it becomes apparent after three months of

CLINICAL CONCEPT: Domains of Outcomes

There are many dimensions, or domains, of outcomes for our consideration. We could argue that any of the following are appropriate outcomes to address clinically, so as you can see, we have a large and diverse collection of domains to choose from:

- Listening effort
- Use time
- Quality of life
- Naturalness of sound
- Sound quality (especially for music)
- Annoyance for loud environmental sounds
- Sound awareness (especially for soft environmental sounds)
- Social interaction
- Satisfaction with device
- Reduced burden for the significant other(s)
- Speech understanding

TIPS AND TRICKS: Other Uses for Outcome Measures (Beyond Individual Patient Management)

1. Comparison of different dispensing sites or personnel: If you are the manager of a clinic that has several different offices, you might want to compare the patient-reported outcomes as a form of quality control.
2. Comparison of different fitting procedures across groups of patients: If you always fit your hearing aids to the NAL-NL2 targets with careful verification and adjustment using probe microphone measures, and another audiologist defers to the manufacturers first-fit setting, will both groups of patients have the same benefit and satisfaction with hearing aids in the real world?
3. Comparison of circuitry across groups of patients: As new circuitry and features become available, it is important to know in your own setting whether "new means better," especially when the newer circuitry adds several hundred dollars to the cost of the hearing aids. If your patients were fitted with that feature, would they observe/report improved speech understanding in noise in their everyday use situations?
4. Counseling effectiveness across groups of patients: Does extra effort result in improved real-world satisfaction and benefit with hearing aids? That is, if you have changes in counseling techniques or time commitments, do the outcomes change for your patients load?
5. Documentation of service effectiveness: You know you do a good job, but do you have data to prove it? Are your patients more satisfied than the average person fitted with hearing aids? For example, how often do their IOI-HA scores exceed national norms? How often are their COSI goals obtained?
6. Research has shown that patients are significantly more satisfied with their hearing aids when they have been given a formalized outcome measure asking them if they are satisfied with their hearing aids. That's right, you can improve patient outcomes simply by measuring them!

use, the patient is not using the hearing aids as he or she had hoped. More counseling regarding the difficulties encountered, as well as ways to achieve more successful use of the hearing aids could be key to future success.

- Assist in determining need for post-fitting adjustment. The patient's post-fitting results revealed that he has a low tolerance for loud sounds with his new hearing aids (e.g., he judges sounds to be "uncomfortably loud" that most individuals wearing hearing aids consider "loud but okay"). This was not the case on the pre-fitting assessment. This information might suggest adjusting the hearing aid MPO settings again, but might also represent a newfound perception of loudness that will be only appreciated after a few weeks of adjustment, and maybe some extra counseling.

Most of the earlier outcome inventories were more general assessments of success, whereas current tools focus on specific domains of benefit or success and are typically developed to be used as open-ended (or user-specified) or closed-ended tools, or both. Open-ended self-report measures allow patients to nominate and target their own areas of expected improvement with amplification. The assumed advantage of an open-ended scale is that it can be tailored to the true communication needs of the individual patient. That is, if you and your patient work together carefully, the items selected will represent true, difficult listening situations for that patient, rather than arbitrary listening situations collected from average patients. One disadvantage with this type of inventory is that it is difficult to compare your patient's performance to a large pool of other hearing aid users because the specific listening situations they nominate might be quite unique.

Bentler et al. (2016) review in detail eight different self-assessment scales that easily can be used for real-world validation of the fitting. We have selected three of our favorites to discuss here. Because each inventory provides somewhat different information, each one is uniquely useful in specific situations. Here is a brief summary (with details to follow):

- Client Oriented Scale of Improvement (COSI): Measures early and final abilities for specific communication situations important to the patient; used as a pre-test to define goals and to plan management and quantify expectations, and as a post-test to assess the success of the management in meeting the patient's goals.
- Abbreviated Profile of Hearing Aid Benefit (APHAB): Provides "percent of problems" the patient has for three different listening conditions involving speech understanding (in quiet, in background noise, and in reverberation) and problems related to annoyance of environmental sounds (aversiveness scale). These values can be obtained as a pre-fitting or unaided measure, as an aided measure, or—by looking at the aided to unaided difference score—as a benefit measure.
- International Outcome Inventory for Hearing Aids (IOI-HA): Covers a minimal set of seven core outcome items that are sufficiently general to apply to many different types of investigations carried out in different countries in the world.

Client Oriented Scale of Improvement (COSI)

The COSI is one of the most frequently used self-assessment tools utilized in the pre-fitting stage of auditory habilitation, and is probably the most commonly used post-fitting outcome measure. In fact, as

> ***AUDIOID: Comfortable with Your COSI?***
>
> It has been suggested that the COSI outcome measure has become popular in part because of the positive warm feeling the name suggests—after all, who wouldn't want to be "cozy"? Of interest, however, is that the COSI was developed in Australia, and in Australia, "cossie" (or "cozzie") is a term sometimes used to refer to ones swimsuit—a shortened version of costume, as in "swimming costume." Let's take a look at your "COSI" might take on a somewhat different meaning!

a pre-test and post-test, this tool has both efficiency and specificity (to the individual)! One issue related to most all standardized self-assessment scales is that the items must be relevant for the hearing aid user. This is the main strength of the COSI.

The COSI concept was first introduced in an article by Harvey Dillon and colleagues in 1997. In short, the COSI allows patients to design their own questionnaire. This tool is an open-ended scale in which patients target listening situations for improvement with amplification. The goal of the COSI is for the patient to target up to five specific listening situations and to report the degree of benefit obtained compared to that expected for the population in similar listening situations. Many hearing aid manufacturers now include the COSI in their fitting software. Dillon, James, and Ginis (1997) recommend the COSI for routine clinical use for five reasons:

- It fits into a well-conducted clinical interview in a nonintrusive manner, by finding out what problems the patient is having, how much these problems are alleviated by the hearing aid fitting and counseling, and how well the patients are now doing in situations that are important to them.
- It is useful to the audiologist for formulating a treatment plan and determining whether additional action needs to be taken. Likewise, the patients view the measure as being relevant and as providing individual attention.
- The correlation between the COSI improvement measure and other longer scales assessing improvement with hearing aids is reasonable.
- The test–retest reliability is reasonable, especially when considering it is only three to five items.
- Clinicians rate the COSI method as useful and convenient for them to use.

As we mentioned, the clinician usually starts out with a blank sheet (see Appendix I)! The process begins by having the patient identify up to five specific listening situations in which he or she would like to hear better. Some patients will happily list six or seven; other patients struggle to come up with two or three. We suggest having at least three whenever possible. It is important to make each item as specific as possible. "Hearing in background noise" is not specific enough. After some questioning, this item might be narrowed to, "Hearing my friends while playing in the pool league in the Ryder bar." Once one situation is identified, you then move on and establish other situations. After all situations are identified, it is then helpful to go back and review and rank all situations. Simply place a "1" for most important, "2" for second most important, and so on in the box to the left of the item. Often, the item that the patient mentions first is something that just happened recently, but is not the most important.

We suggest that what we just described be conducted on the day of the fitting, or even on the day that the hearing aids are ordered. It's also possible to measure the patient's expectations for these nominated items, something we recommend, as it might lead to meaningful counseling if expectations are not realistic. In Figure 6–11, we show the five items selected by this patient, and to the left of each item is the importance rating given to that item. We have modified the original COSI form, so now the ratings that you see to the right of each item are the patient's *expected outcomes*, rather than actual degree of change. This form was completed on the day of the fitting.

Notice that understanding grandchildren, was the last item this patient thought of, yet after some thought and discussion with his wife, it was given #1 priority. Conversely, the first thing he mentioned was

NAL
CLIENT ORIENTED SCALE OF IMPROVEMENT

National Acoustic Laboratories
A division of Australian Hearing

Name : Kirby Mueller Category. New ____ Return ____
Audiologist : ____
Date : 1. Needs Established ____
2. Outcome Assessed ____

SPECIFIC NEEDS

Indicate Order of Significance

Specific Needs	Aided Expectations: Worse	No Difference	Slightly Better	Better	Much Better	CATEGORY	Final Ability (with hearing aid) Person can hear: Hardly Ever 10%	Occasionally 25%	Half the Time 50%	Most of Time 75%	Almost Always 95%
#5 Hearing friends while shooting pool in Ryder Bar.					✓						
#4 Understanding numbers called during Bingo.				✓							
#2 Understanding wife when she is in another room.				✓							
#3 Not have to turn the TV up so loud.				✓							
#1 Understanding soft voices of grandchildren when they visit.				✓							

Figure 6–11. The pre-fitting COSI for a patient. The patient selected five areas for improvement, rated them in priority, and then rated his expectations following the fitting of hearing aids.

understanding at his favorite watering hole (an event that had just happened the night before), yet this ultimately was given #5 priority, as upon reflection, he realized he only visits the Ryder bar a couple times a month—a very small percentage of his total communication needs. (Bingo, however, is every Friday night in the school gym!) Note that overall, his expectations are fairly high, maybe a little unrealistic. We tell him this, but assure him we will give it our best shot.

Regardless of whether expectations were initially assessed, when the patient returns for his or her post-fitting visit, the previously completed COSI form is then brought out for the patient's ratings. It is common that the patient doesn't remember all of the exact items he or she selected (and may have new items based on recent listening experiences). Mormer and Palmer (2001) report that after three weeks of hearing aid use, 96% nominated two items the same, but no patient who originally nominated four items, nominated the same four items on the return visit. Although this lack of consistency can slow down the process a little, because the COSI is such a flexible instrument, item selection can be dealt with quite easily. It is easy to cross out listening tasks that are no longer meaningful, add new ones, or simply have the patient rate only the situations that are consistently on the list.

Benefit on the COSI can be assessed in two different ways: Degree of Change (improvement provided by the hearing aids) and Final Hearing Ability with Hearing Aids (an absolute measure of communication ability). It is typical to see a similar pattern for these two different ratings, but sometimes a difference is noted. For example, a patient with a fairly severe hearing loss who works in a demanding listening situation might rate his Degree of Change as "Much Better," but have only a Final Hearing Ability of 50%. We suggest having the patient rate both categories because doing so may bring up key issues that need to be addressed.

Illustrative Case Study

Our pool-playing grandfather is back in our office after using his hearing aids for three weeks. The first thing he said when he walked in the door was "these things are great"—that's the news we want to hear, but we still move forward and sit down with him to complete the COSI. We don't show him the sheet he completed earlier regarding his expectations—we'll bring that out later. His completed COSI is shown in Figure 6–12.

The good news—he reports doing "much better" in three of the five categories. He notes some improvement with hearing his wife from a different room, but we are falling below his expectations for this category (see Figure 6–9). It may be that given his degree of hearing loss, and the difficulty of this listening situation, this might be as good as it gets. We already have soft sounds programmed to NAL-NL2 fitting targets, but we could try increasing them a few dB. Overall, we would consider this a successful fitting, and indeed we met or exceeded expectations for most of the nominated categories. Moreover, the use of the COSI in this manner facilitates post-fitting counseling.

The form for the COSI can be downloaded from: http://www.nal.gov.au/pdf/COSI-Questionnaire.pdf (also see Appendix I).

Abbreviated Profile of Hearing Aid Benefit (APHAB)

The APHAB was developed by Robyn Cox and her colleagues at the University of Memphis (Cox & Alexander, 1995; Appendix G). It is composed of 24 items that are scored

National Acoustic Laboratories
A division of Australian Hearing

NAL
CLIENT ORIENTED SCALE OF IMPROVEMENT

Name : Kirby Mueller — Category. New X / Return ___
Audiologist : ___
Date : 1. Needs Established ___
2. Outcome Assessed ___

SPECIFIC NEEDS

Indicate Order of Significance

Specific Needs	Degree of Change: Worse	No Difference	Slightly Better	Better	Much Better	CATEGORY	Final Ability (with hearing aid), Person can hear: Hardly Ever (10%)	Occasionally (25%)	Half the Time (50%)	Most of Time (75%)	Almost Always (95%)
#5 Hearing friends while shooting pool in Ryder Bar.			X						X		
#4 Understanding numbers called during Bingo.					X						X
#2 Understanding wife when she is in another room.			X					X			
#3 Not have to turn the TV up so loud.					X						X
#1 Understanding soft voices of grandchildren when they visit.					X					X	

Figure 6–12. The post-fitting COSI for a patient. Prior to the fitting, the patient selected five areas for improvement and rated them in priority. Shown here are the patient ratings of benefit obtained with the hearing aids for each communication situation.

AUDIOID: "Acronym Jim" Has Serious Competition

At the evening banquet, the last night of the Academy of Audiology meeting in April 1993, noted audiologist Chuck Berlin entertained us at the piano (a very common occurrence), and for one song, he sang along (a very uncommon occurrence). It was a song with special lyrics that he had written in honor of James Jerger for the 5th Anniversary of the Academy. The song was "Acronym Jim," sang to the tune of "It had to be you." Jerger of course is known for his acronyms for tests, so Chuck cleverly worked in many of these, such as SPAR, SISI, SPIN, SAL, SWAMI, RASP, and so on. While Jerger may have once been the king of acronyms, today we have a *queen*—Robyn Cox. A good acronym is something that sounds like a real word when you say it—the "ANL" for example, is not a good acronym for more than one reason. In this section, you're reading about the APHAB (pronounced "AYE-FAB), but that is just one of many of Robyn Cox's famous acronyms—nearly all of which are actual tests that you can administer. We can immediately think of the PHAP, IRIS, ECHO, SADL, VIOLA, DOSO, and SIR. There is also the CST—we could ask Robyn if we could buy a vowel, but for now, let's just go with the Spanish "*sieste*."

in four subscales (six questions each). The subscales are as follows:

- Ease of Communication (EC): The strain of communicating under relatively favorable conditions. *When I am in a small office, interviewing or answering questions, I have difficulty following the conversation.*
- Reverberation (RV): Communication in reverberant rooms such as classrooms. *It is hard for me to understand what is being said at lectures or in church services.*
- Background Noise (BN): Communication in settings with high background noise levels. *I have trouble understanding others when an air conditioner or fan is on.*
- Aversiveness (AV): The unpleasantness of environmental sounds. *The sound of a fire engine siren close by is so loud that I need to cover my ears.*

The APHAB can be administered as a paper-and-pencil test or by using a computer software version (e.g., the APHAB is included in the Questionnaire Module of the Noah software). The 24 items of the APHAB are scored on a 7-point scale—the scoring is the same whether the scale is used as a pre-fitting test or an outcome measure. Unaided and/or aided difficulty can be compared to published norms, which is a powerful counseling tool. Perhaps the most common use is in calculating benefit with amplification. To do this, we must first have the unaided baseline for comparison, which hopefully was obtained during the pre-fitting testing discussed earlier. For each subscale a "percent of problems" value is obtain from the answers to the six questions (0 to 100%), both unaided and aided. The benefit is then the reduction in percent of problems, when using hearing aids for each subscale.

Illustrative Case Study

When using the APHAB results for counseling, it is helpful to examine the scores for each one of the four subscales. Following are the results for a new hearing aid user, a 68-year-old golfing buddy of the patient we just met a few pages earlier. He also has a mild-to-moderate downward sloping hearing loss—dropping to 80 dB in the 3000 to 4000 Hz area. He does a lot of volunteer work at the local VA hospital, which involves considerable communication with others, sometimes in background noise. Here are his average *unaided* APHAB percent of problems for each subscale, (which we collected during the pre-fitting appointment):

- EC: 34%
- RV: 58%
- BN: 67%
- AV: 20%

Following three months of hearing aid use, the APHAB was administered again. Here are his current percent of problems for each subscale in the aided condition:

- EC: 14%
- RV: 19%
- BN: 35%
- AV: 53%

We can consider these scores by themselves or compare them to the unaided scores, which allows us to consider the benefit afforded by the new hearing aids. The most current 2010 norms can be found in Table 6–2 for global scores (the average of EC, RV, and BN), as well as for each of the four subtests independently.

We have actually four different ways to evaluate our patient's APHAB scores, so let's go through them one by one:

- We'll first look at his unaided findings, shown in Figure 6–13. The percentiles shown in this chart are takes from Table 6–2. It is apparent that he doesn't have many problems in quiet environments (EC subscale) or with aversive sounds (AV subscale). His real area of concern is background noise (BN subscale), where his problems are at the 50th percentile. Not an unexpected finding, given that his hearing loss is fairly "average" for someone obtaining hearing aids for the first time.
- Next we can examine his aided results, which are shown in Figure 6–14. Both ease of communication and problems in reverberation are in the 20th percentile, and background noise issues are also better. It appears he is having some problems with loud sounds, as his aversiveness scale ratings are higher than average. This is something we will look into—maybe we need to adjust the MPO.
- If we want to think in terms of benefit, we can subtract the unaided from the aided, and this is shown in Figure 6–15. We see his benefit for both reverberation and background noise is about average. As we would predict, there is little benefit for ease of communication, simply because he didn't start with many problems for this subscale.
- Finally, we can compare his aided results to people with normal hearing, and this is shown in Figure 6–16. These findings show that he compares very well, and even for background noise, he is doing better than 20% of people with normal hearing. This good news needs to be passed along to the patient.

Table 6–2. Normative Data for WDRC-Capable Hearing Aids with Current Technology and Fitting Practices Shown for Global Score (GS) and Each Subscale for the APHAB: Ease of Communication (EC), Reverberation (RV), Background Noise (BN), and Aversiveness (AV). Data Are Given for Each Response Mode: Unaided, Aided, and Benefit

	Subscale				
Percentile	*EC*	*RV*	*BN*	*AV*	*GS*
Unaided					
95	99	99	99	70	99
80	83	87	89	35	86
65	75	81	81	21	79
50	63	71	75	14	70
35	56	65	67	9	63
20	46	58	58	3	54
5	26	47	41	1	38
Aided					
95	86	79	82	82	82
80	39	57	58	64	51
65	29	46	49	53	41
50	23	37	40	38	33
35	17	29	32	23	16
20	12	21	22	14	18
5	5	12	14	2	10
Benefit					
95	76	70	56	16	67
80	52	52	47	0	50
65	46	41	39	–8	42
50	38	34	33	–13	35
35	29	27	23	–25	26
20	19	16	12	–41	16
5	10	–3	–1	–61	–5

Source: From Johnson, Cox, and Alexander, 2010.

You can obtain complete APHAB information, including forms and score sheets, at Robyn Cox's website: http://www.memphis.edu/csd/harl. The APHAB scoring software is also available. Some hearing aid manufacturers include the APHAB as part of their software, and the APHAB is part of the Questionnaire Module of Noah, a free add-on for registered Noah users, available for download at http://www.himsa.com.

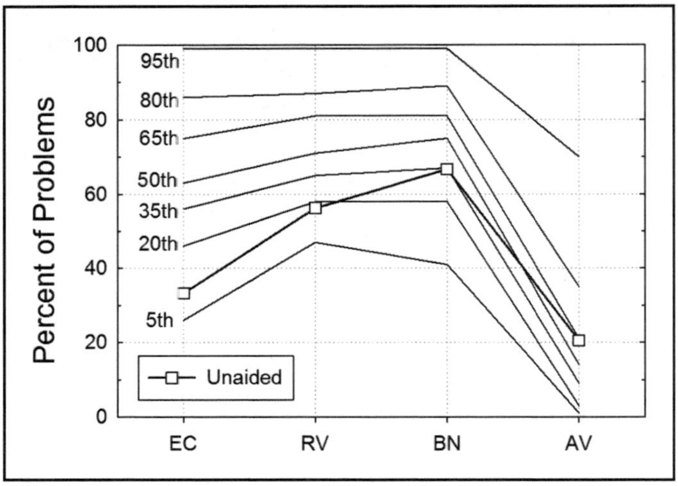

Figure 6–13. Comparison of patient's unaided APHAB scores to unaided norms as provided by Johnson, Cox, & Alexander, 2010.

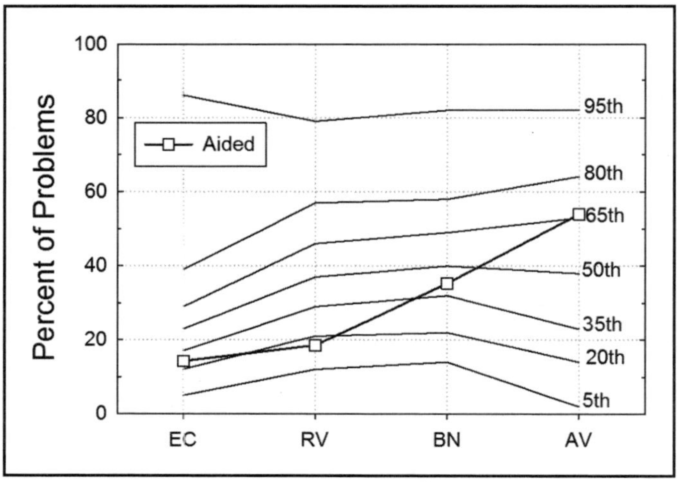

Figure 6–14. Comparison of patient's aided APHAB scores to aided norms as provided by Johnson et al., 2010.

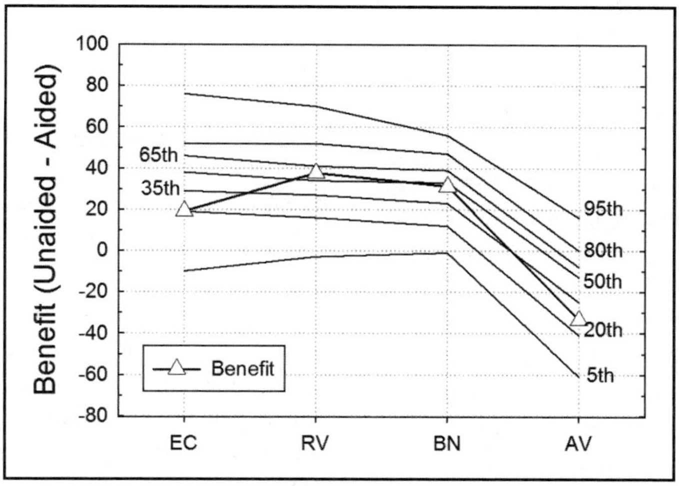

Figure 6–15. Comparison of this patient's benefit, as determined by the APHAB, to the benefit norms as provided by Johnson et al., 2010.

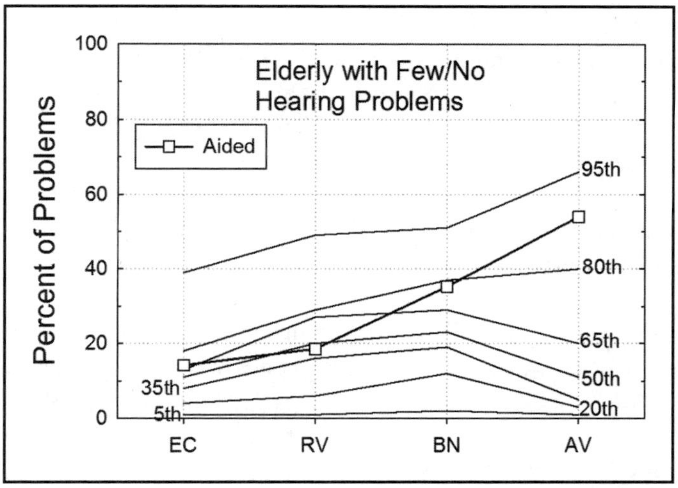

Figure 6–16. Comparison of patient's aided scores to the unaided norms for "Elderly with few/no hearing problems" from Cox, 1997. This information may be useful in counseling the patient.

The International Outcome Inventory for Hearing Aids (IOI-HA)

The IOI-HA is a short inventory used to quantify the effectiveness of hearing aid treatment (Cox & Alexander, 2002). This inventory is unique in that it addresses several domains related to hearing aid use, and is the outcome measure that is available in the greatest number of different languages, allowing for hearing aid outcome comparisons around the world (Appendix L).

It can be useful for clinical comparisons across groups based on differences in clinical setting, treatment option, or specific clinician. Alternatively, it can be used as a very quick way to evaluate patient outcomes to reinforce the positive impact of our clinical services.

While many self-assessment inventories have several questions related to only one domain, the IOI-HA consists of seven items that focus on different domains of hearing aid outcomes, but only one question/domain. The domains assessed are:

- Benefit from hearing aids
- Daily use
- Satisfaction with amplification
- Impact of using hearing aids on significant others
- Residual activity limitation
- Residual participation restriction
- Impact on quality of life

Each of the IOI-HA items has five answers that range from the worst outcome on the left to the best outcome on the right. Answer choices are equidistant in meaning in English. The inventory is meant to be given in paper-and-pencil form. It is very self-explanatory, and there are no formal instructions. To score the outcome, each answer is given a number value 1 (worst) through 5 (best). For this measure, a higher score is indicative of a better outcome. For example, item 4 asks, "Considering everything, do you think your present hearing aids are worth the trouble?" The choices are

- Not at all worth it (1 point)
- Slightly worth it (2 points)
- Moderately worth it (3 points)
- Quite a lot worth it (4 points)
- Very much worth it (5 points)

The norm templates for the IOI-HA are shown in Figures 6–17 and 6–18 (Appendix M) and also in Table 6–3. Referring to the norm templates, if a patient answered the preceding question as "slightly worth it," whether it fell within the norms depends on how much difficulty he or she perceived when not wearing his or her hearing aids. If the patient responded as having mild difficulty, then the response is within the norms, whereas a response of moderately-severe hearing difficulty indicates dissatisfaction. In general, if a patient reports a score of 3 or lower, it is indicative of a poor treatment outcome.

Depending on the personality of the patients, they might or might not let the clinician know when they are having issues with their hearing aids.. The IOI-HA is a quick way to get a general overview of how the patients feel about their hearing aid settings and how they are doing with them. For example, you might consider having every patient in your clinic fill out the IOI-HA each time they come into the office for follow-up visits while they are waiting for their appointments. By looking over the survey before seeing patients, you can focus your questions on their specific problem areas.

Take, for example, item #3, "Think again about the situation where you most wanted to hear better. When you use your present hearing aids, how much difficulty do you

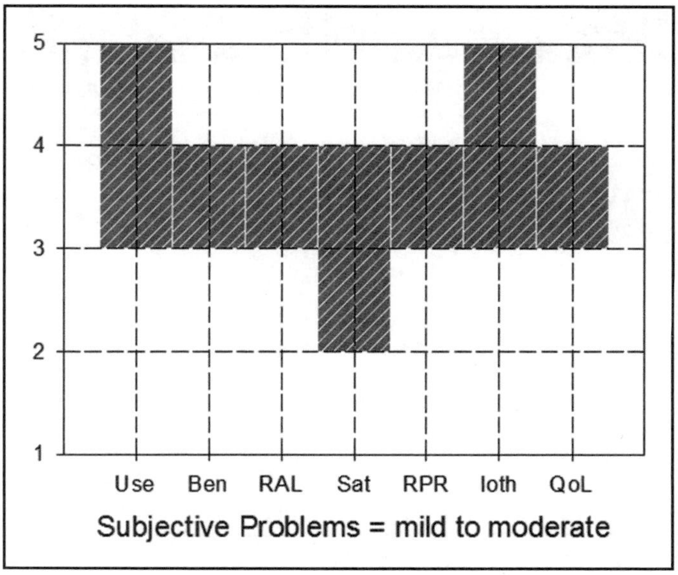

Figure 6–17. Normative data for the IOI-HA for persons with mild-to-moderate degrees of hearing loss. The shaded boxes indicate acceptable outcomes for each of the subscales.

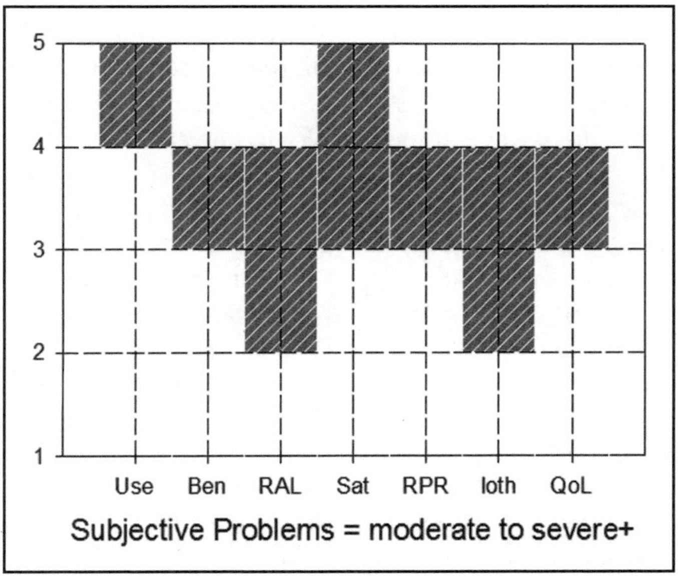

Figure 6–18. Normative data for the IOI-HA for persons with moderate-to-severe degrees of hearing loss. The shaded boxes indicate acceptable outcomes for each of the subscales.

Table 6–3. Normative Data for the IOI-HA Shown for Persons with Mild-To-Moderate Loss and Moderate-To-Severe Loss

	Mild to Moderate		***Moderate to Severe***	
Item	***Mean***	***SD***	***Mean***	***SD***
Daily Use	3.73	1.17	4.50	0.96
Benefit	3.39	0.98	3.52	1.08
Residual Activity Limitation	3.40	0.95	3.19	1.05
Satisfaction	3.20	1.21	3.84	1.17
Residual Participation Restriction	3.57	1.13	3.38	1.11
Impact on Others	3.79	1.13	3.38	1.10
Quality of Life	3.19	0.93	3.68	1.02

Source: From Cox, Alexander, and Beyer, 2003.

still have in that situation?" Patients often write out the reasons why they chose a certain answer in addition to answering the question. They might write, "I still have trouble hearing the TV," or "I cannot understand my grandchildren as well as I would like to." The survey can help clinicians go straight to their patients' issues and spend more time on counseling after adjusting the hearing aid settings. Remember the point we made earlier—simply giving your patients an outcome measure and asking about satisfaction improves satisfaction. This particular scale requires very little time to administer and score.

A PDF version of the scale in English and for all translations can be downloaded from the following source: Link to Questionnaire/Norms: http://www.memphis.edu/ausp/harl/downloads/IOIfiles/EnglishNormsVersion.pdf

In Closing

While the focus of this book is the use of speech mapping and probe microphone measures, we do want to emphasize that this testing is simply part of the overall process of selecting and fitting hearing aids. Real-ear verification of gain and output is critical, but so too is the assessment of the patient's needs, evaluation of his or her hearing handicap, and the use of outcome measures to facilitate post-fitting counseling. In this chapter we have given you a brief overview of how some of these other tests and procedures can be used in conjunction with the real-ear measures. You can find many of the sample forms in the Appendix section. For details regarding the implementation of a complete fitting protocol, see Mueller et al. (2014) and Bentler et al. (2016).

7 Frequently Asked Questions

It's not that I'm so smart; I just stay with the questions much longer.

—Albert Einstein

Asking questions is an important part of life, and certainly a big part of understanding hearing aid fittings. Probe microphone measures seem to generate more questions than most other aspects of the fitting process, probably because of the unique equipment, the use of different terminology, and the overall concept of determining what is the best ear canal SPL for each patient. Some questions have easy answers—"yes, it's good to have the tip of the probe tube close to the eardrum." But as Einstein says, some questions you have to stay with much longer—"Do you use a measured or average REUG for REIG calculation?" We've conducted several hearing aid fitting workshops over the years, and always end with a question and answer period. We have saved many of the questions raised by the attendees, some we hear year after year, and we will do our best to answer them in this chapter.

Equipment Setup and Procedures

Is it necessary to calibrate the room? I have seen that feature on some probe systems.

This feature is available to assure that you do not have reflective surfaces in the test area that could be altering how the test signal is calibrated. Most office/clinic areas are okay, so if you're not doing room calibration measure, you're probably not making serious mistakes. But, it only takes a few seconds to conduct this measure, so if you have that feature available, we'd suggest you go ahead and use it. It is probably not necessary to repeatedly perform this measure, unless you frequency change your environment.

Does the equipment have to be in the middle of a room, or can it be placed against a wall?

This relates to our previous question. For convenience, most of us do have the equipment along a wall, or reasonably close to a wall. The issue of concern relates more to reflections from side walls, which should not be close to the patient. Again, some equipment offers a "room calibration" feature to address this issue.

If I'm using concurrent equalization, is it then okay for the patient to move their head during testing?

Yes and no—depends on what you mean by "move." The concurrent equalization will account for head movements of a few degrees, but no, the patient still cannot turn their head 45 degrees to watch the monitor while you're doing the test run! As we showed back in Chapter 3 (Figure 3–16), even small head turns can make a significant difference in the measured output. We use the very same stern "do not move your head while the sound is on" statement regardless if we are doing concurrent or stored equalization. This also somewhat depends on the specific equipment you use. At least one device performs frequency specific concurrent equalization. In such systems, some changes in frequency response shape due to head turn can be accounted for. Other systems only adjust the total signal level during concurrent equalization and, therefore, will be more negatively affected by moderate changes in head angle.

If I forget to do stored equalization for an open fitting, will it really make much difference in the results?

The magnitude of the "mistake" that you will make is related to many factors (see Chapter 5). What will probably have the greatest influence is the amount of gain that you have programmed for the higher frequencies. The exact value where leakage will have an effect will depend on the patient's ear canal resonance and the openness of the eartip, but in general, once the gain is at 15 to 18 dB, you will have enough leakage to the regulating microphone to alter the measurement. It's fairly unusual to have an open fitting, and not have at least 15 dB of gain in the high frequencies, so yes, there will probably always be a mistake. Now, if there isn't much gain, the mistake might only be a few dB. But if you have 25 to 30 dB of gain, the mistake could be 15 to 20 dB.

What is the best input signal to use?

Well, it depends on what you are assessing. The best for matching targets isn't the best for assessing the magnitude of the noise reduction algorithm, which isn't the best for assessing MPO. But assuming you're talking about matching prescriptive targets, the "best" is the one that has been synchronized with the targets that appear on the screen. Different input signals have slightly different spectrums, and the target must change accordingly. This might vary somewhat among manufacturers, but the ISTS would be our choice for target verification. We would minimally suggest the signal has the spectral and temporal properties of speech or it is made up of speech or speech segments, (which takes us back to our original recommendation of the ISTS).

When do you use ICRA signals?

We don't—in part because many modern hearing aids would classify them as noise. We describe these signals in Chapter 3, and there may be some uses for them for research purposes. As we said earlier, for clinical prescriptive verification, we prefer the ISTS. It is shaped to mimic the ILTASS, the spectrum used in the development of the NAL prescription, and is very similar to the LTASS used with the DSL.

I've recently started using the ISTS. I've noticed, however, that when I run an REUR, the values on the screen are not very close to what I have selected. For example, when I select 65 dB SPL, the measured values are way below 65 dB SPL. Why is this?

Ha! Like many of us, you probably became used to using (and seeing displayed) signals that were equalized—65 dB input was 65 dB on the screen. This was okay for insertion gain measurements, but this is not what we want when we use the REAR for verification. We want a signal that represents average speech, referred to as the LTASS. Now, when you select 65 dB SPL, you will have a speech signal with an *overall rms* of 65 dB—but the frequency specific values are considerably less. This might be more information than you'd like, but we have included a table (Table 7–1) that gives you some specific numbers for the LTASS for speech of different loudness levels.

Table 7–1. Mean Sound Pressure Levels in One-Third-Octave Bands for Speech at Five Vocal Efforts by Three Groups of Talkers

Frequency (kHz)	*.125*	*.160*	*.200*	*.250*	*.315*	*.400*	*.500*	*.630*	*.800*	*1.0*	*1.25*	*1.6*	*2.0*	*2.5*	*3.15*	*4.0*	*5.0*	*6.3*	*8.0*
Females																			
Casual	26	36	47	44	39	45	45	44	39	36	36	36	35	31	30	30	30	32	33
Normal	26	37	48	47	42	49	50	48	46	42	43	42	38	36	38	40	36	36	34
Raised	25	35	48	53	49	53	57	55	54	52	53	52	47	45	45	45	42	40	39
Loud	20	34	45	55	55	55	59	62	62	61	62	62	57	54	53	53	49	47	45
Shouted	20	30	40	50	55	61	64	68	70	72	74	74	70	67	67	64	60	57	55
Males																			
Casual	44	42	46	46	44	47	48	45	38	37	39	39	35	33	33	35	34	33	32
Normal	48	43	48	52	51	53	54	52	46	45	47	44	40	41	41	38	34	35	32
Raised	51	49	51	56	55	58	60	58	54	53	54	51	47	47	46	44	40	41	38
Loud	50	55	57	60	62	65	68	69	66	65	67	64	59	59	57	55	49	48	46
Shouted	42	42	57	66	68	69	74	78	78	78	80	78	73	72	70	68	62	61	59
Children																			
Casual	23	25	42	47	39	43	49	48	43	39	37	38	38	33	33	33	33	33	33
Normal	24	29	42	51	47	47	53	52	49	44	43	43	41	38	39	40	38	36	37
Raised	25	30	41	51	54	53	55	58	57	54	54	54	50	46	47	48	45	43	43
Loud	24	29	41	51	54	58	60	60	63	61	62	63	60	54	54	54	52	49	48
Shouted	24	45	43	49	53	61	66	66	67	72	72	72	71	65	66	66	63	57	54

Source: Tabular data from Pearsons, Bennett, and Fidell, 1977.

Does it really matter if the patient sits at a 0 or 45-degree azimuth to the loudspeaker?

You could probably do equally accurate testing using either azimuth, but there are some practical reasons why you want to use 0 degree. First, since you are mostly doing bilateral fittings, the patient now doesn't have to move (or the loudspeaker doesn't have to move), when you go from ear to ear —you can simply work behind the patient. Secondly, it is becoming more common to conduct simultaneous right and left measures. This requires the signal to be calibrated by two different regulating microphones, one on each side of the head, and this is only going to work effectively if the signal is coming from a 0-degree azimuth.

I've heard that it's okay if your loudspeaker is too low or too high, as the system will calibrate for any location?

To some extent, yes it will, but we have seen some strange results when the loudspeaker wasn't positioned at a 0-degree vertical azimuth, especially when it's placed too low. Given the minimal effort to arrange things so that a 0-degree vertical azimuth is always used (a patient chair that can be raised and lowered is helpful), we recommend always using this azimuth.

What are the pros and cons of doing unilateral versus bilateral measures?

The only "con" we can think of for using bilateral, is that if the patient cannot sit still, it would be difficult to keep both sides within calibration; these systems use a simultaneous calibration approach. The advantage of bilateral is that it could save you some time. The downside is that you will have to continually switch your thinking between the right and left ear—remember which ear needs gain tuned up or down at what frequency. Let's assume it's going to take you four runs to get things set correctly for each of the three input levels. What you can do then, in-between runs, is to alter programming as needed for both the left and right ear (even in symmetrical losses, it's unlikely that you would be making the same programming changes for each ear). Then do your next bilateral run. Let's say each run takes about 30 seconds (10 to 15 seconds of signal, another 15 for fiddling), the bilateral approach would maybe save you 6 minutes (4 runs x 30 seconds x 3 input levels = 360 seconds/60 = 6 minutes). Of course, you might lose some time switching back and forth during programming, and there are some of us who might lose even more time by programming the wrong ear because we can't think about two ears at the same time!

Probe Tube Use and Placement

Are there any tricks to getting the probe placed at the correct depth?

We talk about four different methods for doing this in Chapter 3, but the most common method involves no tricks, just a little bit of math. If we consider the length of the average adult ear canal, and the distance of the intertragal notch of the pinna from the opening of the ear canal, our calculations suggest this distance should be around 35 mm. We want the tip of our probe tube to be about 5 mm from the TM, so if we put the probe-tube marker 30 mm from the end, and place this marker at the intertragal notch, all should be well. If you want to be a little conservative, or you have a hunch the person has a shorter-than-average ear canal length, use 28 mm. For children, different rules apply. See Chapter 3.

I have heard about using a "notch" approach for getting the right placement of the probe tube. How does that work?

Well, assuming your equipment has a good frequency resolution of the signal, you will likely observe a negative anti-resonance notch in the REUR when the probe tip reaches a certain distance from the TM— as you move the probe toward the TM the notch will move to a higher frequency, or disappear. As you move the tip of the probe tube away from the TM the notch will likely get bigger and occur at a lower frequency. The goal is to have the probe tip deep enough that the notch has moved above 6000 Hz (or no longer visible) and no longer has an effect on the measured REUG. When the notch is gone, or where you want it, adjust your sleeve marker accordingly. Shown in Figure 7–1 are three different outputs. The probe tip was first placed around 5 mm of the TM, and then moved back in 3-mm steps. Observe, that there is no high frequency notch in the top curve (correct placement). As the tube was pulled away from the TM, we first see a notch appear, and then become larger and at a lower frequency for the farthest distance. Note that we also are losing high frequencies when the placement isn't correct.

I tend to have a problem with the probe tube being springy and popping out of the ear. Solution?

There are a few solutions that might work. Some manufacturers have a device for holding the probe tube, this usually keeps it more rigid and "pointed" in the right direction. You might be able to slide the probe tube behind the cord that is holding the regulating microphone, which will generally hold it in place. Or, putting a little gel on tube (staying away from the very end, of course) will help it adhere to the canal.

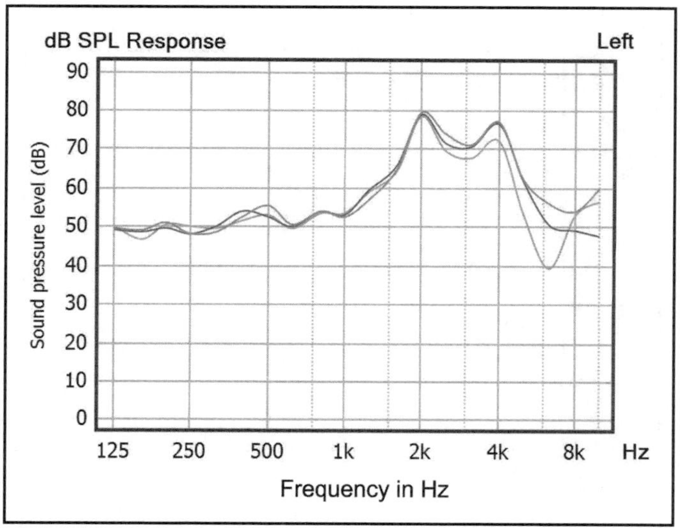

Figure 7–1. Illustration of using the notch in the response to determine a correct probe-tube placement. The upper curve is a deep placement, about 5 mm from the TM. The lower curves were the result of pulling the tube back 3 mm, and then another 3 mm.

One other method some clinicians like is to use hypoallergenic tape (e.g., toupee tape) to help hold the tube in place by either taping the tube to the intertragal notch or to the earmold itself (using very thin tape). See Figure 3–23 for an example of a probeholder on the probe assembly.

If I don't have the probe tube in deep enough, what is the likely mistake I will observe?

Let's assume you are doing REAR speech mapping. If the probe tube is too shallow, the main effect will be in the higher frequencies—it will appear that your output is less than it really is. If you are trying to match target, you will then program in more gain than appropriate for this frequency range. It would be easy to make a 5 dB mistake in the 3000 to 4000 Hz range, which would likely be noticeable for the patient. Now that we have hearing aids with significant gain in the 5 to 8 kHz region, and prescriptive targets for this extended frequency region, the chance of an overfit due to tube placement that is too shallow has only increased. If you are using REIG calculations, however, and you used a *measured* REUG, you might not make a mistake at all if you kept the probe depth the same for both the REUR and REAR measurements (see Chapter 5).

How do I know if the probe tube is plugged?

If the tube is truly plugged, you'll know, as the output displayed will be less than the input signal. What you will see looks something like that shown in Figure 7–2 (bottom curve). Note that the output falls well below the aided (average speech of 65 dB), consid-

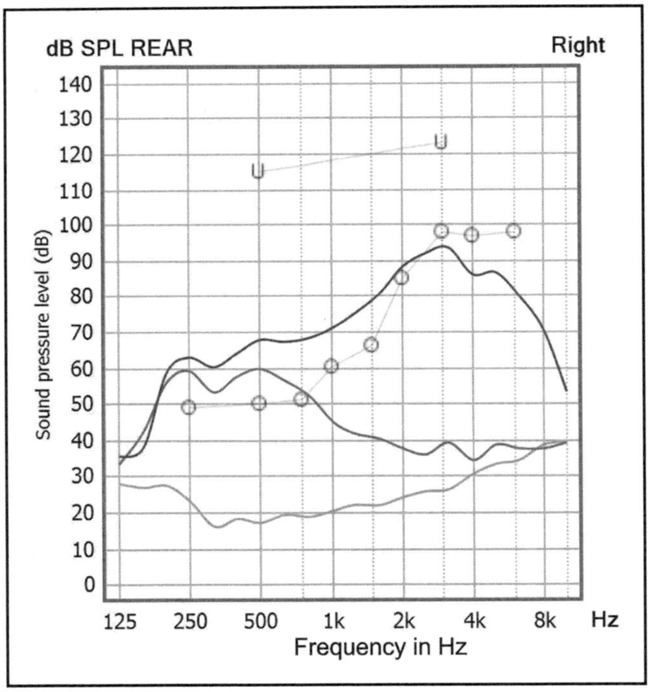

Figure 7–2. An example of the resulting plot if the probe tube is plugged (*lowest curve shown*). Note that the output from the measure is considerably below the threshold values, and significantly lower than the REOR (*middle curve*).

erably less output than if you simply forget to unmute the hearing aid (middle curve). Fortunately, the tube is usually either totally plugged or totally open—there isn't an in-between stage, which would be more difficult to detect. There are times, however, when things don't look quite right, and we wonder if this is the case. An easy way to check is to take the probe out of the ear, and place it next to the regulating microphone, as you would for calibration. Run a curve using an equalized signal, and you should see a flat line (output = input). If you do, the probe is okay. If you don't, grab a new tube, calibrate, and go at it again.

Do you always need a new tube when the tube is plugged?

A plugged tube usually is a throwaway situation, and if you are dealing with a patient with gooey cerumen, a persistent clinician can go through many tubes during a single test session. Cleaning the tubes does not work very well (you do not want moisture in the tube), but if your clinic is on a tight budget, there could be a solution. If your probe microphone system calibrates the probe tube as we talked about earlier (and most do), then you simply could snip off the tip that is plugged, recalibrate the tube, and continue to use it for testing. As we mentioned previously, this is not recommended by some probe microphone manufacturers, but it will likely work for one or two shortcuts.

Can one manufacturer's tubes be used with the equipment from a different manufacturer?

We would recommend using the tubes provided by the manufacturer of the equipment you are using, but in a pinch, this probably would work, if you were using equipment that requires calibration of the tube. If you do the calibration with the rogue tube, and you see a flat line on recheck (input = output), then you may be good-to-go. A potential problem with this approach, however, is that the probe tube may not seal tightly to the microphone. As we mentioned earlier, use of a nonstandard tube may also result in a warning that the tube is not within tolerances and may not be able to be used.

Should probe tubes be thrown away after each use?

Yes. Infection control is a concern in any office or clinic. We certainly hope that no one would use the same tube on different people, but we have heard of clinics that have a protocol that recommends taping the tube in the patient's chart for use on follow-up visits. Not good. This simply allows time for the growth of bacteria. The last time we checked, probe tubes were selling for less than $2.00 each. Because that they are normally used for testing hearing aids that sell for thousands of dollars, a $2.00 investment for infection control does not seem like an unreasonable expenditure.

What about probe tube placement when there is cerumen in the ear?

Well, the first choice of course would be to remove the cerumen, but we recognize that that is not always possible. If it is gooey, you are in for a battle. You may have to hope that your manufacturer's software will get you close, and then do your probe microphone measures on a repeat visit. We usually give it two or three tries before we give up. If it is hardened cerumen, however, your otoscopic exam will usually reveal a good path to get by it. Often, the cerumen ledge is about midway down the canal, and once you get by, the ear canal is clean. Does this cerumen in the canal change your findings? Not by much, and certainly not to the degree that you would skip verification. A little error due to cerumen is likely much less than using a manufacturer first fit!

Is it okay to place the probe tube through the hearing aid vent?

It sure is tempting to put it there, isn't it? If your tube is small and your vent is big, it's okay. Remember, however, that one thing that is being measured when we conduct probe microphone testing is the acoustic effects of venting. If the probe tube fills all or most of the vent, the resulting measurement will not represent true gain (the greatest mistake will be in the low frequencies). On the other hand, if the vent is larger than 2 mm, and you're using one of today's thin probe tubes, placing the probe tube through the vent will not influence the test results significantly.

For patients, such as children, who are followed every three months or so, is it worth ordering a probe tube vent for their earmold?

Your earmold manufacturer can place a vent in the earmold for the purpose of conducting RECD and other important probe microphone measures (since probe tubes come in different diameters, it might be good to send a sample tube of what you use along with the ear impression). When you do the testing, the probe tube is threaded through this vent (it is usually difficult to do—you will need to use a good lubricant) and can be held in place with Fun-Tak during testing. This procedure helps ensure that that the tip of the probe tube extends beyond the tip of the earmold. A second advantage is that you have only one thing to hold on to when you place the earmold in the ear. When testing is completed, the vent is plugged. Is it worth the time and effort? We know people who frequently test children who do not use this approach, and rather use a very thin tape to keep the probe in place on the inferior portion of the earmold when using it to measure individual RECD. If you are fairly new to pediatric evaluations, it might add some comfort to the test procedure knowing that you have a good placement of the probe-tube tip, if you can manage to get it through the vent!

For a tight fitting, is it common that the probe tube gets squashed and gives unreliable results?

We have heard that this happens, but we wonder if maybe it is that the clinician just didn't have the tip of the tube past the end of the hearing aid. Or, it was deep and then curled in the canal. In general, this should not be a problem. Consider that back in the 1990s, there were two studies that compared REIG to functional gain for deep, tightly fitted CICs (Mueller & Ebinger, 1997; Seewald et al., 1997). This is the type of fitting where you might expect some "squash effect" to occur, and if it did occur, you would expect it to show up in the higher frequencies. In both of these studies, mean REIG was equal to mean functional gain at 4000 Hz.

Verification of Prescriptive Targets

For my adult patients, does it matter if I select NAL-NL2 or DSL 5.0? Is there much of a difference?

There are small differences, and the differences change for different audiometric configurations. We have an example of some comparative findings in Chapter 2. You will see that for most audiometric configurations, for most frequencies, for a 65-dB input the prescribed differences are less than 5 dB. Our guess is that if you programmed memory 1 to the NAL-NL2, memory 2 to the DSL 5.0, and had your patients switch back and forth, they would not hear much difference between the two. Something you might want to try out just for fun! Importantly, for children, the differences are larger.

The rep from my favorite company told me that with their new product, there is no need to conduct real-ear measures, as there are no fitting targets, and the processing is "dynamic." He said that if I must do probe-mic, I should just look at their on-screen simulation for guidance? Does this seem reasonable?

No. First, we don't quite understand why there wouldn't be targets. The desired ear canal SPL is not based on how the sound gets there—it could be via a new fancy circuit, or from an oxen horn—the targets are still the same! It sounds to us like someone doesn't want you to see what the output really looks like. And, there are considerable data to show that what is on the fitting screen is not accurate, so no, we certainly would not recommend using that as a guideline.

For open fittings, how do I separate the acoustic effects of the hearing aid path versus the open-ear path?

Usually you don't, but true, you often are looking at both when you view the REAR. Depending on the openness of the fitting, the crossing point is often around 1200 to 1500 Hz, and there might be a little summation and cancelation in this range, but this shouldn't have much effect. These effects often occur as narrow notches and peaks that are smoothed out by the 1/3th or 1/12th-octave analysis of the probe microphone system. This is okay though, because the human auditory system is not very sensitive to narrow notches and peaks. What you could do to see the more general effect, using the standard ISTS input, is first conduct an REAR with the hearing aid muted, which actually would be an REOR. This would give you a good idea of what part of the REAR might be from the open-ear path.

Why is it that sometimes the fittings targets in the high frequencies are below the patient's thresholds? This has to be some calculation mistake, right?

Well, at first glance it might look like a mistake, but we're quite certain that after 30 to 40 years of research with thousands of people, the developers of the DSL 5.0 and the NAL-NL2 know what they are doing. You indeed will see this for both the NAL and DSL, particularly for steeply downward-sloping audiometric configurations. Figure 7–3 shows targets for an average input for both the NAL and the DSL, and note that for both procedures, the fitting target falls below the patient's thresholds for 3000 Hz and above. This is addressed by Mueller (2017) and we explain it in a couple of our chapters, but here are the main points to consider:

- Don't just look at the LTASS, look at the full-amplified spectrum, or speech banana. It might be that the peaks are above threshold. Remember, the peaks are about 15 dB higher than the LTASS line.
- Prescriptive methods were designed to deliver the "correct" amount of loudness. Boosting the loudness in these high frequencies will likely necessitate reducing gain elsewhere, where audibility has a greater impact on intelligibility—it's a compromise—use your dB allotment carefully. For most hearing losses, we would not want to sacrifice audibility at 2000 Hz for audibility at 4000 Hz.
- There is this thing called "effective audibility." More gain for this region might not mean increased speech understanding.
- The amplified signal must have acceptable sound quality. Increasing gain in this region might have a negative impact.

So while it might be tempting to boost gain in these cases, we're going to hang our hat on the research that developed the targets, and stick with them.

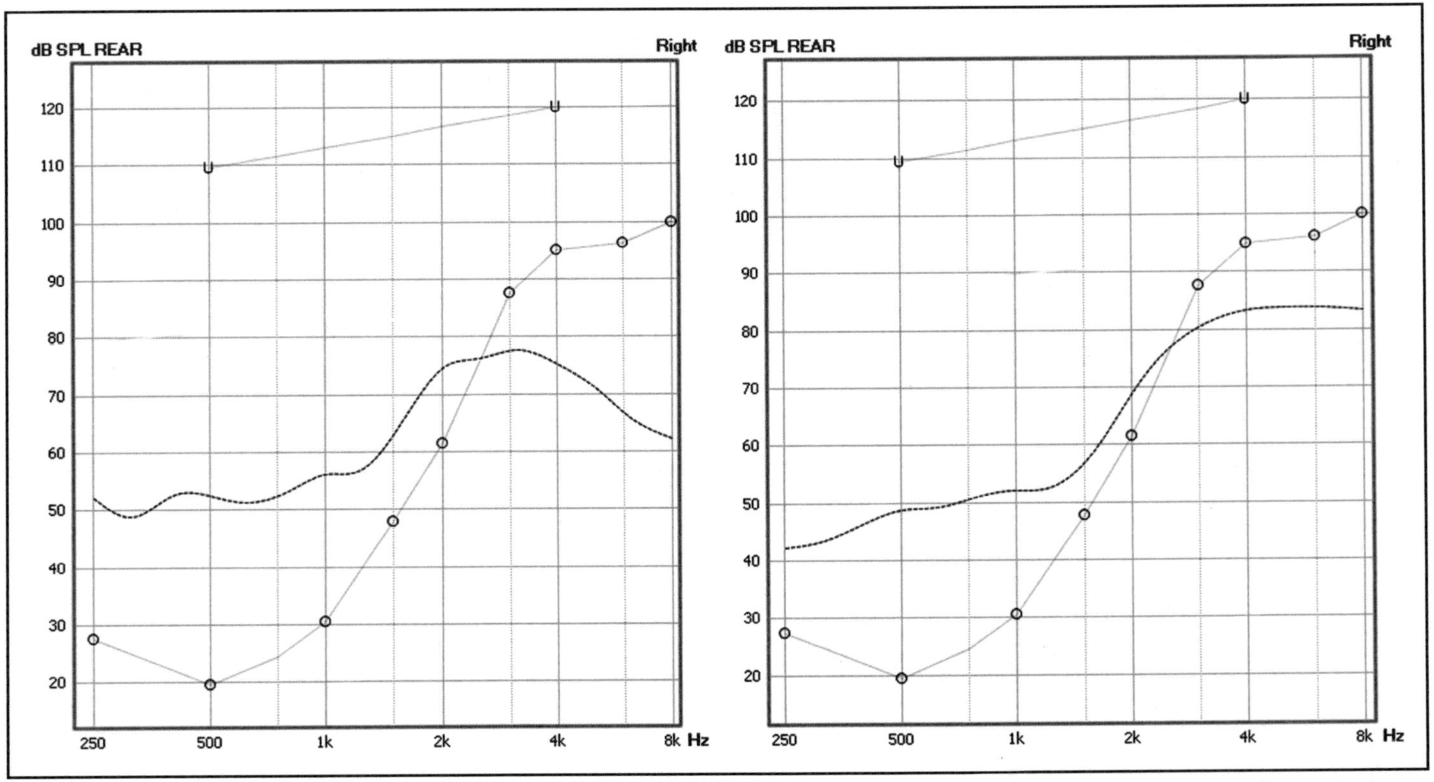

Figure 7–3. Example of the targets for the NAL (*left*) and DSL (*right*) falling below the patient's thresholds in the high frequencies. fitting was used.

I have a colleague who uses probe-mic measures, but doesn't believe in fitting targets. She doesn't put targets on the screen, and just looks at the patient's thresholds and then makes adjustments accordingly. Is this okay?

Okay? No. Better than not doing probe-mic at all? Probably. Our guess is that she is simply trying to place the aided speech signal above the thresholds—that is, provide good audibility. This is something that is, of course, important, especially for soft speech, and as we discuss in Chapter 1, something that won't happen if you stick with the manufacturer's first fit. The problem is how much of the 30 dB of the average soft-speech signal do you want to place above threshold? 50%?, 75%?, 100%? How does this percentage change as a function of frequency in a downward sloping hearing loss (as most are)? If your colleague has all those answers, for soft, average, and loud inputs, she might want to publish her own fitting method. If she doesn't have all the answers, it's much simpler to use the data from the people who already have done all the heavy lifting—those who developed the DSL and NAL fitting methods!

Can't I simply use the "speech banana" as the target—that is, making sure it is audible for the different levels.

No. This relates to the previous two questions—see those answers. Making the entire spectrum audible will result in too much audibility/loudness. It is a good technique to use however, if your goal is to end up with the hearing aid rejected and in the drawer!

I seem to get better fit-to-target when I use NAL-NL1 than when I use NAL-NL2. It is okay to keep using NL-NL1?

It's probably "okay"—the NAL-NL1 was a good friend of ours for 10 years, and as reviewed by Johnson and Dillon (2011), the differences between the NL1 and NL2 are not huge—but the differences are large enough to make a noticeable change in the fitting. Our question to you is, if Harvey Dillon and his NAL colleagues spent several years conducting research with the NAL-NL1 to "improve" the fitting outcome, then applied the results of all this research to develop the NAL-NL2, why wouldn't you want the improved version? We know it's tempting to keep using Windows ME, but Windows 10 is really better, trust us.

How close do I have to be to target to consider it a good (or okay) fitting?

Good question—we talk about this in Chapter 4. There is some research to suggest that patients notice a 5-dB change, so one answer could be that +/−3 or so would be okay. But, this assumes that the target is a very distinct point for that patient, and it isn't. Because of the potential for a variety of measurement and calculation errors, and the differences in preferred loudness among patients with the same hearing loss, the target is really a range, not a specific value, so we could live with +/−5 dB. We say this, however, with the assumption that your REAR is following the general output spectrum detailed by the targets. That is, we would consider falling below targets a consistent 3 to 5 dB for 1000 to 3000 Hz to be a much better fitting than being under target by 5 dB at 1000 Hz, over target by 5 dB at 2000 Hz, and then back under target by 5 dB at 3000 Hz. And of course, if your patient has a way to control the volume, you really don't know what your fit to target is once they leave your office—which again is why you want to provide the best shaping of the amplified speech signal.

When I fit to REAR targets using probe-mic, and then I look back at the fitting screen, the curve on the fitting screen is bizarre, and usually not even close to target. Why is this?

Well . . . we indirectly go into this in Chapter 1, and we encourage you to go back and review the findings of Sanders et al. (2015).

Recall that these data showed that when you select the NAL-NL2 in the fitting software, and there is a perfect match to target on the fitting screen, on average you will be making mistakes of 10 dB or more in the real-ear. So if you turn things around, and make a perfect (or near perfect) match in the rea-ear, it stands to reason that what you then see on the fitting screen *will not* be a match to target. And, because the mismatch is considerably greater in the high frequencies, what you see will indeed be a bizarre looking response. Hopefully, you are 100% certain regarding which of the two displays you should believe!

I saw the data from Sanders et al. (2015) showing that a NAL-NL2 fit in the fitting software is not likely to be a NAL-NL2 fit in the real-ear. Is the same true for the DSL v5.0? Would I expect to see average mistakes of 10 dB or more in the high frequencies for that algorithm also?

We are not aware of similar research that has been conducted for the DSL v5. Susan Scollie, PhD, from DSL HQ (University of Western Ontario) tells us, however, that when they transfer DSL v5 for implementation, the hearing aid company signs a license agreement that specifies a list of "minimum implementation requirements." This means that the manufacturer has to create software menus and/or behind-the-scenes software corrections that will calculate the DSL target using the correct definitions of transforms, headphone types, input signal, and so forth. The manufacturer must also agree to send in their software and a sample hearing aid for testing at DSL HQ before the software can be released. During this evaluation process, the accuracy of the targets and the software-based fit is checked for every implementation, and the manufacturer is then provided feedback regarding accuracy. Susan mentions that it sometimes takes more than one version of the software to meet the whole list of requirements. Our best guess is that this protocol would lead to a pretty good match between what you see on the fitting screen and the *average* real-ear finding. Of course, that does not mean you will be correct for any individual listener! With all that said, the bottom line is that if you verify using probe microphone measures, you really have little reason to care if what is on the screen agrees perfectly with what is in the ear canal. Of course, if you are at least starting at the correct average, it will be a little quicker to make the adjustments to fit individual patients accurately. But true, there are some patients where you just can't conduct real-ear testing (e.g., gooey ear canal, uncooperative patient) and for those cases, it would be nice if the screen display were at least close.

I've heard that if I do an RECD, I can then simply do my entire fitting in the 2-cc coupler using these corrections. True?

Usually no. If your mix of products is average, you're probably fitting 50 to 75% of your patients with open fittings. The approach you are referring to using RECD corrections works very well with closed fittings, but would lead to fairly large mistakes with open fittings. It's obvious why this is true in the low frequencies, but you'll also be making mistakes in the high frequencies because of the residual REUG. We talk about all this in detail in Chapter 4.

Why have I been told by a company rep that I can't do probe-mic testing with some of their products?

Assuming you are referring to conventional hearing aids, that simply isn't true. Could be there is something that is meant to be kept secret (like minimal gain in the highs)? All the more reason to actually DO the measures!

I usually start off in the manufacturer's default fitting, but then verify to the NAL-NL2 targets when I do speech mapping. Is that what you would recommend?

Typically no. Not sure why you prefer this approach, but we would always suggest starting off with the fitting method that you will be verifying to, the NAL-NL2 or the DSL v5.0. Some manufacturers use different parameters if they know your goal is to meet specific targets. A good example of this is shown in Figure 7–4. On the left panel, you see our best fit to NAL-NL2 targets for the 55 and 75 dB SPL inputs when we started by selecting NAL-NL2. We first fit to the 55 dB SPL input, and then adjusted compression to match the 75 dB input targets. Note a good match for the 75 dB inputs from 1500 to 4000 Hz (sorry about the dip just before 1000 Hz, we'll talk about that later). Knowing that our desire was to meet NAL-NL2 targets, the software used compression parameters that would facilitate this (shorter release times).

In the right panel of Figure 7–4, you see what happened when we started in the default proprietary mode, and fitted to the 55 dB input signal, then tried to fit to the 75 dB SPL input signal. What you see is the best fit we could obtain, even when the input compression was adjusted to the maximum. We were still over target by about 5 dB. This is because the default algorithm uses a much slower compression release time.

This is a common dilemma for audiologists who want to use a slow release time, fit to NAL-NL2 targets, and are fitting a patient with considerable high-frequency hearing loss (narrow dynamic range). To illustrate how release time can impact the speech banana (and the LTASS) take a look at Figure 7–5. These are two real-speech measures with the same hearing aid. Every-

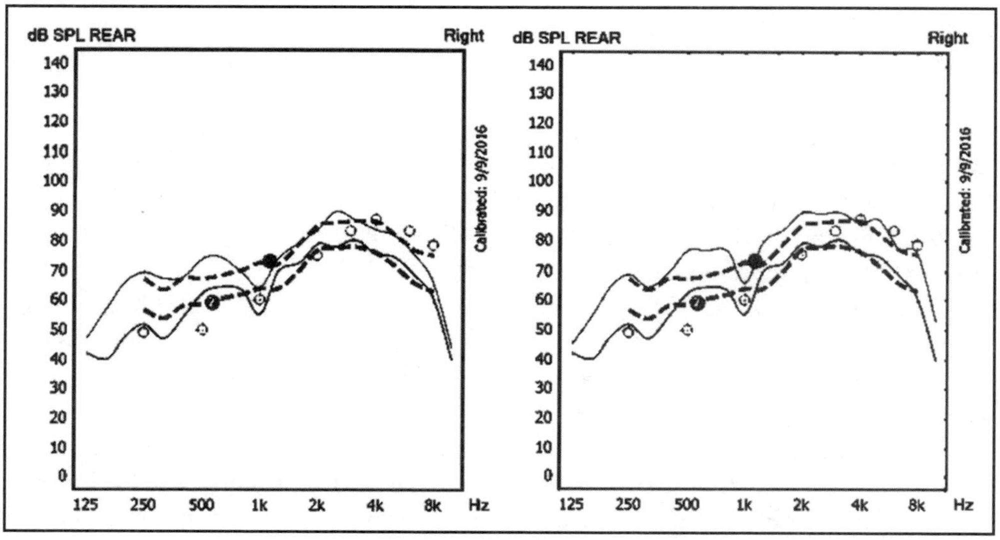

Figure 7–4. Illustration of the effects on the final fitting when either the default fitting or the NAL-NL2 is selected in the fitting software. The left panel is the "best-fit-to-target" when the NAL-NL2 was selected in the software. The right panel is the best-fit-to-target when the default fitting was initially selected. Note differences for the upper curve (75 dB SPL input).

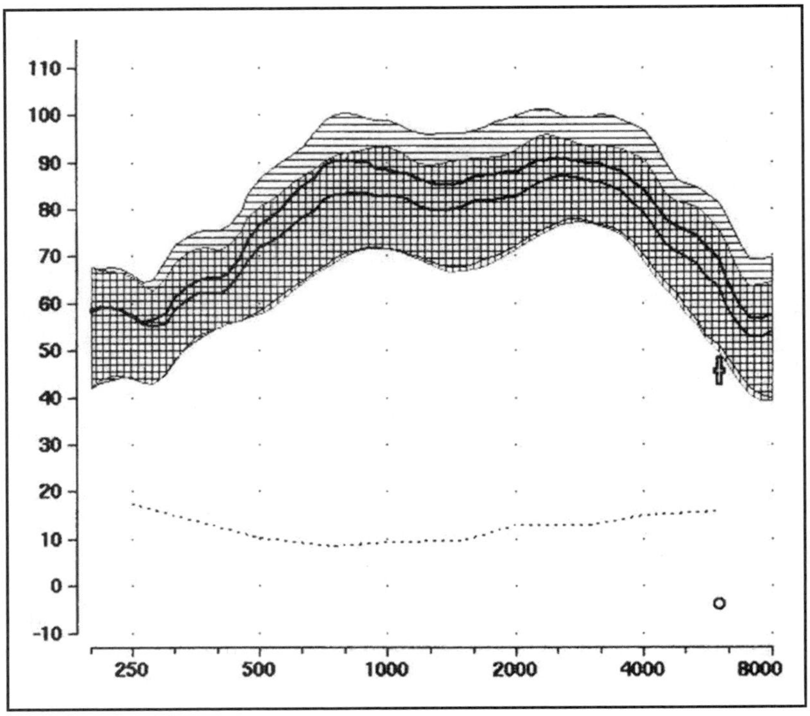

Figure 7–5. Aided real-ear output for real speech (30th to 99th percentiles). All hearing aid setting were the same except for the compression release time (fast versus slow).

thing was held constant (3:1 compression ratio), except the compression release time (adjustable on this hearing aid), which first was set to "short" (about 60 msec) and then to "long" (about 2 seconds). The 30 to 99th percentile for the short release (the checkerboard shading), shows a range in the mid frequencies of about 22 to 24 dB. The range for the long release for the same frequencies is about 30 dB, and notice that the LTASS also is about 5 dB higher. This clearly can impact match to target.

With all this said and getting back to the question, there have been rare instances when, a manufacturer's default fitting will be closer to NAL-NL2, than their "NAL-NL2" fitting. Even though this seems like a fairly serious math error on the part of the manufacturer, it may be faster to start with their default if you run into this.

My colleague first does speech mapping verification, but then follows up with insertion gain testing as a cross-check. Is this something you would recommend?

No. Well, if you had a lot of time and cooperative patients, it might be mildly interesting and maybe even a little educational, but for the most part, unnecessary. We assume when you say "speech mapping" you mean verification using the REAR (technically, when you use real speech, insertion gain measures are also speech mapping). If a patient has an unusual REUG, and your colleague uses a *measured* REUG for the REIG calculations, then it's possible that you would adjust the hearing aid somewhat differently, depending on what procedure you use. It's not that one is a cross-check of the other, just two different approaches. For the most part, a good fit is a good fit and a bad fit is a bad fit, regardless if you use the REAR or the REIG to reach this conclusion.

The hearing aids that I fit are user-trainable, and I also use the automatic gain increase (AGI) feature. So, does it really matter much if I start at a verified target?

Yes, it matters very much. Research with trainable hearing aids has shown that the starting point will impact the ending point, for both new and previous users, so you need to start at a good place (see Mueller, Hornsby, & Weber, 2008; Mueller & Hornsby, 2014). Your question also prompts us to comment on the combined use of user training and AGI to establish the best fitting, as you will continue to use your probe microphone measures during this approach.

As reviewed by Mueller (2014b), we really have three choices if you want to use both user training and AGI:

1. We could implement both patient training and AGI at the time of the fitting. That seems like a poor choice to us because you have two different things going on, which could be working in opposite directions. Moreover, for user training, the user needs to be in control of the gain. For AGI to be effective, the user *cannot* be in control of the gain (or they would simply override the AGI changes).
2. We could use AGI first. This might help us push gain to a higher level than patients might initially accept, which might take a couple of months. Then after they arrive at that higher level, we could implement training to fine-tune compression and obtain preferred gain for different listening situations. This seems reasonable to us and would be good for the patient who initially is not fond of much gain.
3. Our third option is to use patient-training first for patients who initially accepted an appropriate amount of gain—recall that the gain starting point does influence the ending point. We allow the patient to settle on a preferred gain for different listening situations, which might take a couple of weeks. Once preferred gain is established, we conduct probe microphone testing to determine how the fitting looks. If audibility is not optimal, we could then implement AGI. Although this might make sense for some patients and some clinicians, it seems less efficient to us because it may require multiple office visits to recheck the fitted gain values.

AGI is something that you have in your back pocket to pull out for either Option #2 or Option #3, and the use seems to depend on the patient's first perceptions or the outcome of training. We are mostly talking about new hearing aid users for these scenarios. We assume that experienced users are fairly settled on their preferences. This might not be true, however, if they were underfit for gain initially and have been using hearing aids that did not have gain adjustments (Mueller & Hornsby, 2014). Implementing these training procedures usually involves a few more trips back to your office, but that is not necessarily a bad thing. Furthermore, given current advances in distance-based telehealth technologies, it is likely that completing follow-up services related to trainable hearing aids may be increasingly less cumbersome for both patients and clinicians.

Verification and Assessment of Special Feature

I rarely do speech-mapping verification as I was told that special features only work in the default fitting, and there are no real-ear targets for the default fitting, right?

Your last statement is indeed correct, but we have some problems with the rest of your question. First, we know of no product where changing from proprietary to NAL or DSL impacts the function of directional technology, noise reduction, and so forth. In fact, if you look at the research published on these features, in most cases the hearing aids were programmed to a validated prescriptive method. Secondly, you *could* start off in the default proprietary program, and then still fit to NAL or DSL targets using speech mapping. There are some minor issues regarding doing this, which we discussed in an earlier question, but it certainly would be better than not doing verification at all.

If special features are turned off during probe microphone measures, then do we really know how the hearing aids are working when the features are turned on?

Okay, let's start from the beginning on this one. While indeed it was necessary 15 years ago or so, we no longer have to, or want to turn off special features during probe-mic verification. The need to turn off those features was eliminated when we started using recorded real-speech inputs. The exception might be frequency lowering, which you might want to evaluate independently after your initial verification to NAL or DSL targets (see Chapter 5). But, regarding feedback reduction, noise reduction, directional features, bilateral beamforming, and so forth, we recommend doing your verification with these features set the way each individual patient will be using them in the real world.

I find testing DNR using probe microphone measures provides a great counseling opportunity with a new patient, so I do it often. I'd like to make it as real-world as possible. What input levels do you think I should use?

The demonstration will most likely be the most impressive using a fairly high noise signal without introducing any speech—many products increase the amount of noise reduction as the overall level increases. There are several recorded environmental noises you can use for this. If you want to make it more real-world (but maybe not as impressive), you might also try testing at a common SNR or noise level your patient experiences (presenting speech and noise at the same time; DNR on versus DNR off). This will tell you if there really is noise reduction for a given SNR (don't be surprised if you don't see any) and will also help you confirm that the noise reduction doesn't reduce the speech signal. For your patients who are handy with their smartphone, have them use a sound level meter app during their next outing, and they can then tell you the level of the background noise at their favorite club or restaurant. Smeds, Wolters, and Rung (2015) published some average SNR values of different listening situations, which are shown in Figure 7–6.

I have had some patients who have complained about background noises, such as car noise, and I've changed the DNR from mild to strong, and they say they don't hear any difference? Is there some probe microphone measure that I should be doing that would help me with this programming?

Yes. Well, it might not help you with programming per se, but it will help both you and the patient understand the problem. Our bet is that you are talking about open fittings. If the ear is open, background noise goes directly to the eardrum. With an open ear, the effects of DNR in the low frequen-

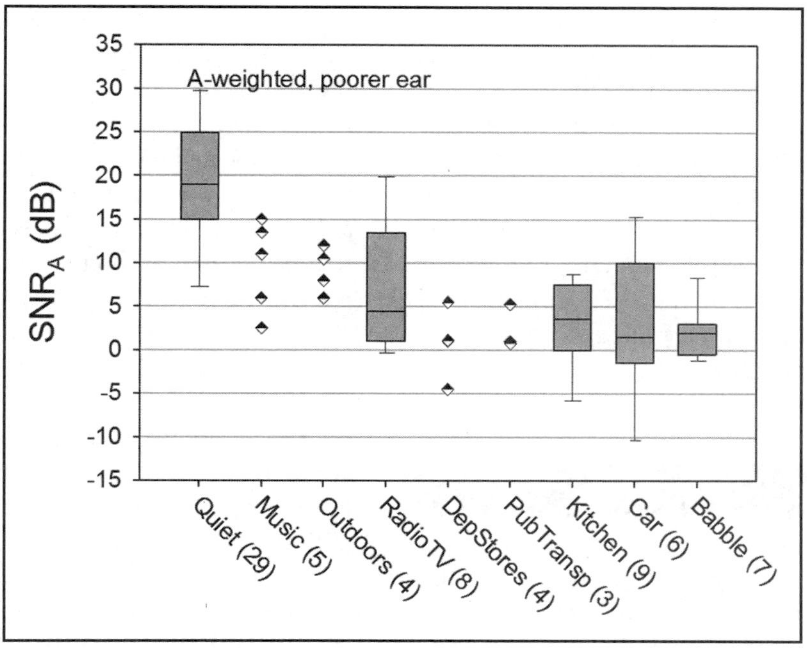

Figure 7–6. Signal-to-noise ratios for the poorer ear for each of the noise categories. For noise categories with five recordings or less, the actual SNR estimates are plotted. For noise categories greater than five recordings, box plots are shown. The central mark in each boxplot shows the median across the recordings, the box the interquartile range, and the whiskers extend to the most extreme data points. The number in brackets after each noise category name gives the number of recordings in that category. Adapted from Smeds, Wolters, and Rung, 2015.

cies will be exactly the same for "min" versus "max"—0 dB! To state the obvious, you can't reduce a signal that wasn't amplified in the first place. So, yes, conducting real-ear testing of DNR will give both you and the patient a good idea of when (and at what frequencies) DNR will be effective, and when it will not be.

For fitting frequency lowering, should I use specialized signals, or the standard ISTS?

A signal such as the ISTS will tell you if frequency lowering has been activated (see Chapter 5), but it won't tell you what you really need to know—the frequency location and the intensity of the lowered signal. You must use specialized signals to determine this—we suggest the ISTS excised /s/ and /sh/ signals that were developed by the Western Ontario group.

I have seen charts showing a directional effect of 20 dB or so for the front-to-back difference, but when I measure it using my real-ear equipment, it's never that big. Am I doing something wrong?

Probably not. The reason you are seeing the smaller differences relates to how compression works, assuming that you are not presenting the front and back signal simultaneously. We talk about this in Chapter 5, and Mueller (2001c) has a longer description complete with math. There are many reasons to look at directionality in the real-ear (see

Chapter 5), but if you are concerned about the true front-to-back difference, we suggest you use the special application designed for your test box. Some probe microphone equipment might also have the capability for simultaneous measures, although you'd need two loudspeakers. Another approach for the real-ear would be to program your hearing aid to linear processing (e.g., compression ratios of 1:1), which will give you a better idea of the true directivity.

Unusual Outcomes

After I fit to target, I sometimes take a look at the resulting compression ratios. Often they are 3.0 or higher? Could this cause distortion of the speech signal?

It's quite unlikely. You might be thinking of some older research warning against using high compression ratios for WDRC. This was before the days of multiple overlapping channels that we have today, and usually involved ratios of 4.0 or higher. Manufactures today typically do not allow you to program a ratio higher than about 3.0 to 3.5. A ratio this high could impact music quality, which is why you typically will have a separate program for that.

Why do I sometimes not see a change in the REAR when I make increases in the fitting software up to 6 dB or so?

Hmm. This is sort of one of those "you have to be there" kind of questions, but we can think of three different things that could be happening.

- If you're talking about the low frequencies, this easily could happen if you have a very open fitting and have little or no gain in the instrument. What you might be seeing in the REAR is the direct sound, not the amplified signal. The amplified signal is leaking out of the ear, and even when you continue to increase gain, the majority is still leaking out, and the in-flow direct signal SPL stays the same. Take a look at Figure 7–7. The top curve is our best fit to target, and the bottom curve is the patient's REOR (hearing aid muted). We were having problems getting rid of the more-than-desired output in the 1000 to 2000 Hz range. The REOR clearly tells us why! Note that what we are seeing, until we reach 2000 Hz, is the direct input signal, not the output of the hearing aid. We know this because the REAR and REOR are identical below 2000 Hz. No wonder changes in the fitting software didn't get rid of the unwanted output.
- If you are referring to the higher frequencies, then it could be that you are using concurrent rather than stored equalization for your open fittings. As you increase gain, you have a 1:1 increase in leakage to the monitor microphone, which then lowers the input signal, which counteracts your increase in gain, and the net result is no change in the REAR (see Chapter 5).
- A final thought is that some manufacturers set a very low MPO (e.g., 90 dB SPL) for their default fitting. If you don't override this, it could be that for louder inputs (e.g., 75 dB SPL) the output is being limited by the MPO. In this case, increasing gain would not show a noticeable difference in the REAR.

In some fittings, my REAR is over target in the low frequencies (around 500 Hz) and even when I remove all the gain from the hearing aid (according the software, anyway), the REAR is still over target? What's happening and what do I do?

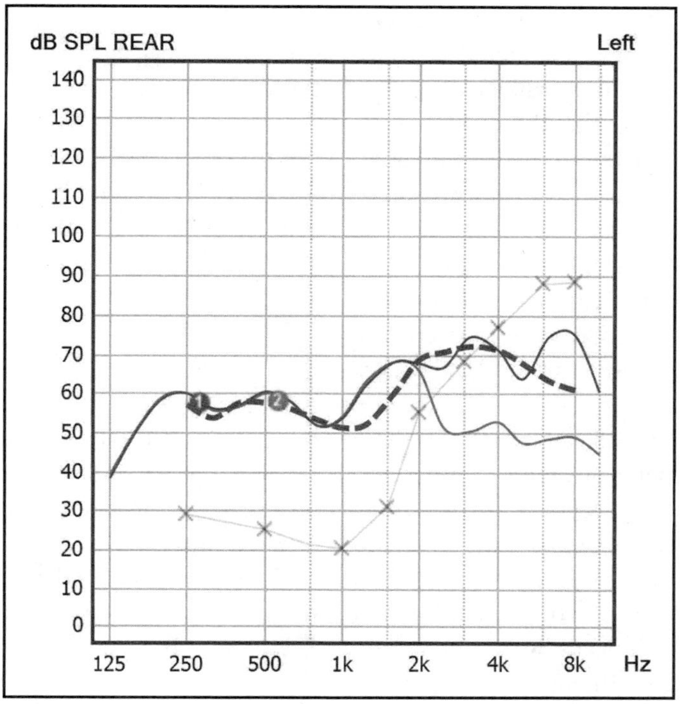

Figure 7–7. Illustration of the contribution of the REOR (direct sound to TM; *lower curve*) in an open fitting (*upper curve* is REAR best-match to target). Note that up to 2000 Hz, the output is due to the REOR (the direct sound path), not the amplified signal of the hearing aid.

This is not uncommon for an open fitting when the patient's thresholds are 0 to 20 dB in the low frequencies. What you are seeing in the REAR is the direct signal, not the amplified signal, and indeed, sometimes it exceeds the REAR target. This is very similar to what we showed in Figure 7–7. Running an REOR is a quick troubleshooting check to see if that is the problem. If you were to view everything in the REIG mode, you would see that 0 dB of gain was prescribed, and 0 dB of gain was present, and all would be well—so that is one option. If this REAR/target discrepancy really bothers you, you could fit an occluding eartip, which would attenuate the input signal enough that you would then match the REAR target. Probably a bit extreme. We simply think of this as a quirk of the REAR verification procedure. No harm done—it's simply the low-frequency SPL the patient is used to hearing prior to being fitted with hearing aids.

When conducting REAR85 measurements and the real-ear output is too high, there have been times when I have lowered the MPO by 10 dB or more, to a point below the REAR85 curve, but there has been no lowering of the REAR85 output?

Keep in mind that what you are seeing on the screen is output in real-ear SPL, and in the software the MPO is referenced to 2-cc coupler, so there isn't a one-to-one relationship for the adjustments you are referring to (but you could use an average RECD to get a general idea). Regardless, our best guess is that you are referring to an open fitting, and the ear canal SPL output that you are seeing is the direct signal of the REAR85 input. As we showed in Chapter 4, with some open fitting tips, the patient retains nearly all of their ear canal resonance, which can be as large as 15 to 20 dB. Add that onto your 85 dB SPL signal and you can see some fairly high ear canal SPLs that are unrelated to the hearing aid itself. An easy check of what is going on would be to mute the hearing aid, and conduct a REAR85—if you see the same high values, then you know why changing the MPO has no effect. To illustrate, that is exactly what we did with a patient, and the findings are in Figure 7–8. This is an open fitting, but with the hearing aid muted. While technically, we are measuring an REOR, because the tip is very open, it's very similar to the patient's REUR. Note that without the hearing aid on, the input signal exceeds his LDL in the 3000 Hz region.

Okay, thanks, that makes sense—here is a follow-up REAR85 question. There are times when the REAR85 measurement shows that the real-ear output is too low. Sometimes 15 dB or so below the patient's LDLs. In these cases, I raise the MPO (AGCo kneepoints) but the real-ear output doesn't change. Why is that?

This finding is usually related to the input compression (WDRC). Usually, for good reasons, the REAR85 verification is conducted after the hearing aids have been fitted to prescriptive targets. You probably worked hard to assure that ear canal output was at least close to targets for your 75 dB SPL inputs. To accomplish this, you probably had to use compression ratios of 3:1 for

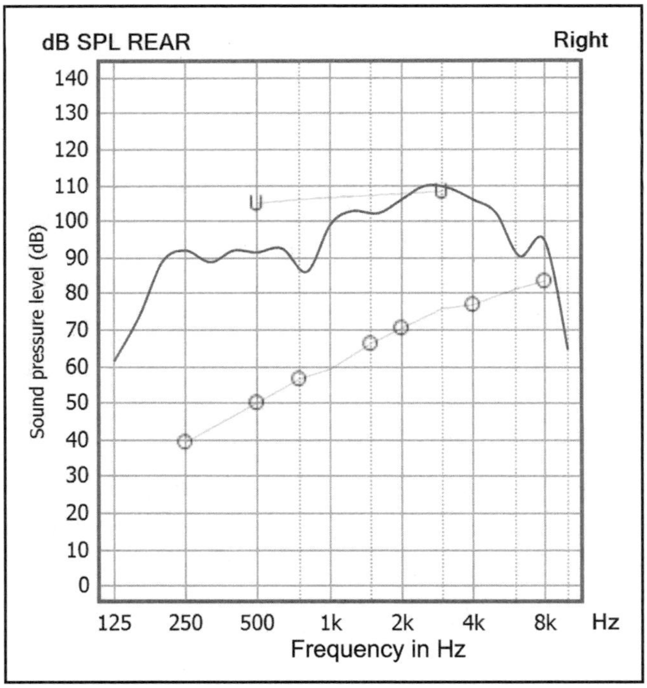

Figure 7–8. Example of output of REOR for REAR85 measure for open fitting. Note that although the hearing aid was muted, the output exceeds the patient's LDL.

the higher frequencies. With relatively low kneepoints, and relatively aggressive compression ratios, it is possible, if not probable, that the WDRC will be limiting the output, not the AGCo. This means that to move the MPO up, and provide the patient with some welcome headroom, you probably will need to reduce the WDRC compression for loud inputs (some products have more than one AGC kneepoint, so this might make it easier). Of course, this means that you probably will be overshooting the REAR targets for loud speech—with the patient's help, you should be able to reach a compromise.

Not all the time, but often, I see a notch in the REAR around 1000 to 1500 Hz of 5 dB or so. It seems to be unrelated to the gain I have programmed, which has more or less equal gain for all frequencies in that region. Is this due to probe placement?

We have seen this also and it's sometimes difficult to fix. An example is shown in Figure 7–9 from a recent patient. For this patient, we are using the ISTS, and had equal gain programmed from 500 to 1500 Hz, yet this nasty dip of almost 10 dB appeared, present for the same degree for the 55 and 75 dB input signals. It is tempting to think that it's some kind of anti-resonance in the ear canal, which could be related to the location of the tip of the probe tube or the eartip itself. That is possible, but we know that in at least some cases, the dip remains, even when we have changed probe placement and eartips. Another possibility in an open fit is that there is little or no real ear gain from the hearing aid and the amplified signal mixes with the direct signal coming in around the eartip which might be out of phase causing a cancellation. If this is it, the dip should go away when you either

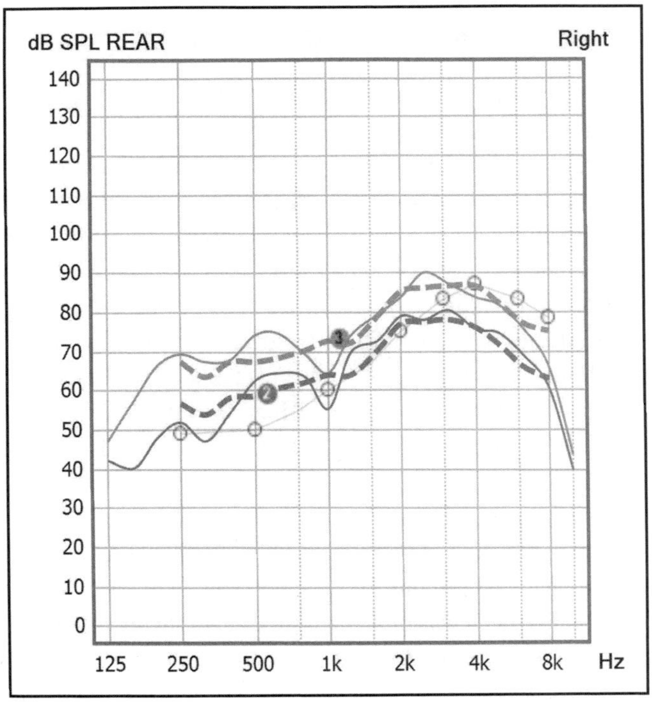

Figure 7–9. Example of unexplainable unusual dip in the REAR in the 1000 Hz region.

increase *or* decrease gain significantly. Our best guess, when the latter is *not* the case, is that it is related to the filters of the hearing aid, and there is some type of interaction happening at the filter crossover frequency region. A good possibility would be split-band feedback suppression. You might see that it occurs at slightly different regions for different manufacturers. It's annoying, but usually fixable by adding extra gain to this region.

The Big Picture

How does acclimatization fit into the process of target verification?

If you mean acclimatization using the audiologic definition, it doesn't! A consensus conference was held in Copenhagen, Denmark, in 1995, at which the following statement was formulated by the 15 international researchers in participation: "Auditory acclimatization is a systematic change in auditory performance with time, linked to a change in the acoustic information available to the listener. It involves an improvement in performance that cannot be attributed to task, procedural, or training effects." (Arlinger et al., 1996, p. 87S) Some early research (with flawed design) did show an improvement in speech understanding following continued hearing aid use after the initial fitting. A recent, well-controlled study, however, by Dawes, Munro, Kalluri, and Edwards (2014) addressed several of the earlier design flaws and found no evidence for acclimatization. That is, when gain and output are held constant, there is no improvement in speech understanding.

Now, hearing aid manufacturers like to toss around the word acclimatization when

AUDIOID: Acclimatization and Old Records

Our question about auditory acclimatization reminded us of a frequently told anecdote about one of the great hearing scientists of the 1900s, Harvey Fletcher. The following version of the story was kindly provided by Mead Killion, although we have added a few of our own embellishments. Back in the 1940s, wideband high-fidelity phonograph consoles were just becoming available. Because of his interest in high-quality audio, noted acoustic scientist Harvey Fletcher bought one for his home. Harvey enjoyed listening to this new high-fidelity system, but unfortunately, the enjoyment was not shared by his wife. After listening to an old 78-rpm record, with the surface noise made particularly prominent by the extended bandwidth of this new high-fidelity system, she said, "That sounds awful. I don't really like having that screechy sound in my home." Always the creative thinker, the next day, when his wife was out of the house, Harvey went into the living room and soldered twenty capacitors across the loudspeaker terminals, which had the effect of rolling off the high frequencies. (Remember that amplifiers were high impedance back then, so the trick worked.) That evening, when the music played, his wife was happy. One night each week, while his wife was sleeping, Harvey would sneak downstairs and clip one capacitor. After twenty weeks, when the music played, they were *both* happy.

they probably mean adjustment. So regarding your question, it is possible that your patients will indeed "adjust" to the loudness levels provided by the hearing aid, and because of this, they might use more gain. In most cases, more audibility means better speech understanding. There are software designs for facilitating the use of more gain. This is one reason why you would want to check use-gain via probe microphone measures on repeat visits.

What about the patient who loves his old hearing aids and simply wants the new hearing aids to sound like the old ones?

We usually ask these patients if they also request that their new cars drive like their old one. But, we know what you mean, we've been there, and usually the old fitting isn't very good. We try to counsel away this notion, and usually are successful. We are reminded of a Mueller and Hornsby study (2014) where individuals who were happy users, and were fitted to around 10 dB below target for soft sounds, were fitted with new hearing aids programmed to NAL-NL2. However, they were given trainable hearing aids with a +/−16 dB range, so they easily could have trained back to their old fitting. They didn't! But, if the patient simply won't accept anything but what is close to his old fitting, and you feel you need to buy into that, at least one manufacturer has made that simple for you, by allowing you to use the gain from the old hearing aid as the new fitting target.

Given that my probe microphone system automatically calculates an SII, I am trying to use those values in my counseling. Can I assume that a 10% improvement in the SII will improve the patient's discrimination [word recognition] by that amount?

It's not that simple. There is not a 1:1 relationship between the SII and speech recognition. The effects of a 10% change in SII on speech recognition are highly dependent on the starting point (patient's unaided SII) and the speech material or content. Take a look at Figure 7–10. Notice that going from an SII (AI) of .60 to .70 would indeed give you a predicted speech recognition improvement of about 10% for monosyllable words. But notice that for words in sentences, and for the even easier sentences and spondees, there is essentially no improvement. Now, if the patient had started off at .20, then 10% would make a sizeable different for these latter two speech materials.

I work in a busy clinic. If you only have time to run one probe microphone measure, which one is the most important?

Wow, that's like asking us to name our favorite child! If you know the software well for your favorite product, it shouldn't take more than 2 to 3 minutes to match prescriptive targets for a given input level. If you do three inputs/ear, and a verification REAR85 for each ear, you should still finish a bilateral fitting in less than 20 minutes. That is not much of a time investment when you consider the magnitude of the expenditure by the patient. How much of your time did he or she buy? But, to answer your question, we'd probably do a speech mapping match-to-target for a 65 dB input, and just hope we got lucky with all the other inputs. And, you really do need to follow this measure with a quick REAR85 to ensure you are not exceeding the patient's measured LDLs. You're right, we just named two probe microphone measures, but we couldn't help ourselves!

When is the best time to conduct probe microphone measures?

We have heard that some audiologists start off by fitting to the manufacturer's first fit (no verification), send the patient out

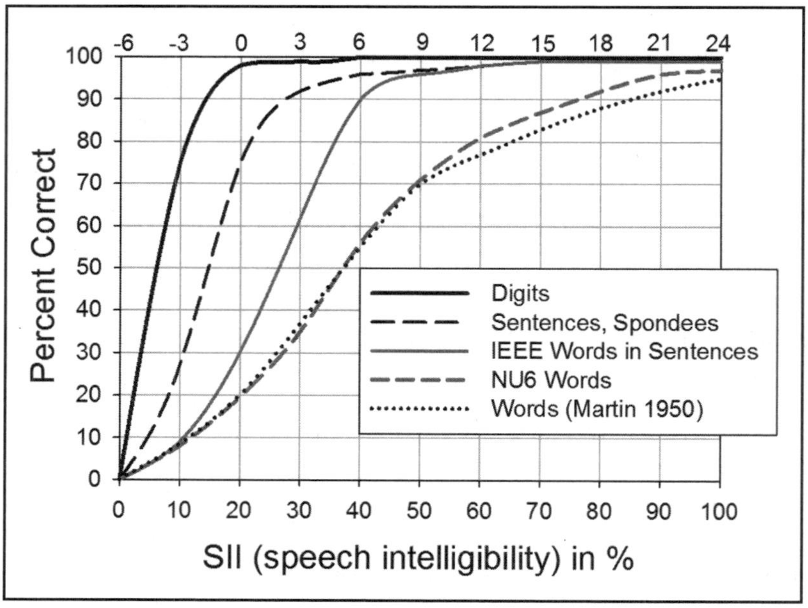

Figure 7–10. Predicted speech recognition performance as a function of SII for different types of speech materials. As contextual content increases, a lower SII will result in higher speech recognition performance. Adapted from Killion and Mueller, 2010.

the door, and then do speech mapping a few weeks later on a return appointment. Strange. That's like a dentist sending you out with a new crown that prevents you biting down, only to give you the "correct" crown fitting two weeks later? Why not make things right from the beginning? So yes, the best time is always on the day of the fitting. You want to send the patient out the door with the best chance to be successful, and the evidence tells us that happens when they have been fitted to a validated prescriptive method. If you make fitting changes on follow-up visits, then of course you would document this with real-ear measures.

What if after going through all the trouble to match to targets, the patient doesn't like it?

If it's a new user, we wouldn't really expect them to be delighted. We are giving them a fair amount of audibility that they probably haven't heard for 10, 20, or more years. We have often found that when you adjust the output to reach something that a new user likes, the resulting response is very similar to their REUR, which of course would be 0 dB gain. Previous users often want the new hearing aids to sound like their old ones, which very likely weren't programmed well. Therefore, we are generally looking for a fitting that the patient is willing to "accept," try for a while, not necessarily something they "like." (As a last resort, you can use the automatic gain increase strategy; start the patient with a little less gain and bring them up to targets over a period of several weeks—this of course will only work if they don't have a means to control the volume themselves.) With that said, we would expect that some patients would consider a verified prescriptive fitting too loud, others would think it's too soft, as their loudness judgments might be somewhat different from average. Altering the fitting from a loudness standpoint would be expected, but we would keep the same aided spectrum, tracking the REAR targets.

I'm a firm believer in patient counseling—is there any way to use the speech mapping process for counseling the patient?

Most certainly. That's a big part of the overall verification. Here's a brief outline of how we work counseling into the measurement process:

- We start by showing the patient the average speech banana compared to his or her thresholds on the speech mapping fitting screen. We show the patient all the high-frequency sounds that are inaudible for him or her, explaining that this is why he or she can "hear, but not understand." The patient normally gives us a "now I get it" nod.
- Once we have the targets on the screen, we point out to the patient that this is our goal for what we are going to accomplish today. This is a "prescription" just for him or her, just like he or she has prescriptions for his or her hypertension and high cholesterol. We emphasize that this prescription is based on 40 years of research, and is used around the world.
- We next talk about the fact that real-world listening has many different levels of sounds, some soft, some loud. Therefore, we need to have a different prescription for different loudness levels—we point them out on the screen.
- We then start with programming soft inputs, describing why these are so important, but also that these might be the most annoying, as he or she will be hearing many things that he or she is not used to hearing. We will probably toss out the phrase, "You have to hear what you don't want to hear to know what you don't want to hear" (maybe even adding a short story about people living near the airport or a railroad track). We might talk to the patient a little at this time, pointing out that our speech should now have more audible high frequencies, what he or she is going to have to get used to hearing if he or she wants to understand speech well. The patient normally gives us a "now I get it" nod.
- We then program the hearing aids for loud and average inputs, describing why we need to make loud sounds loud, but not uncomfortably loud. We point to the match to his or her prescription on the screen.
- At the conclusion, we again emphasize that he or she now has his hearing aids programmed based on years and years of research evidence. We also just might point out, that this is a service he or she is not going to get everywhere. It's a lucky patient that came to see us. The patient normally gives us a "now I get it" nod.

Is it all really worth it?

As we've said many times, there is evidence to support the fact that your patients will have better outcomes if they are fitted to a validated prescriptive method. There is no other way than real-ear measures to accomplish this. Moreover, allowing someone to walk out your door with their hearing aids programmed to poor audibility goes against all of our Best Practice statements, and would be considered unethical practice by some. And, there is something to be said about going home each day knowing that you did the best you could to provide the highest level of service to your patients. How much is a good night's sleep worth?

References

Aarts, N. L., & Caffee, C. S. (2005). Manufacturer predicted and measured REAR values in adult hearing aid fitting: Accuracy and clinical usefulness. *International Journal of Audiology*, *44*(5), 293–301.

Aazh, H., & Moore, B. C. (2007). The value of routine real-ear measurement of the gain of digital hearing aids. *Journal of the American Academy of Audiology*, *18*(8), 653–664.

Aazh, H., Moore, B. C., & Prasher, D. (2012). The accuracy of matching target insertion gains with open-fit hearing aids. *American Journal of Audiology*, *21*(2), 175.

Abrams, H. B., Chisolm, T. H., McManus, M., & McArdle, R. (2012). Initial-fit approach versus verified prescription: Comparing self-perceived hearing aid benefit. *Journal of the American Academy of Audiology*, *23*(10), 768–778.

Alexander, J. M. (2013, April). The highs and lows of frequency lowering amplification. *AudiologyOnline*, Article #11772. Retrieved from: http://www.audiologyonline.com/

Alexander, J. M. (2016, September). 20Q: Frequency lowering ten years later—new technology innovations. *AudiologyOnline*, Article 18040. Retrieved from http:www.audiologyonline.com

American Academy of Audiology. (2006). Guidelines for the audiological management of adult hearing impairment. *Audiology Today*, *18*(5), 32–36.

Amlani, A. M., Pumford, J., & Gessling E. (2016). Improving patient perception toward clinical services through the provision of real-ear measures. *Hearing Review*, *23*(12), 12.

ANSI. (1996). Specification for audiometers *(ANSI S3.6-1996)*. New York, NY: American National Standards Institute.

ANSI. (1997). Methods of measurement of real-ear characteristics of hearing instruments (*ANSI S3.46-1997)*. New York, NY: American National Standards Institute.

ANSI. (2013). Methods of measurement of real-ear characteristics of hearing instruments (*ANSI S3.46-2013)*. New York, NY: American National Standards Institute.

Arlinger, S., Gatehouse, S., Bentler, R. A., Byrne, D., Cox, R. M., Dirks, D. D., . . . Willott, J. F. (1996). Report of the Eriksholm Workshop on Auditory Deprivation and Acclimatization. *Ear and Hearing*, *17*(Suppl. 3), 87S–98S.

Bagatto, M., Moodie, S., Scollie, S., Seewald, R., Moodie, S., Pumford, J., & Liu, K.P.R. (2005). Clinical protocols for hearing instrument fitting in the desired sensation level method. *Trends in Amplification*, *9*(4), 199–226.

Bagatto, M. P., Scollie, S. D., Seewald, R. C., Moodie, K. S., & Hoover, B. M. (2002). Real-ear-to-coupler difference predictions as a function of age for two coupling procedures. *Journal of the American Academy of Audiology*, *13*(8), 407–415.

Bentler R. A. (2004). *Advanced hearing aid features: Do they work?* Paper presented at the convention of the American Speech-Language-Hearing Association, Washington, DC.

Bentler, R. A., & Cooley, L. J. (2001). An examination of several characteristics that affect the prediction of OSPL90 in hearing aids. *Ear and Hearing*, *22*(1), 58–64.

Bentler R. A., Mueller, H. G., & Ricketts, T. A. (2016). *Modern hearing aids: Verification, outcome measures, and follow-up*. San Diego, CA: Plural.

Bentler R. A., Wu, Y. H., & Jeon, J. (2006). Effectiveness of directional technology in open-canal hearing instruments. *The Hearing Journal*, 59(11), 40–42.

Berger, K. (1976). Prescription of hearing aids: A rationale. *Journal of the American Audiology Society*, *2*(3), 71–78.

Berger, K., Hagberg, E., & Rane, R. (1984). *Prescription of hearing aids: Rationale, procedures and results*. Kent, OH: Herald.

Bess, F. H., Chase, P. A., Gravel, J. S., Hedley-Williams A, Seewald. R. C., Stelmachowicz, P. G., & Tharpe, A. M. (1996). Amplification for infants and children with hearing loss. Reprinted, with permission, from *American Journal of Audiology* *5*(1), 66.

Burney, P. A. (1972) A survey of hearing aid evaluation procedures. *ASHA*, *14*(9), 439–444.

Byrne, D. J. (1982). Theoretical approaches for hearing aid selection. In G. A. Studebaker & F. H. Bess (Eds.), *The Vanderbilt hearing-aid report: State of the art—research needs* (pp. 175–179). Upper Darby, PA: Monographs in Contemporary Audiology.

Byrne, D. (1996). Hearing aid selection for the 1990s: Where to? *Journal of the American Academy of Audiology*, *7*(6), 377–395.

Byrne, D., & Dillon, H. (1986). The National Acoustic Laboratories' new procedure for selecting the gain and frequency response of a hearing aid. *Ear and Hearing*, *7*(4), 257–265.

Byrne, D., Dillon, H., Tran, K., Arlinger, S., Wilbraham, K., Cox, R., . . . Ludvigsen, C. (1994). An international comparison of long-term average speech spectra. *Journal of the Acoustical Society of America*, *96*(4), 2108–2120.

Byrne, D., Parkinson, A., & Newall, P. (1990). Hearing aid gain and frequency response requirements for the severely/profoundly hearing impaired. *Ear and Hearing*, *11*(1), 40–49.

Byrne, D., & Tonisson, W. (1976). Selecting the gain of hearing aids for persons with sensorineural hearing impairments. *Scandinavian Audiology*, *5*(2), 51–59.

Carhart, R. (1946). Tests for the selection of hearing aids. *Laryngoscope*, *56*(12), 780–794.

Chasin, M. Pirzaniski, C., Hayes, D., & Mueller, H. G. (1997). Real-ear occluded gain as a clinical predictor. *Hearing Review*, *4*(4), 22–26.

Ching, T., Dillon, H., & Byrne, D. (1998). Speech recognition of hearing-impaired listeners: Predictions from audibility and the limited role of high frequency amplification. *Journal of the Acoustical Society of America*, *103*, 1128–1140.

Ching, T. Y., Dillon, H., Katsch, R., & Byrne, D. (2001). Maximizing effective audibility in hearing aid fitting. *Ear and Hearing*, *22*(3), 212–224.

Consumer Reports. (2009). How to buy a hearing aid. Retrieved from http://www.consumerreports.org/cro/hearing-aids/buying-guide.htm

Convery, E., Keidser, G., & Dillon, H. (2005). A review and analysis: Does amplification experience have an effect on preferred gain over time? *Australian and New Zealand Journal of Audiology*, *27*(1), 18.

Cornelisse, L. E., Seewald, R. C., & Jamieson, D. G. (1995). The input/output formula: A theoretical approach to the fitting of personal amplification devices. *Journal of the Acoustical Society of America*, *97*(3), 1854–1864.

Cox, R. M. (1988). The MSUv3 hearing instrument prescription procedure. *Hearing Instruments*, *39*(1), 6–10.

Cox, R. M. (1995). Using loudness data for hearing aid selection: The IHAFF approach. *Hearing Journal*, *48*(2), 10, 39–44.

Cox, R. M. (1997). Administration and application of the APHAB. *Hearing Journal*, *50*(4), 32–48.

Cox, R. M. (2009). Verification and what to do until your probe-mic system arrives: The second of two parts. *Hearing Journal*, *62*(10), 10–14.

Cox, R. M., & Alexander, G. C. (1995). The abbreviated profile of hearing aid benefit. *Ear and Hearing*, *16*(2), 176–183.

Cox, R. M., & Alexander, G. C. (2002). The International Inventory for Hearing Aids (IOI-HA): Psychometric properties of the English version. *International Journal of Audiology*, *41*(1), 30–35.

Cox, R. M., Alexander, G. C., & Beyer C. M. (2003). Norms for the international outcome inventory for hearing aids. *Journal of the American Academy of Audiology*, *14*(8), 407–417.

Cox, R. M., Goff, C. M., Martin, S. E., & McLoud, L. L. (1994b, April). *The contour test: Normative data.* Presented at the American Academy of Audiology Convention, Richmond, VA.

Cox, R. M., Johnson, J. A., & Alexander, G. C. (2012). Implications of high-frequency cochlear dead regions for fitting hearing aids to adults with mild to moderately severe hearing loss. *Ear and Hearing*, 33(5), 573–587.

Cox, R. M., Matesich, J. S., & Moore, J. N. (1988). Distribution of short-term rms levels in conversational speech. *Journal of the Acoustical Society of America*, *84*(3), 1100–1104.

Cox, R. M., & Moore, J. N. (1988). Composite speech spectrum for hearing aid gain prescriptions. *Journal of Speech and Hearing Research*, *31*(1), 102–107.

Cox, R. M., Taylor, I. M., Gray, G. A., & Brainerd, L. E. (1994a, April). *The contour test: Applications to hearing aid selection and fitting.* Presented at the American Academy of Audiology Meeting, Richmond, VA.

Davies-Venn, E., Souza, P., Brennan, M., & Stecker, G. C. (2009). Effects of audibility and multichannel wide dynamic range compression on consonant recognition for listeners with severe hearing loss. *Ear and Hearing*, *30*(5), 494.

Davis, H., Hudgins, C. V., Marquis, R. J., Nichols, R. H., Peterson, G. E., Ross, D. A., & Stevens, S. S. (1946a). The selection of hearing aids. *Laryngoscope*, *56*(3), 85–115.

Dawes, P., Hopkins, R., & Munro, K. J. (2013). Placebo effects in hearing-aid trials are reliable. *International Journal of Audiology*, *52*(7), 472–477.

Dawes, P., Munro, K. J., Kalluri, S., & Edwards, B. (2014). Acclimatization to hearing aids. *Ear and Hearing*, *35*; 203–212.

De Jonge, R. (1996). Real-ear measures: Individual and measurement error. In M. Valente (Ed.), *Hearing aids: Standards, options, and limitations* (pp 72–125). New York, NY: Thieme Medical.

Deming, W. E. (1986). *Out of the crisis*. Cambridge, MA: MIT Center for Advanced Engineering Study.

Dillon, H. (1999). NAL-NL1: A new procedure for fitting non-linear hearing aids. *Hearing Journal*, *52*(4), 10–12.

Dillon, H. (December, 2001). The research of Denis Byrne at NAL: Implications for clinicians today. *AudiologyOnline*. Retrieved February 3, 2015, from http://www.audiologyonline.com/articles/research-denis-byrne-at-nal-1200

Dillon, H., James, A., & Ginis, J. (1997). The Client Oriented Scale of Improvement (COSI) and its relationship to several other measures of benefit and satisfaction provided by hearing aids. *Journal of the American Academy of Audiology*, *8*(1), 27–43.

Dirks, D. D., Ahlstrom, J. B., & Eisenberg, L. S. (1994). Effects of probe insertion depth on real-ear measurements. *Otolaryngology-Head and Neck Surgery*, *110*(1), 64–74.

Dirks, D. D., & Kincaid, G. E. (1987). Basic acoustic considerations of ear canal: Probe measurements. *Ear and Hearing*, *8*(5), 60S–67S.

Dreschler, W. A., Verschuure, H., Ludvigsen, C., & Westermann, S. (2001). ICRA noises: Artificial noise signals with speech-like spectral and temporal properties for hearing instrument assessment. *International Journal of Audiology*, *40*(3), 148–157.

Erickson, F. N., & Van Tasell, D. J. (1991). Maximum real-ear gain of in-the-ear hearing aids. *Journal of Speech, Language, and Hearing Research*, *34*(2), 351–359.

Feigin, J. A., Kopun, J. G., Stelmachowicz, P. G., & Gorga, M. P. (1989). Probe-tube microphone measures of ear-canal sound pressure levels in infants and children. *Ear and Hearing*, *10*(4), 254–258.

Frye Electronics (2013) *Fonix hearing aid test system: Operators manual*, Version 2.41. http://www.frye.com/wp/wp-content/uploads/2013b/manuals/8000v2.41.pdf

Harford, E. R. (1980). The use of a miniature microphone in the ear canal for the verification of hearing aid performance. *Ear and Hearing, 1*(6), 329–337.

Hawkins, D. B., Alvarez E., & Houlihan, J. (1991). Reliability of three types of probe tube microphone measurements. *Hearing Instruments, 42*, 14–16.

Hawkins, D. B., Beck, L. B., Bratt, G. W., Fabry, D. A., Mueller, H. G., & Stelmachowicz, P. G. (1991). Vanderbilt/VA Hearing Aid Conference 1990 consensus statement. Recommended components of a hearing aid selection procedure for adults. *ASHA, 33*(4), 37–38.

Hawkins, D. B., & Cook, J. A. (2003). Hearing aid software predictive gain values: How accurate are they? *Hearing Journal, 56*(7), 26–28.

Hawkins, D., & Mueller, H. G. (1992). Procedural considerations in probe-microphone measurements. In H. G. Mueller, D. Hawkins, & J. Northern (Eds.), *Probe microphone measurements: Hearing aid selection and assessment* (pp. 67–91). San Diego, CA: Singular.

Hellman, R. P., & Meiselman, C. H. (1990). Loudness relations for individuals and groups in normal and impaired hearing. *Journal of the Acoustical Society of America, 88*(6), 2596–2606.

Hellman, R. P., & Meiselman, C. H. (1993). Rate of loudness growth for pure tones in normal and impaired hearing. *Journal of the Acoustical Society of America, 93*(2), 966–975.

Holube, I., Fredelake, S., Vlaming, M., & Kollmeier, B. (2010). Development and analysis of an international speech test signal (ISTS). *International Journal of Audiology, 49*(12), 891–903.

Holube, I. (2015, February). 20Q: getting to know the ISTS. *AudiologyOnline*, Article 13295. Retrieved from http://www.audiology online.com.

Hornsby, B., & Mueller, H. G. (2013, July). Monosyllabic word testing: Five simple steps to improve accuracy and efficiency. *AudiologyOnline*, Article #11978. Retrieved from http://www.audiologyonline.com/

Institute of Electrical and Electronics Engineers. (1969). *IEEE recommended practice for speech quality measurements* (IEEE Report No. 297, Appendix C). Boulder, CO: Global Engineering Documents.

IHAFF. (1994). *A comprehensive hearing aid fitting protocol.* Retrieved from http://www.frye .com/wp/wp-content/uploads/2013b/manu als/IHAFF.pdf

International Society of Audiology. (2005). *Good practice guidance for adult hearing aid fittings and services.* Retrieved January 28, 2015, from http://www.isa-audiology.org/members/pdf/ gpg-adaf.pdf

Jenstad, L. M., Van Tasell, D., & Ewert, C. (2003). Hearing aid troubleshooting based on patients' descriptions. *Journal of the American Academy of Audiology, 14*(7), 347–360.

Jespersen, C. T., Groth, J., Kiessling, J., Brenner, B., & Jensen, O. D. (2006). The occlusion effect in unilateral versus bilateral hearing aids. *Journal of the American Academy of Audiology, 17*(10), 763–773.

Johnson, E. E. (April, 2012). Comparing the latest NAL and DSL prescriptive targets. *AudiologyOnline.* Retrieved February 3, 2015, from http://www.audiologyonline.com/arti cles/20q-same-or-different-comparing-769 ?report=reader

Johnson, E. E., & Dillon, H. (2011). A comparison of gain for adults from generic hearing aid prescriptive methods: Impacts on predicted loudness, frequency bandwidth, and speech intelligibility. *Journal of the American Academy of Audiology, 22*, 441–459.

Johnson, J. A., Cox, R. M., & Alexander, G. C. (2010). Development of APHAB norms for WDRC hearing aids and comparisons with original norms. *Ear and Hearing, 31*(1), 47–55.

Keidser, G., & Alamudi, K. (2013). Real-life efficacy and reliability of training a hearing aid. *Ear and Hearing, 34*(5), 619–629.

Keidser, G., Brew, C., & Peck, A. (2003). Proprietary fitting algorithms compared with one another and with generic formulas. *Hearing Journal, 56*(3), 28–32.

Keidser, G., & Dillon, H. (2006). What's new in prescriptive fittings down under. In C. Palmer & R. Seewald (Eds), *Hearing care for adults* (pp. 133–142). Stäfa, Switzerland: Phonak AG.

Keidser, G., & Dillon, H. (2012, October). NAL-NL2—principles, background data, and comparison to other procedures. *AudiologyOnline*. Retrieved February 4, 2015, from http://www.audiologyonline.com/articles/siemens-expert-series-nal-nl2-11355

Keidser, G., O'Brien, A., Carter, L., McLelland, M. & Yeend, I. (2008). Variation in preferred gain with experience for hearing aid users. *International Journal of Audiology 47*(10), 621–635.

Killion, M. C. (1994). *Hearing aid fitting targets for 40, 65 and 95 dB SPL inputs. (Version 1.01D)* [Fig6.exe software:]. Elk Grove Village, IL: Etymotic Research.

Killion, M. C., & Monser, E. L. (1980). CORFIG: Coupler response for flat insertion gain. In G. A. Studebaker & I. Hochberg (Eds.), *Acoustical factors affecting hearing aid performance.* Baltimore, MD: University Park Press.

Killion, M. C., & Mueller, H. G. (2010). Twenty years later: A new count-the-dots method. *Hearing Journal, 63*(1), 10–17.

Killion, M. C., Niquette, P. A., Gudmundsen, G. I., Revit, L. J., & Banerjee, S. (2004). Development of a quick speech-in-noise test for measuring signal-to-noise ratio loss in normal-hearing and hearing-impaired listeners. *Journal of the Acoustical Society of America, 116*(4), 2395–2405.

Killion, M. C., & Revit, L. J. (1987). Insertion gain repeatability versus loudspeaker location: You want me to put my loudspeaker WHERE? *Ear and Hearing, 8*(5), 74s.

Killion, M. C. & Revit, L. (1993). CORGIG and GIFROC: Real ear to coupler and back. In G. A. Studebaker & I. Hochberg (Eds.), *Acoustical factors affecting hearing aid performance-2* (pp. 65–85). Boston, MA: Allyn & Bacon

Kochkin S. (2009). MarkeTrak VIII: 25-year trends in the hearing health market. *Hearing Review, 16*(10), 12–31.

Kochkin, S. (2010). Marketrak VIII: Consumer satisfaction with hearing aids is slowly increasing. *Hearing Journal, 63*(1), 19–27.

Kochkin, S. (2011). MarkeTrak VIII: Reducing patient visits through verification and validation. *Hearing Review, 18*(6), 10–12.

Kochkin, S. (2014). A comparison of consumer satisfaction, subjective benefit, and quality of life changes associated with traditional and direct-mail hearing aid use. *Hearing Review, 21*(1), 16–26.

Kochkin, S., Beck, D. L., Christensen, L. A., Compton-Conley, C., Fligor, B. J., Kricos, P. B., . . . Turner, R. (2010). MarkeTrak VIII: The impact of the hearing healthcare professional on hearing aid user success. *Hearing Review, 17*(4), 12–34.

Leavitt R., & Flexer, C. (2012). The importance of audibility in successful amplification of hearing loss. *Hearing Review, 19*(13), 20–23.

Libby, R. (1986). The 1/3–2/3 insertion gain hearing aid selection guide. *Hearing Instruments, 37*(3), 27–28.

Lybarger, S. F. (1944). *US. Patent application SN 5320 278.* July 3, 1944.

Lybarger, S. F. (1953). *U.S. Patent No. 2,656,421.* Washington, DC: U.S. Patent and Trademark Office.

Lybarger, S. F. (1963). *Simplified fitting system for hearing aids.* Canonsburg, PA: Radioear.

MacKenzie, D. L. (2006). Open-canal fittings and the hearing aid occlusion effect. *Hearing Journal, 59*(11), 50–56.

McArdle, R. A., & Wilson, R. H. (2006). Homogeneity of the 18 QuickSIN[TM] lists. *Journal of the American Academy of Audiology, 17*(3), 157–167.

McCandless, G. A., & Lyregaard, P. E. (1983). Prescription of gain/output (POGO) for hearing aids. *Hearing Instruments, 34*(1), 16–21.

Moodie, S., Pietrobon, J., Rall, E., Lindley, G., Eiten, L., Gordey, D., . . . Scollie, S. (2016). Using the real-ear-to-coupler difference within the American Academy of Audiology Pediatric Amplification Guideline: Protocols for applying and predicting earmold RECDs. *Journal of the American Academy of Audioiology, 27*(3), 264–275.

Moodie, K. S., Seewald, R. C., & Sinclair, S. T. (1994). Procedure for predicting real-ear hearing aid performance in young children. *American Journal of Audiology, 3*(1), 23–31.

Mormer, E., & Palmer, C. V. (2001). *Reliability of hearing aid expectation responses.* Paper presented at the annual meeting of the American Academy of Audiology.

Mueller, H. G. (1989). Individualizing the ordering of custom instruments. *Hearing Instruments, 40*, 18–22

Mueller, H. G. (1990). Probe tube microphone measures: Some opinions on terminology and procedures. *Hearing Journal, 41*(1), 1–5.

Mueller, H. G. (1992a). Terminology and procedures. In H. Mueller, D. Hawkins, & J. Northern (Eds.), *Probe microphone measures* (pp. 41–66). San Diego, CA: Singular.

Mueller, H. G. (1992b). Insertion gain measures. In H. Mueller, D. Hawkins, & J. Northern (Eds.), *Probe microphone measures* (pp. 113–144). San Diego, CA: Singular.

Mueller, H. G. (1994a). CIC hearing aids: What is their impact on the occlusion effect? *Hearing Journal, 47*(11), 29–30.

Mueller, H. G. (1994b). Getting ready for the IHAFF protocol. *Hearing Journal, 47*(6), 10, 46–48.

Mueller, H. G. (1995). Probe-microphone measurements: Unplugged. *Hearing Journal, 48*(1), 10–34.

Mueller, H. G. (1999). Experts debate key fitting issues. *Hearing Journal, 52*(10), 21–32.

Mueller, H. G. (2001a). Probe-mic assessment of digital hearing aids? Yes, you can! *Hearing Journal, 54*(1), 10–12.

Mueller, H. G. (2001b). Probe microphone measures: 20 years of progress. *Trends Amplification, 5*(2),35–68

Mueller, H. G. (2001c, February). Directionality and WDRC. *AudiologyOnline*. Retrieved from http://www.audiologyonline.com/ask-the-experts/directionality-and-wdrc-763

Mueller, H. G. (2003a). In the words of Shakespeare: Fitting test protocols are "more honored in the breach than the observance." *Hearing Journal, 56*(10), 19–20.

Mueller, H. G. (2003b). There is less talking in barrels, but the occlusion effect is still with us. *Hearing Journal, 56*(8), 10.

Mueller, H. G. (2005a). Fitting hearing aids to adults using prescriptive methods: An evidence-based review of effectiveness. *Journal of the American Academy of Audiology, 16*(7), 448–460.

Mueller, H. G. (2005b). Probe-mic measures: Hearing aid fitting's most neglected element. *Hearing Journal, 58*(10), 21–22.

Mueller, H. G. (2006). Hearing aid verification: Old concepts and new considerations. In C. Palmer & R. Seewald (Eds.), *Hearing care for adults* (pp. 155–165). Staefa, Switzerland: Phonak AG.

Mueller, H. G. (2009). A candid round table discussion on open-canal fittings. *Hearing Journal, 62*(4), 19–26.

Mueller, H. G. (2012, April). Sondenschlauchmessung zur Horgerateeinstrellung und Fehlerbehaebung [Probe tube measurement for hearing aid adjustment and troubleshooting]. *Horakustic (In-situ special)*, pp. 25–30.

Mueller, H. G. (2014a). Real-ear probe-microphone measures—30 years of progress? *AudiologyOnline*, Article 12410. Retrieved from http://www.audiologyonline.com

Mueller, H. G. (2014b, July). Trainable hearing aids—friend or foe for the clinician? *AudiologyOnline*, Article 12774. Retrieved from http://www.audiologyonline.com

Mueller, H. G. (2015). Today's use of validated prescriptive fittings—What would Denis say? *AudiologyOnline*, Article 14101. Retrieved from http://www.audiologyonline.com

Mueller, H. G. (2016). Speech-in-noise testing for selection and fitting of hearing aids: Worth the effort? *AudiologyOnline.* Retrieved from http://www.audiologyonline.com/articles/signia-expert-series-speech-in-18336

Mueller, H. G. (2017, February). Why are prescriptive fitting targets below the patient's thresholds? *AudiologyOnline*. Retrieved from http://www.audiologyonline.com

Mueller, H. G., Alexander, J. M., & Scollie, S. (2013). 20Q: Frequency lowering—The whole shebang. *AudiologyOnline*, Article 11913. Retrieved from http://www.audiologyonline.com/articles/20q-frequency-lowering-whole-shebang-11913

Mueller, H. G., & Bentler, R. A. (2005). Fitting hearing aids using clinical measures of loudness discomfort levels: An evidence-based review of effectiveness. *Journal of the American Academy of Audiology*, 16(7), 461–472.

Mueller, H. G., Bentler, R. A., & Wu, Y. H. (2008). Prescribing maximum hearing aid output: Differences among manufacturers found. *Hearing Journal*, 61(3), 30–36.

Mueller, H. G., Bright, K. E., & Northern, J. L. (1996). Studies of the hearing aid occlusion effect. In *Seminars in Hearing*, 17(01), 21–31.

Mueller, H. G., & Ebinger, K. A. (1997). Verification of the performance of CIC hearing aids. In M. Chasin (Ed.), *CIC handbook* (pp. 101–126). San Diego, CA: Singular.

Mueller, H. G., Fabry, D., Kirkwood, D., Smaka, C., Strom, K., & Taylor, B. (2016, January). Hearing aids—the future ain't what is used to be! *AudiologyOnline*, Article 16150. Retrieved from http://www.audiologyonline.com.

Mueller, H. G., & Hall, J. W. (1998). *Audiologists' desk reference* (Vol. 2). San Diego, CA: Singular.

Mueller, H. G., Hawkins, D. B., & Northern, J. L. (1992). *Probe microphone measurements: Hearing aid selection and assessment*. San Diego, CA: Singular.

Mueller, H. G., & Hornsby, B. (2014). Trainable hearing aids: The influence of previous use-gain. *AudiologyOnline*. Retrieved Feb. 3, 2015, from http://www.audiologyonline.com/articles/trainable-hearing-aids-the-influence-12764

Mueller, H. G., Hornsby, B. W., & Weber, J. E. (2008). Using trainable hearing aids to examine real-world preferred gain. *Journal of the American Academy of Audiology*, *19*(10), 758–773.

Mueller, H. G., & Picou, E. M. (2010). Survey examines popularity of real-ear probe-microphone measures. *Hearing Journal*, *63*(5), 27–28.

Mueller, H. G., & Ricketts, T. A. (2006). Open-canal fittings: Ten take-home tips. *Hearing Journal*, *59*(11), 24–26.

Mueller, H. G., Ricketts, T. A., & Bentler, R. A. (2014). *Modern hearing aids book one: Prefitting testing and selection considerations*. San Diego, CA: Plural.

Mueller, H. G. & Strouse, A. L. (1995). Survey shows that user judgment remains dispensers' favorite fitting procedure. *Hearing Journal*, *48*(10), 25–31.

Mueller, H. G., & Sweetow, R. W. (1987). A clinical comparison of probe microphone systems. *Hearing Insruments*, *38*, 19–21, 57.

Nielsen, H. B., & Rasmussen, S. B. (1984). New aspects in hearing aid fittings. *Hearing Instruments*, *35*(1), 18–20.

Painton, S.W. (1993). Objective measure of low frequency amplification reduction in canal hearing aids with adaptive circuitry. *Journal of the American Academy of Audiology*, *4*(3), 152–156.

Palmer, C. V. (2009). Best practice: It's a matter of ethics. *Audiology Today*, *21*(5), 31–35.

Palmer, C. V. (2012, August). Implementing a gain learning feature. *AudiologyOnline*, Article 11244. Retrieved from http://www.audiologyonline.com

Pavlovic, C. V., Studebaker, G. A., & Sherbecoe, R. L. (1986). An articulation index–based procedure for predicting the speech recognition performance of hearing-impaired individuals. *Journal of the Acoustical Society of America*, *80*(1), 50–57.

Pearsons, K., Bennett, L., & Fidell, S. (1977). *Speech levels in various noise environments*. (Report No. EPA-600/1-77-025). Washington, D.C.: U.S. Environmental Protection Agency.

Picou, E. M., & Ricketts, T. A. (2011). Comparison of wireless and acoustic hearing aid–based telephone listening strategies. *Ear and Hearing*, *32*(2), 209–220.

Picou, E. M., & Ricketts, T. A. (2013). Efficacy of hearing-aid based telephone strategies for listeners with moderate-to-severe hearing loss. *Journal of the American Academy of Audiology*, *24*(1), 59–70.

Plomp, R. (1984). Perception of speech as a modulated signal. In A. Cohen & M. P. R. van de Broecke (Eds.), *Proceedings of the Tenth International Congress of Phonetic Sciences* (pp. 29–40).

Protocol for the Provision of Amplification. (2014). M Bagatto & S. Scollie (Eds.). Retrieved from https://www.dslio.com/wp-content/uploads/2015/05/DSL5-Pediatric-Protocol.2014.01.pdf

Pumford, J., & Sinclair, S. (2001). Real-ear measurement: Basic terminology and procedures.

AudiologyOnline, Article 1229. Retrieved from http://www.audiologyonline.com

Revit L. (1991). New thinking on the proper application of real-ear unaided response measurements to prescriptions and fittings. *New Zealand Audiological Society Bulletin*, *1*, 1–17.

Revit, L. (1997). The circle of decibels: Relating the hearing test, to the hearing instrument, to real-ear response. *Hearing Review*, *4*, 35–38.

Ricketts, T., Johnson, E., & Federman, J. (2008). Individual differences within and across feedback suppression hearing aids. *Journal of the American Academy of Audiology*, *19*(10), 748–757.

Ricketts, T., Lindley, G., & Henry, P. (2001). Impact of compression and hearing aid style on directional hearing aid benefit and performance. *Ear and Hearing*, *22*(4), 348-361.

Sachs, R. M., & Burkhard, M. D. (1972). *Earphone pressure response in ears and couplers* (Report No. 20021-2). Elk Grove Village, IL: Industrial Research Products.

Sanders, J., Stoody, T. M., Weber, J. E., & Mueller, H. G. (2015). Manufacturer's NAL-NL2 fittings fail real-ear verification. *Hearing Review*, *21*(3), 24.

Saunders, G. H., & Morgan, D. E. (2003). Impact on hearing aid targets of measuring thresholds in dB HL versus dB SPL. *International Journal of Audiology*, *42*(6), 319–326.

Schwartz, D., Lyregaard, P., & Lundh, P. (1988). Hearing aid selection for severe-to-profound hearing loss. *Hearing Journal*, *41*(2), 13–17.

Schweitzer, H. C., Sullivan, R. F., Beck, L. B., & Cole, W. A. (1990). Developing a consensus for "real ear" hearing aid terms. *Hearing Instruments*, *41*(2) 28, 46.

Scollie, S. (2007, January). DSL version v5.0: Description and early results in children. *AudiologyOnline*. Retrieved from http://www.audiologyonline.com/articles/dsl-version-v5-0-description-959

Scollie, S. (2013, May). The ins and outs of frequency lowering amplification. *AudiologyOnline*, Article 11863. Retrieved from http:www.audiologyonline.com/

Scollie, S., Glista, D., Seto, J., Dunn, A., Schuett, B., Hawkins, M., . . . Parsa, V. (2016). Fitting frequency-lowering signal processing applying the American Academy of Audiology pediatric amplification guideline: Updates and protocols. *Journal American Academy Audiology*, *27*(3), 219–236.

Scollie, S., & Seewald, R. (2002). Evaluation of electroacoustic test signals I: Comparison with amplified speech. *Ear and Hearing*, *23*(5), 477–487.

Scollie, S., Seewald, R., Cornelisse, L., Moodie, S., Bagatto, M., Laurnagaray, D., . . . Pumford, J. (2005). The desired sensation level multistage input/output algorithm. *Trends in Amplification*, *9*(4), 159–197.

Seewald, R. C., Cornelisse, L. E., Richert, F. M., & Block, M. G. (1997). Acoustic transforms for fitting CIC instruments. In M. Chasin, (Ed), *CIC handbook* (pp. 83–100). San Diego, CA: Singular.

Seewald, R. C., Moodie, S., Scollie, S., & Bagatto, M. (2005). The DSL method for pediatric hearing instrument fitting: Historical perspective and current issues. *Trends in Amplification*, *9*(4), 145–157.

Seewald, R. C., Moodie, K. S., Sinclair, S. T., & Scollie, S. D. (1999). Predictive validity of a procedure for pediatric hearing instrument fitting. *American Journal of Audiology*, *8*(2), 143–152.

Seewald, R. C., Ramji, K. V., Sinclair, S. T., Moodie, K. S., & Jamieson, D. G. (1993). *A computer-assisted implementation of the desired sensation level method for electroacousticselection and fitting in children: User's manual.* London, ON: Hearing Health Care Research Unit.

Seewald, R. C., Ross, M., & Spiro, M. K. (1985). Selecting amplification characteristics for young hearing-impaired children. *Ear and Hearing*, *6*(1), 48–53.

Shaw, E. A. G. (1974). Transformation of sound pressure from the free field to the eardrum in the horizontal plane. *Journal of Acoustical Society of America*, *56*, 1848–1861.

Shaw, E. A. G., & Vaillancourt, M. M. (1985). Transformation of sound-pressure level from the free field to the eardrum presented in numerical form. *Journal of the Acoustical Society of America, 78*(3), 1120–1123.

Smeds, K., Wolters, F., & Rung, M. (2015). Estimation of signal-to-noise ratios in realistic sound scenarios. *Journal of the American Academy of Audiology, 26*(2), 183–196.

Souza, P. E., Arehart, K. H., Kates, J. M., Croghan, N. B., & Gehani, N. (2013). Exploring the limits of frequency lowering. *Journal of Speech, Language, and Hearing Research, 56*(5), 1349–1363.

Stelmachowicz, P. (1991). *Clinical issues related to hearing aid maximum output*. In G. Studebaker, F. Bess, & L. Beck (Eds.), *The Vanderbilt Hearing Aid Report II* (pp 141–145). Parkton, MD: York Press.

Stender, T., & Appleby, R. (2009). Occlusion effect measures: Are they all created equal? *Hearing Journal, 62*(7), 21–24.

Storey, L., & Dillon, H. (2001). Estimating the location of probe microphones relative to the tympanic membrane. *Journal of the American Academy of Audiology, 12*(3), 150–154.

Sullivan, R. F. (1988). Probe tube microphone placement near the tympanic membrane. *Hearing Instruments, 39*(7), 43–50.

Tecca, J. (1991). Real-ear vent effects in ITE hearing instrument fittings. *Hearing Instruments, 42*(12), 10–12.

Thornton, A. R., & Raffin, M. J. M. (1978). Speech discrimination scores modeled as a binomial variable. *Journal of Speech and Hearing Research*, 21(3), 507–518.

Vaisberg, J.M., Macpherson, E.A., & Scollie, S. D. (2016). Extended bandwidth real-ear measurement accuracy and repeatability to 10 kHz. *International Journal Audiology. 55*(10), 580–586.

Valente, M. (1990). Intratester and test-retest reliability of insertion gain measures. *Ear and Hearing, 11*,181–184.

Valente, M., Oeding,K., Brockmeyer, A., Smith, S., & Kallogieri, D. (2017). *Differences in word recognition in quiet, sentence recognition in noise, and subjective preference between manufacturer first-fit and hearing aids programmed to NAL-NL2 using real-ear measures.* Manuscript submitted for publication.

Valente, M., Potts, L. G., Valente, M., & Goebel, J. (1995). Wireless CROS versus transcranial CROS for unilateral hearing loss. *American Journal of Audiology, 4*(1), 52–59.

Watson, L., & Tolan, T. (1949). *Hearing tests and hearing instruments*. Baltimore, MD: Williams and Wilkins.

Wiener, F. M., & Ross, D. A. (1946). The pressure distribution in the auditory canal in a progressive sound field. *Journal of the Acoustical Society of America, 18*(2), 401–408.

Wilson, R. H., & McArdle, R. (2008). A change is in the air. *Hearing Journal, 61*(10), 10–15.

Appendix A

SII 2010 Revision of the 1990 Mueller and Killion Count-The-Dots Audiogram

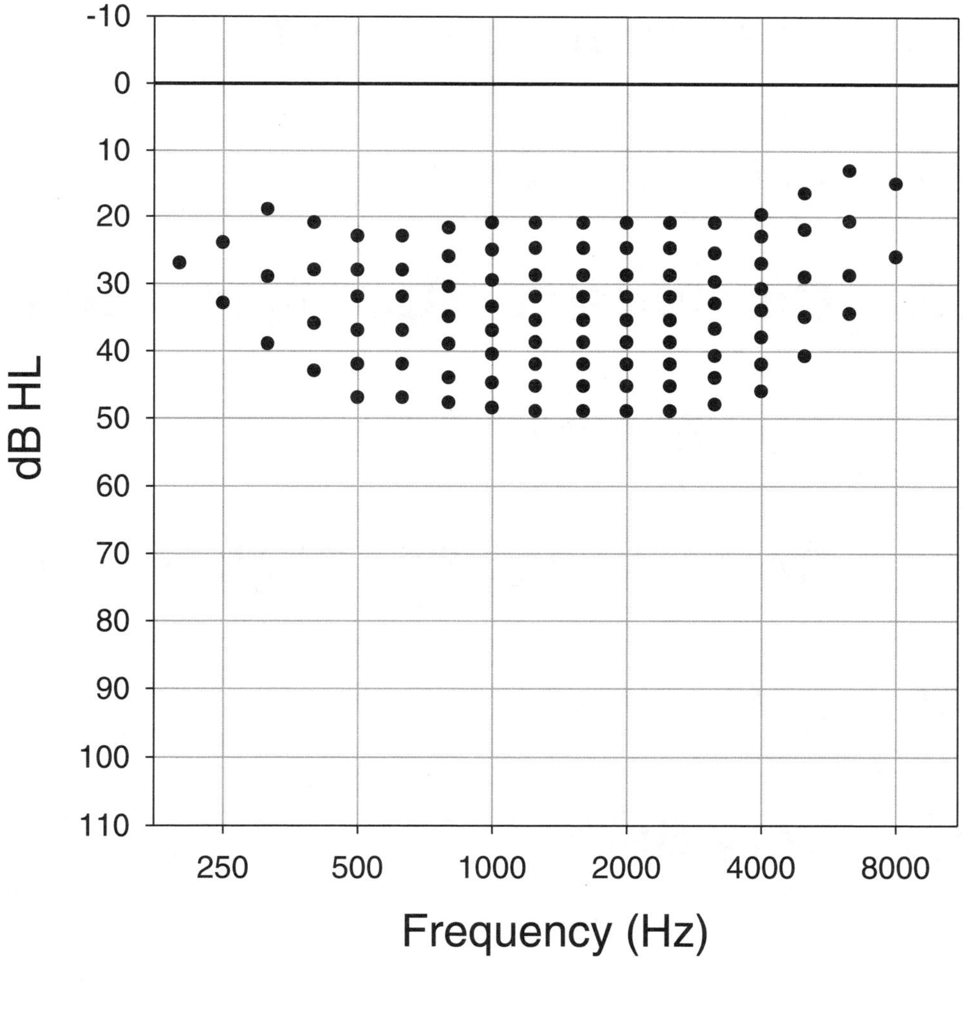

Appendix B

LDL Loudness Anchors

#7. Uncomfortably Loud

#6. Loud, But Okay

#5. Comfortable, But Slightly Loud

#4. Comfortable

#3. Comfortable, But Slightly Soft

#2. Soft

#1. Very Soft

Appendix C

LDL Instructions

The purpose of this test is to find your judgments of the loudness of different sounds.

You will hear sounds that increase and decrease in volume. You must make a judgment about how loud the sounds are. Pretend you are listening to the radio at that volume. How loud would it be?

After each sound, tell me which of these categories best describes the loudness. It is okay to repeat a loudness category, and it is okay to skip a category.

Keep in mind that an uncomfortably loud sound is louder than you would ever choose on your radio no matter what mood you are in.

Appendix D

Thornton and Raffin (1978) Binomial Model Critical Differences at the .05 Confidence Level

Score %	*N* = 50	*N* = 25	Score %	N = 50	N = 25
0	0–4	0–8	52	34–70	28–76
2	0–10		54	36–72	
4	0–14	0–20	56	38–74	32–80
6	2–18		58	40–76	
8	2–22	0–28	60	42–78	36–84
10	2–24		62	44–78	
12	4–26	4–32	64	46–80	40–64
14	4–30		66	48–82	
16	6–32	4–40	68	50–84	44–88
18	6–34		70	52–86	
20	8–36	4–44	72	54–86	48–92
22	8–40		74	56–88	
24	10–42	8–48	76	58–90	52–92
26	12–44		78	60–92	
28	14–46	8–52	80	64–92	56–96
30	14–48		82	66–94	
32	16–50	12–56	84	68–94	60–96
34	18–52		86	70–96	
36	20–54	16–60	88	74–96	68–96
38	22–56		90	76–98	
40	22–58	16–64	92	78–98	72–100
42	24–60		94	82–98	
44	26–62	20–68	96	86–100	80–100
46	28–64		98	90–100	
48	30–66	24–72	100	96–100	92–100
50	32–68				

Appendix E

Hearing Handicap for the Elderly (HHIE)–Screening

Name: ______________________________ Date: ______________

The purpose of this scale is to identify the problems your hearing loss may be causing you. Check "Yes," "Sometimes," or "No" for each question. Do not skip any questions. If you use a hearing aid, please answer the way you hear without a hearing aid.

	Yes	Sometimes	No
1. Does a hearing problem cause you to feel embarrassed when meeting new people?			
2. Does a hearing problem cause you to feel frustrated when talking to members of your family?			
3. Do you have difficulty hearing when someone speaks in a whisper?			
4. Do you feel handicapped by a hearing problem?			
5. Does a hearing problem cause you difficulty when visiting friends, relatives, or neighbors?			
6. Does a hearing problem cause you to attend religious services less often than you would like?			
7. Does a hearing problem cause you to have arguments with family members?			
8. Does a hearing problem cause you difficulty when listening to TV or radio?			
9. Do you feel that any difficulty with your hearing limits or hampers your personal or social life?			
10. Does a hearing problem cause you difficulty when in a restaurant with relatives or friends?			

Appendix F

Hearing Handicap for Adults (HHIA)-Screening

Name: ______________________________ Date: ____________________

The purpose of this scale is to identify the problems your hearing loss may be causing you. Check "Yes," "Sometimes," or "No" for each question. Do not skip any questions. If you use a hearing aid, please answer the way you hear without a hearing aid.

	Yes	Sometimes	No
1. Does a hearing problem cause you to feel embarrassed when meeting new people?			
2. Does a hearing problem cause you to feel frustrated when talking to members of your family?			
3. Does a hearing problem cause you difficulty hearing/understanding co-workers, clients, or customers?			
4. Do you feel handicapped by a hearing problem?			
5. Does a hearing problem cause you difficulty when visiting friends, relatives, or neighbors?			
6. Does a hearing problem cause you difficulty in the movies or theater?			
7. Does a hearing problem cause you to have arguments with family members?			
8. Does a hearing problem cause you difficulty when listening to TV or radio?			
9. Do you feel that any difficulty with your hearing limits or hampers your personal or social life?			
10. Does a hearing problem cause you difficulty when in a restaurant with relatives or friends?			

Appendix G

Abbreviated Profile of Hearing Aid Benefit

NAME: ______________________________ ☐ Male ☐ Female TODAY'S DATE: ___/___/___
Last *First*

INSTRUCTIONS: Please circle the answers that come closest to your everyday experience. Notice that each choice includes a percentage. You can use this to help you decide on your answer. For example, if a statement is true about 75% of the time, circle "C" for that item. If you have not experienced the situation we describe, try to think of a similar situation that you have been in and respond for that situation. If you have no idea, leave that item blank.

A Always (99%)
B Almost Always (87%)
C Generally (75%)
D Half-the-time (50%)
E Occasionally (25%)
F Seldom (12%)
G Never (1%)

	Without Hearing Aid	With Hearing Aid
1. When I am in a crowded grocery store, talking with the cashier, I can follow the conversation.	A B C D E F G	A B C D E F G
2. I miss a lot of information when I'm listening to a lecture.	A B C D E F G	A B C D E F G
3. Unexpected sounds, like a smoke detector or alarm bell are uncomfortable.	A B C D E F G	A B C D E F G
4. I have difficulty hearing a conversation when I'm with one of my family at home.	A B C D E F G	A B C D E F G
5. I have trouble understanding the dialogue in a movie or at the theater.	A B C D E F G	A B C D E F G
6. When I am listening to the news on the car radio, and family members are talking, I have trouble hearing the news.	A B C D E F G	A B C D E F G
7. When I'm at the dinner table with several people, and am trying to have a conversation with one person, understanding speech is difficult.	A B C D E F G	A B C D E F G
8. Traffic noises are too loud.	A B C D E F G	A B C D E F G
9. When I am talking with someone across a large empty room, I understand the words.	A B C D E F G	A B C D E F G
10. When I am in a small office, interviewing or answering questions, I have difficulty following the conversation.	A B C D E F G	A B C D E F G
11. When I am in a theater watching a movie or play, and the people around me are whispering and rustling paper wrappers, I can still make out the dialogue.	A B C D E F G	A B C D E F G
12. When I am having a quiet conversation with a friend, I have difficulty understanding.	A B C D E F G	A B C D E F G

continues

A **Always (99%)**
B **Almost Always (87%)**
C **Generally (75%)**
D **Half-the-time (50%)**
E **Occasionally (25%)**
F **Seldom (12%)**
G **Never (1%)**

	Without Hearing Aids	With Hearing Aids
13. The sounds of running water, such as a toilet or shower, are uncomfortably loud.	A B C D E F G	A B C D E F G
14. When a speaker is addressing a small group, and everyone is listening quietly, I have to strain to understand.	A B C D E F G	A B C D E F G
15. When I'm in a quiet conversation with my doctor in an examination room, it is hard to follow the conversation.	A B C D E F G	A B C D E F G
16. I can understand conversations even when several people are talking.	A B C D E F G	A B C D E F G
17. The sounds of construction work are uncomfortably loud.	A B C D E F G	A B C D E F G
18. It's hard for me to understand what is being said at lectures or church services.	A B C D E F G	A B C D E F G
19. I can communicate with others when we are in a crowd.	A B C D E F G	A B C D E F G
20. The sound of a fire engine siren close by is so loud that I need to cover my ears.	A B C D E F G	A B C D E F G
21. I can follow the words of a sermon when listening to a religious service.	A B C D E F G	A B C D E F G
22. The sound of screeching tires is uncomfortably loud.	A B C D E F G	A B C D E F G
23. I have to ask people to repeat themselves in one-on-one conversation in a quiet room.	A B C D E F G	A B C D E F G
24. I have trouble understanding others when an air conditioner or fan is on.	A B C D E F G	A B C D E F G

Please fill out these additional items.

HEARING AID EXPERIENCE:	DAILY HEARING AID USE	DEGREE OF HEARING DIFFICULTY (without wearing a hearing aid):
☐ None	☐ None	☐ None
☐ Less than 6 weeks	☐ Less than 1 hour per day	☐ Mild
☐ 6 weeks to 11 months	☐ 1 to 4 hours per day	☐ Moderate
☐ 1 to 10 years	☐ 4 to 8 hours per day	☐ Moderately-Severe
☐ Over 10 years	☐ 8 to 16 hours per day	☐ Severe

HARL
Hearing Aid Research Lab

Appendix H

ECHO Questionnaire

NAME ______________________ GENDER M F DATE OF BIRTH ___/___/___ TODAY'S DATE ___/___/___

INSTRUCTIONS
Listed below are statements about hearing aids. Please circle the letter that indicates the extent to which you agree with each statement. Use the list of words on the right to determine your answer.

A Not At All
B A Little
C Somewhat
D Medium
E Considerably
F Greatly
G Tremendously

How much do you agree with each statement?

1. My hearing aids will help me understand the people I speak with most frequently.	A B C D E F G
2. I will be frustrated when my hearing aids pick up sounds that keep me from hearing what I want to hear.	A B C D E F G
3. Getting hearing aids is in my best interest.	A B C D E F G
4. People will notice my hearing loss more when I wear my hearing aids.	A B C D E F G
5. My hearing aids will reduce the number of times I have to ask people to repeat.	A B C D E F G
6. My hearing aids will be worth the trouble.	A B C D E F G
7. Sometimes I will be bothered by an inability to get enough loudness from my hearing aids without feedback (whistling).	A B C D E F G
8. I will be content with the appearance of my hearing aids.	A B C D E F G
9. Using hearing aids will improve my self-confidence.	A B C D E F G

continues

A **Not At All**
B **A Little**
C **Somewhat**
D **Medium**
E **Considerably**
F **Greatly**
G **Tremendously**

How much do you agree with each statement?

10. My hearing aids will have a natural sound.	A B C D E F G
11. My hearing aids will be helpful on most telephones without amplifiers or loudspeakers. (If you hear well on the telephone *without* hearing aids, check here ☐)	A B C D E F G
12. The person who provides me with my hearing aids will be competent.	A B C D E F G
13. Wearing my hearing aids will make me seem less capable.	A B C D E F G
14. The cost of my hearing aids will be reasonable.	A B C D E F G
15. My hearing aids will be dependable (need few repairs).	A B C D E F G

Please respond to these additional items.

LIFETIME HEARING AID EXPERIENCE (includes all old and current hearing aids)	DAILY HEARING AID USE	DEGREE OF HEARING DIFFICULTY (without wearing a hearing aid)
☐ None ☐ Less than 6 weeks ☐ 6 weeks to 11 months ☐ 1 to 10 years ☐ Over 10 years	☐ None ☐ Less than 1 hour per day ☐ 1 to 4 hours per day ☐ 4 to 8 hours per day ☐ 8 to 16 hours per day	☐ None ☐ Mild ☐ Moderate ☐ Moderately Severe ☐ Severe

HARL
Hearing Aid Research Lab.

Appendix I

Client Oriented Scale of Improvement

National Acoustic Laboratories
A division of Australian Hearing

NAL
CLIENT ORIENTED SCALE OF IMPROVEMENT

Name : ______________ **Category.** **New** ____
Audiologist : ______________ **Return** ____
Date : **1. Needs Established** ______
2. Outcome Assessed ______

SPECIFIC NEEDS

Indicate Order of Significance

Specific Needs	Degree of Change: Worse	No Difference	Slightly Better	Better	Much Better	CATEGORY	Final Ability (with hearing aid) — Person can hear: Hardly Ever (10%)	Occasionally (25%)	Half the Time (50%)	Most of Time (75%)	Almost Always (95%)
☐											
☐											
☐											
☐											
☐											

Categories

1. Conversation with 1 or 2 in quiet
2. Conversation with 1 or 2 in noise
3. Conversation with group in quiet
4. Conversation with group in noise
5. Television/Radio @ normal volume
6. Familiar speaker on phone
7. Unfamiliar speaker on phone
8. Hearing phone ring from another room
9. Hear front door bell or knock
10. Hear traffic
11. Increased social contact
12. Feel embarrassed or stupid
13. Feeling left out
14. Feeling upset or angry
15. Church or meeting
16. Other

Appendix J

Profile of Aided Loudness

PROFILE OF AIDED LOUDNESS

Name: ______________________________

Date: ______________________________

Status: __ unaided __ previous hearing aids
___ current hearing aids

Instructions: Please rate the following items by both the level of loudness of the sound and by the appropriateness of that loudness level. For example, you might rate a particular sound as "Very Soft." If "Very Soft" is your preferred level for this sound, then you would rate your loudness satisfaction as "Just Right." If, on the other hand, you think the sound should be louder than "Very Soft", then your loudness satisfaction rating might be "Not Too Good" or "Not Good At All." The Loudness Satisfaction rating is not related to how pleasing the sound is to you, but rather, the appropriateness of the loudness. Here is an example:

The hum of a refrigerator motor:

Loudness rating	Satisfaction rating
0 Do not hear	(5.) Just right
1 Very soft	4. Pretty good
(2) Soft	3. Okay
3 Comfortable, but slightly soft	2. Not too good
4 Comfortable	1. Not good at all
5 Comfortable, but slightly loud	
6 Loud, but OK	
7 Uncomfortably loud	

In this example, the hearing aid user rated the loudness level of a refrigerator motor running as "Comfortable, but slightly soft" and rated his loudness satisfaction for this sound as "Just right." This satisfaction rating indicates that the person believes that it is appropriate for a refrigerator motor to sound "Comfortable, but slightly soft."

Circle the responses that best describe your listening experiences. If you have not experienced one of the sounds listed (or a similar sound), simply leave that question blank.

1. An electric razor:

Loudness rating	Satisfaction rating
0 Do not hear	5. Just right
1 Very soft	4. Pretty good
2 Soft	3. Okay
3 Comfortable, but slightly soft	2. Not too good
4 Comfortable	1. Not good at all
5 Comfortable, but slightly loud	
6 Loud, but OK	
7 Uncomfortably loud	

2. A door slamming:

Loudness rating	Satisfaction rating
0 Do not hear	5. Just right
1 Very soft	4. Pretty good
2 Soft	3. Okay
3 Comfortable, but slightly soft	2. Not too good
4 Comfortable	1. Not good at all
5 Comfortable, but slightly loud	
6 Loud, but OK	
7 Uncomfortably loud	

3. Your own breathing:

Loudness rating	Satisfaction rating
0 Do not hear	5. Just right
1 Very soft	4. Pretty good
2 Soft	3. Okay
3 Comfortable, but slightly soft	2. Not too good
4 Comfortable	1. Not good at all
5 Comfortable, but slightly loud	
6 Loud, but OK	
7 Uncomfortably loud	

4. Water boiling on the stove:

Loudness rating	Satisfaction rating
0 Do not hear	5. Just right
1 Very soft	4. Pretty good
2 Soft	3. Okay
3 Comfortable, but slightly soft	2. Not too good
4 Comfortable	1. Not good at all
5 Comfortable, but slightly loud	
6 Loud, but OK	
7 Uncomfortably loud	

5. A car's turn signal:

Loudness rating	Satisfaction rating
0 Do not hear	5. Just right
1 Very soft	4. Pretty good
2 Soft	3. Okay
3 Comfortable, but slightly soft	2. Not too good
4 Comfortable	1. Not good at all
5 Comfortable, but slightly loud	
6 Loud, but OK	
7 Uncomfortably loud	

6. The religious leader during the sermon:

Loudness rating	Satisfaction rating
0 Do not hear	5. Just right
1 Very soft	4. Pretty good
2 Soft	3. Okay
3 Comfortable, but slightly soft	2. Not too good
4 Comfortable	1. Not good at all
5 Comfortable, but slightly loud	
6 Loud, but OK	
7 Uncomfortably loud	

7. The dryer running:

Loudness rating	Satisfaction rating
0 Do not hear	5. Just right
1 Very soft	4. Pretty good
2 Soft	3. Okay
3 Comfortable, but slightly soft	2. Not too good
4 Comfortable	1. Not good at all
5 Comfortable, but slightly loud	
6 Loud, but OK	
7 Uncomfortably loud	

8. You chewing soft food:

Loudness rating	Satisfaction rating
0 Do not hear	5. Just right
1 Very soft	4. Pretty good
2 Soft	3. Okay
3 Comfortable, but slightly soft	2. Not too good
4 Comfortable	1. Not good at all
5 Comfortable, but slightly loud	
6 Loud, but OK	
7 Uncomfortably loud	

9. Listening to a marching band:

Loudness rating	Satisfaction rating
0 Do not hear	5. Just right
1 Very soft	4. Pretty good
2 Soft	3. Okay
3 Comfortable, but slightly soft	2. Not too good
4 Comfortable	1. Not good at all
5 Comfortable, but slightly loud	
6 Loud, but OK	
7 Uncomfortably loud	

10. A barking dog:

Loudness rating	Satisfaction rating
0 Do not hear	5. Just right
1 Very soft	4. Pretty good
2 Soft	3. Okay
3 Comfortable, but slightly soft	2. Not too good
4 Comfortable	1. Not good at all
5 Comfortable, but slightly loud	
6 Loud, but OK	
7 Uncomfortably loud	

11. A lawn mower:

Loudness rating	Satisfaction rating
0 Do not hear	5. Just right
1 Very soft	4. Pretty good
2 Soft	3. Okay
3 Comfortable, but slightly soft	2. Not too good
4 Comfortable	1. Not good at all
5 Comfortable, but slightly loud	
6 Loud, but OK	
7 Uncomfortably loud	

12. A microwave buzzer sounding:

Loudness rating	Satisfaction rating
0 Do not hear	5. Just right
1 Very soft	4. Pretty good
2 Soft	3. Okay
3 Comfortable, but slightly soft	2. Not too good
4 Comfortable	1. Not good at all
5 Comfortable, but slightly loud	
6 Loud, but OK	
7 Uncomfortably loud	

Take an average score for soft, average, and loud sounds and compare the scores to the average scores of normally hearing individuals. The patient summary sheet is used for this type of scoring. In this manner, the clinician may compare unaided loudness perception to aided loudness perception as well as having a numeric target for the aided condition.

PATIENT SUMMARY
Profile of Aided Loudness (PAL)
Unaided Performance

Soft sounds	Q3	Q4	Q5	Q8	Category average
Loudness	___	___	___	___	____(target = 2)
Satisfaction	___	___	___	___	____

Average sounds	Q1	Q6	Q7	Q12	Category average
Loudness	___	___	___	___	____(target = 4)
Satisfaction	___	___	___	___	____

Loud sounds	Q2	Q9	Q10	Q11	Category average
Loudness	___	___	___	___	____(target = 6)
Satisfaction	___	___	___	___	____

Aided Performance

Soft sounds	Q3	Q4	Q5	Q8	Category average
Loudness	___	___	___	___	____(target = 2)
Satisfaction	___	___	___	___	____

Average sounds	Q1	Q6	Q7	Q12	Category average
Loudness	___	___	___	___	____(target = 4)
Satisfaction	___	___	___	___	____

Loud sounds	Q2	Q9	Q10	Q11	Category average
Loudness	___	___	___	___	____(target = 6)
Satisfaction	___	___	___	___	____

Appendix K

Normative Data for PAL

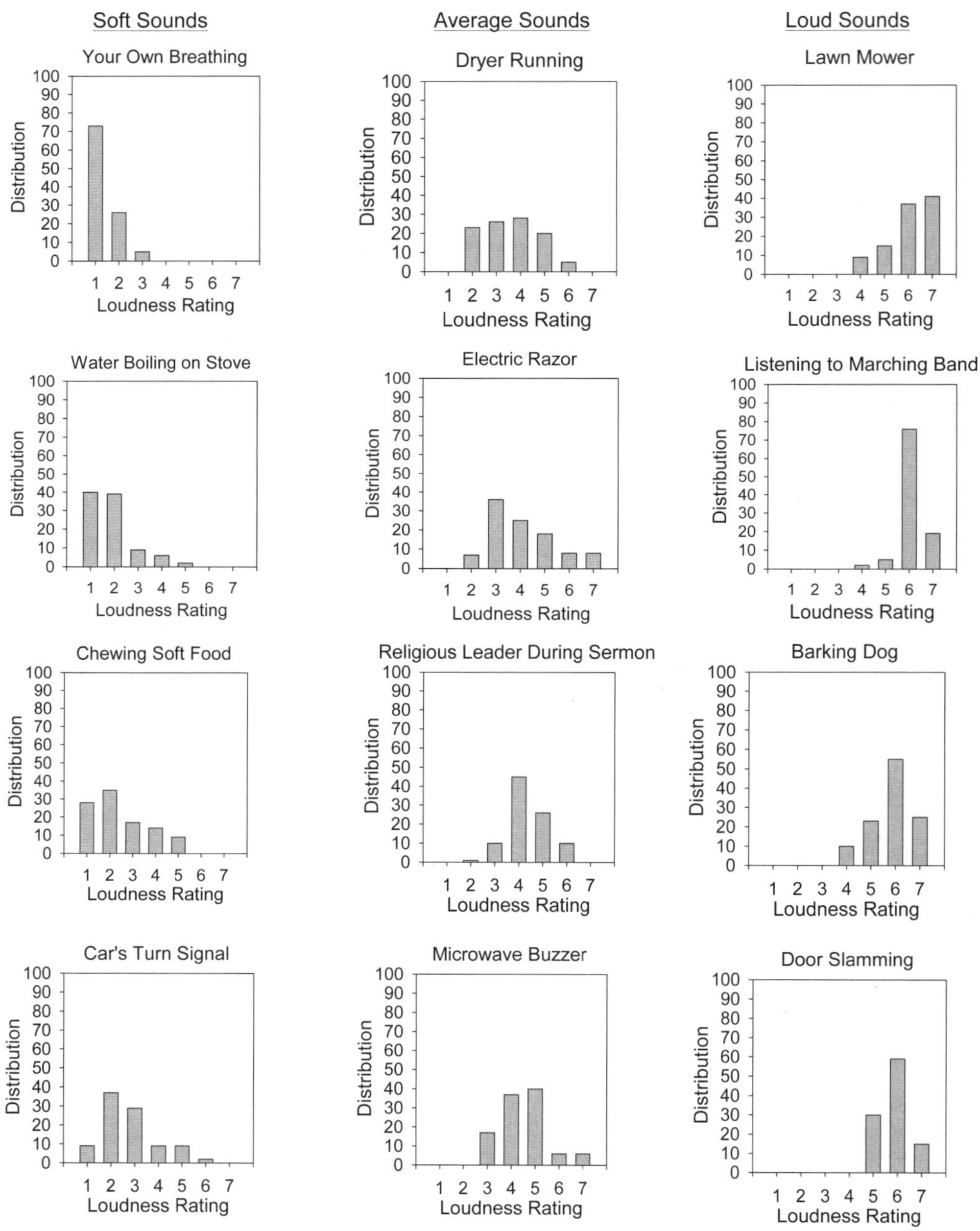

Appendix L

International Outcome Inventory for Hearing Aids (IOI-HA)

1. Think about how much you used your present hearing aid(s) over the past two weeks. On an average day, how many hours did you use the hearing aid(s)?

none	less than 1 hour a day	1 to 4 hours a day	4 to 8 hours a day	more than 8 hours a day
☐	☐	☐	☐	☐

2. Think about the situation where you most wanted to hear better, before you got your present hearing aid(s). Over the past two weeks, how much has the hearing aid helped in those situations?

helped not at all	helped slightly	helped moderately	helped quite a lot	helped very much
☐	☐	☐	☐	☐

3. Think again about the situation where you most wanted to hear better. When you use your present hearing aid(s), how much difficulty do you STILL have in that situation?

very much difficulty	quite a lot of difficulty	moderate difficulty	Slight difficulty	no difficulty
☐	☐	☐	☐	☐

4. Considering everything, do you think your present hearing aid(s) is worth the trouble?

not at all worth it	Slightly worth it	Moderately worth it	quite a lot worth it	very much worth it
☐	☐	☐	☐	☐

5. Over the past two weeks, with your present hearing aid(s), how much have your hearing difficulties affected the things you can do?

affected very much	affected quite a lot	affected moderately	affected slightly	affected not at all
☐	☐	☐	☐	☐

6. Over the past two weeks, with your present hearing aid(s), how much do you think other people were bothered by your hearing difficulties?

bothered very much	bothered quite a lot	bothered moderately	bothered slightly	bothered not at all
☐	☐	☐	☐	☐

7. Considering everything, how much has your present hearing aid(s) changed your enjoyment of life?

worse	no change	slightly better	quite a lot better	Very much better
☐	☐	☐	☐	☐

8. How much hearing difficulty do you have when you are **not** wearing a hearing aid?

severe	moderately-severe	moderate	mild	none
☐	☐	☐	☐	☐

Printed May 3, 2005

Appendix M

IOI-HA Norm Template for Individual Scores

Cox, Alexander, & Beyer, 2002

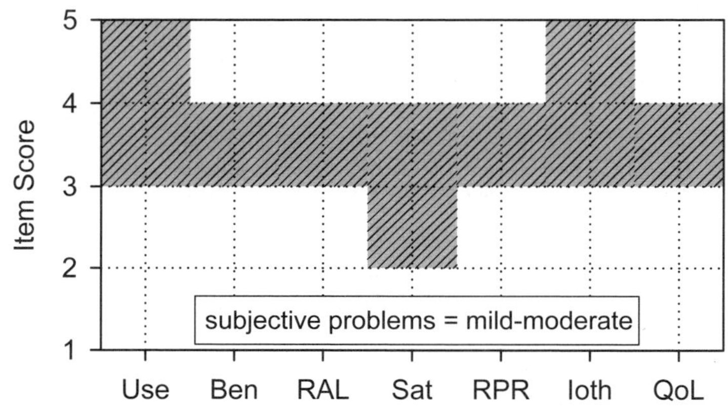

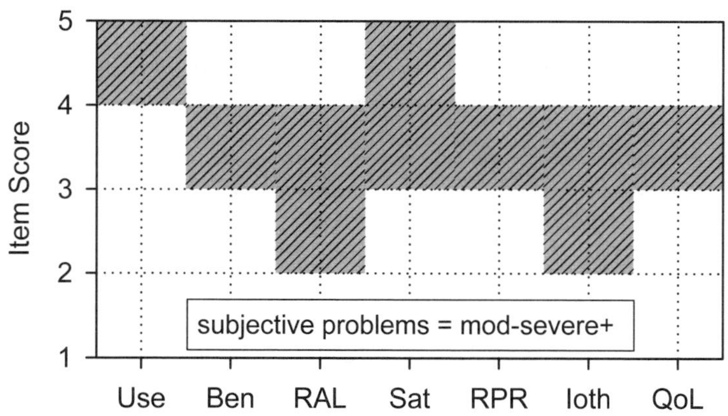

Index

Note: Page numbers in **bold** reference non-text material.

A

Aarts, N.L., 27
Aazh, H., 24, 25
Abbreviated Profile of Hearing Aid Benefit (APHAB)
  about, 216–217, 230
  case study, 236–237, **237–239**
  instrument for, 237, **285–286**
  post-fitting, 21–23, 233, 235–237
  pre-fitting, 230
  scoring of, 237
  subscales of, 235
Abrams, H.B., 21, 22
  subscales of, 235
Acclimatization, 264–265
Acoustic positioning of probe tube, 98–99, 101
Acoustically assisted positioning of probe tube, 99
Acoustimed, probe microphone product, viii
"Acronym Jim," **235**
AGCi/AGCo. *See* Automatic gain control-input (output)
AGI, 257
Aided audiogram, **156**, **157**
Aided speech recognition, 217–221
Air-bone gap, DSL v5.0 vs. NAL-NL2, 56
Alamudi, K., 18
Alexander, G.C., 20
Ambient noise probe microphone measurement and, 89, **90**
American Academy of Audiology (AAA), 4, 7
American Speech-Language-Hearing Association (ASHA), 4, 7, 66
Amlani, A.M., 35
Ampclusion, **190**
ANSI standards, 105
  ANSI S3.46-2013, 83, 105, 106
  ANSI S3.6-2010, 208
  for RECD measurement, **138**, **139–140**
APHAB. *See* Abbreviated Profile of Hearing Aid Benefit
Audibility, 77, **81**, 198, 199
  effective audibility, 77, **155**
  percent audibility, **199**
  REAR for assessment of, 127–128
Audiogram
  count-the-dot audiogram, 198–200, **199**, **279**
  for pre-fitting counseling, 198–200, **199**
  for predicting LDLs, 204–205, **205**
  speech banana, 74, 198–199, **199**, **200**, 253, 267, **279**
Audiologists
  "listening in," 86
  reasons for not using probe microphone measures, 8–10
  training, 9–10, **9**
Audiology, origin of term, **40**
Audiometer, 223–225
Auditory acclimatization, 264–265
Aurora (Nicolet), viii
Automated real-ear verification, **104**
Automatic gain control-input (AGCi), **203**
Automatic gain control-output (AGCo), **203**, 221, 225
Aversiveness subscale, 235

B

Background Noise subscale, 235
Bagatto, M., 47
Bentler, R.A., 11, 202, 204, 205, 226, 230, 242
Berger method, 42
Berlin, Chuck, **235**
Bernafon hearing aids, vii
Berra, Lawrence "Yogi," 37
Best Practice Guidelines, 4–7, **6**, 30
Bilateral CROS, 183
Bilateral fittings, DSL v5.0 vs. NAL-NL2, 55
Bilateral loudness testing, **223**, 246
Bilateral testing, **87**, 93, 246
Binaural (bilateral) summation, 221–222
Binomial Model Critical Differences, **282**
Bosch, probe microphone product, viii
Boyle, Robert, **139**
Boyle's law, **139**
Brew, C., 11
Broadband output limiting thresholds (BOLT), 52
Brockmeyer, A., 22, 23
Brown noise, 68
Bump-and-pull method, 99
Burkhard, M.D., 140
Byrne, Denis, 11, 38, 45, 60, 71, **72**
Byrne and Tonisson method, 45

C

Caffee, C.S., 27
Calibration, of probe tube, 89, 91–92, **92**
Carhart, Raymond, 40, **40**
Carter, L., **56**
CCI-10 (Rastronics), vii
Cerumen, 101, 249
Channel summation, 222
Characteristics of Amplification Tool (COAT), 217
Cherry, Colin, **211**
Children
  probe tube placement, 250
  RECD use with, 137–138, **139–140**, 140, **141**, 142
Chisolm, T.H., 21, 22
Circle of Decibels, 148, **148**
Client Oriented Scale of Improvement (COSI)
  about, 217, **230**, **234**
  case study, 233
  post-fitting, 230–231, **230**, 233, **234**
  pre-fitting, 217, 230–231, **232**
  scale of improvement for, **289**
Closed-loop self-verifying hearing aids, **104**
COAT. *See* Characteristics of Amplification Tool
Cocktail party effect, **211**
Cole, Bill, 3
Connected Speech Test (CST), 211
Constant insertion depth method, 96–97
Contralateral routing of offside signal (CROS) fittings, 182–183
  fitting tips, 185
  sample findings, 183, **184**, 185
  test protocol, 183
Controlling microphone, 83–84, **83**, **84**
Convery, E., **56**
Cook, J.A., 27
Cooley, L.J., 204, 205
CORFIG (coupler response for flat insertion gain), **61**, 62, 112, **118**
Cornelisse, L.E., 48
Correction factors, 60–62
COSI. *See* Client Oriented Scale of Improvement
Counseling. *See* Patient counseling
Count-the-dot audiogram, 198–200, **199**, **279**
Coupler response for flat insertion gain. *See* CORFIG
Cox, R.M., 11, 20, 43, **43**, 44, 165, 205, 206, 233
Cox Contour Chart, **43**, 205, 222, **224**
CROS fittings. *See* Contralateral routing of offside signal (CROS) fittings
CST. *See* Connected Speech Test

D

Davis, Hallowell, **40**
Dawes, P., 264
De Jonge, R., **114**
Deming, W. Edwards, 33
Desensitization, **49**

Deshon Army Hospital (Pennsylvania), 40
DFS. *See* Digital feedback suppression
DigiSpeech, 70
Digital feedback suppression (DFS), 179–182
  fitting tips, 182
  sample findings, 181–182, **182**
  test protocol, 180–181
Digital noise reduction, 171–172
  fitting tips, 173–174
  REAR and, **126**
  sample findings, 172–173, **173**
  test protocol for, 172
  test signals and, 77, 81–82
Digital Speech in Noise, 70
Dillon, Harvey, 38–39, 45, 46, **56**, 57, **59**, 99, 231
Directional microphone technology, 78, **79**, 166–171
  directionality measures, **167**
  fitting tips, 170–171
  sample findings, 168–170, **169**, **170**
  test protocol, 166, **167**, 168
Dirks, on, 96
DNR, 258–259
DSL [i/o] method version 4.1, 48
DSL methods, history of, 47–49, **48**, **49**
DSL Multistage Input/Output v5.0a. *See* DSL v5.0
DSL v5.0, 50–52
  compared to NAL-NL2, 55–62, **57**, **58**, 250–251
    correction factors, 60–62
    outcomes, 57, 59–60
  loudness normalization, **47**
  revisions to, 50–52, **51**
DSL v5.0a, speech spectra, **72**
DSL v5.0b, 50–52, **51**
Dynamic range of speech, 74–77
Dynamic Roving Tone, 70

E

Ear canal
  probe tube placement, 97, **97**
  REUG and, 107–108
Ear canal resonance, 107
Ease of Communication subscale, 235
ECHO. *See* Expected Consequences of Hearing Aid Ownership
Edison, Thomas, 151, 195
Edwards, B., 264
Effective audibility, 77, **155**
EHIMA. *See* European Hearing Instrument Manufacturers Association
Einstein, Albert, 243
Entrainment, 179
Erber, Norm, 48, **49**
Ethics, lack of use of probe microphone testing, 7–8
Etymonic Design Inc., 3
European Hearing Instrument Manufacturers Association (EHIMA), 74
Ewert, C., 202
Expected Consequences of Hearing Aid Ownership (ECHO), 217, **287–288**

F

FBR. *See* Front-to-back ratio
Feigin, J.A., 137
FIG6 strategy, 44–45
Fixed SNR method, 211
Fletcher, Harvey, **69**, **264**
Flexer, C., 12, 15
FM systems, **73**
Free-field to eardrum transfer function, 107
Frequency lowering, 174–179
  fitting tips, 177, **178**, 179
  sample findings, 175, **176**, 177, **178**
  test protocol, 174–175
Fricatives, 79–80, **80**
Front-to-back ratio (FBR), **167**, 168
Frye Electronics, 68

G

Gain, 202
  desensitization and, **49**
  experienced users and, **56**, **58**
  high frequencies and, **154–155**, 251, **252**
  low-frequency gain, **194**
  NAL-NL2 compared to DSL v5.0, 55, **56–58**, 59
  prediction by REOG, 119

Gender
DSL v5.0 vs. NAL-NL2, 55, **58**
occlusion effect and, **191**
Geometric positioning of probe tube, 97–98, **98**, 101
Gessling, E., 35
GIFROC term, **61**
Ginis, J., 231
Gorga, M.P., 137

H

HACTES. *See* Hearing Aid Clinical Test Environment Standardization
Half-gain rule, 41, **42**
Harford, Earl, vii, 65
Harvard Report, 39
HASP. *See* Hearing Aid Selection Profile
Hawkins, D.B., viii, 132, 27, 74
HCL. *See* Highest comfortable level
Headphones, 86
Hearing Aid Clinical Test Environment Standardization (HACTES), 70
Hearing aid fitting
bilateral CROS, 183
bilateral fittings, 55
contralateral routing of offside signal (CROS) fittings, 182–183, **184**, 185
correct fitting statistics, 6
follow-up, 226–242
guidelines for, 2
open-ear canal fittings, 158–159, **160**, 161, **161**
pre-fitting tools, 197–201
software for, 10, 27
testing. *See* Post-fitting testing; Pre-fitting testing
transcranial CROS, 185
See also Prescriptive fitting; Proprietary fitting
Hearing Aid Selection Profile (HASP), 217
Hearing aid testing
during the fitting, 217–242
aided speech recognition, 217–221
loudness comfort, 221–222
outcome measures, 226–242
post-fitting. *See* Post-fitting testing
pre-fitting testing. *See* Pre-fitting testing
Hearing aids
closed-loop self-verifying hearing aids, **104**
MPO of, 77, 78, 163, **163**, 164–165, **165**, 202, **203**, 221
probe tube vent, 250
software, 10, 27, **128**, 200
trainable, 16–20, 257
WDRC instrument, **167**
See also Hearing aid fitting; Hearing aid testing
Hearing Handicap Inventory for the Elderly/Adult (HHIE/A), 216, **283**, **284**
Hearing instrument specialists (HISs), 5–6
Hearing loss desensitization, **49**
HHIE/A. *See* Hearing Handicap Inventory for the Elderly/Adult
High frequencies, **154–155**, 251, **252**
Highest comfortable level (HCL), **43**, **203**
HINT, 211
Holube, I., 75
Hooke, Robert, **139**
Hornsby, B.W., 16, 18, 265

I

ICRA signals, 70, **71**, 244
ILTASS. *See* International long-term average speech spectrum
In situ measurement, 2
Independent Hearing Aid Fitting Forum (IHAFF), 4, 43
Insertion gain optimizer (IGO) (Madsen), viii
Insertion loss, REOG and, **118**
International Collegium of Rehabilitative Audiology, 70
International long-term average speech spectrum (ILTASS), **72**
International Outcome Inventory for Hearing Aids (IOI-HA)
about, 230, 240
instrument, **293**
norm templates, 240, **241**, **242**, **294**
post-fitting, 240, **241**, 242, **242**
International Society of Audiology, 4
International Speech Test Signal (ISTS), 71–74, **72–74**, 75, 244, 259

Intertragal Notch Rule, 96
Invivo (Bosch), viii
IOI-HA. *See* International Outcome Inventory for Hearing Aids
ISTS. *See* International Speech Test Signal

J

Jenstad, L.M., 202
Jeon, J., 11
Jerger, James, **235**
Johnson, E.E., 39, 57, **58**, **59**
Johnson, J.A., 20

K

Kallogieri, D., 22, 23
Kalluri, S., 264
Keidser, G., 11, 18, **56**
Killion, M.C., 15, 44, 45, **61**, 82, 198, **264**, **279**
Kincaid, Gerald, 96
Kirby, John, **40**
Kochkin, S., 28, 29, 31, 32
Kopun, J.G., 137

L

Leavitt, R., 12, 15
Libby, E. Robert "Cy," 43
Libby one-third method, 43, **44**, 104
Ling sounds, 79, 177
Lombardi, Vince, 65
Long-term average speech signal (LTASS), 68, **68**, **69**, 70, 71, 75, 244, **245**
Loudness anchors, 205–206, **206**, **280**
Loudness comfort, verification of during fitting, 221–226
Loudness discomfort
  DSL v5.0 vs. NAL-NL2, 56–57
  predicting from the audiogram, 204–205, **205**
  terminology, **43**, **202**, **203**
  testing, **43**, 201–217, **203**, **280**, **281**
Loudness discomfort level (LDL) testing, **43**, 201–217, **203**
  clinical applications, 208–209
  instructions, 206–207, **206**, **207**, **281**
  loudness anchors, 205–206, **206**, **280**
  measuring, 205–209
  test procedures, 207–208
Loudness equalization, **47**
Loudness level, **154–155**
Loudness measures, open fittings and, **224**
Loudness normalization, **46–47**, 48, 221
Loudspeakers, 82–83, **83**
  placement of, 93, **94**, 102, 246
Low-frequency gain, and occlusion effect, **194**
Lybarger, Samuel, 41, **42**
Lybarger half-gain rule, 41, **42**

M

MacKenzie, D.J., 194
Madsen, probe microphone product, viii
MarkeTrak VIII study, 27–35
  about, ix, 7
  history of, **28**
  loudness comfort, 202
  patient comfort, 202
  patient loyalty, 30–31, 33, **34**
  professionalism and perceptions, 35
  return patient visits, 31–33
  survey process, 28–29
  test protocol and patient satisfaction, 29–31, **29–31**
Matrix Test, 211
Maximum audibility, **81**
Maximum power output (MPO)
  defined, **203**
  REAR 85/90 to verify, 77, 78, 162, **163**, 164–165, **165**, 202, **203**
  verification of, 225–226
McArdle, R., 21, 22, 210
McLelland, M., **56**
McManus, M., 21, 22
Microphones, 83–84, **83**, **84**
Modulated Speech Noise, 70
Monaural summation, 221
Monitor headphones, 86
Monitor microphone, 83–84, **83**, **84**
Monosyllables in quiet, **210**
Monser, Ed, **61**
Moodie, K.S., 142, 145

Moodie, S., 47
Moore, B.C., 24, 25
Mormer, E., 233
MPO. *See* Maximum power output
Mueller, H.G., vii, viii, 2, 5, 6, 13, 15, 16, 18, 24, 25, 35, 37, 38, 66, 84, **118**, **124**, 132, 144, **167**, 188, 198, 213, 216, 242, 257, 259, 265, **279**
Munro, K.J., 264

N

NAL methods
  history of, 45–46, 104
  trusting manufacturer's algorithm, 24–25
NAL-NL1
  about, 53, **54**, 253
  history of, 45–46
  proprietary fitting and, 11–13, **12**, 21
  SNR-Loss and, 12–13, **12**
  speech spectra, **72**
  trainable hearing aids to validate, 16–20, **17**, **19**, **20**, 257
NAL-NL2, 52–55, 253, 254
  compared to DSL v5.0, 55–62, **57**, **58**, 250–251
    correction factors, 60–62
    outcomes, 57, 59–60
  loudness normalization, **47**, 53
  manufacturer's algorithm and, 25, **26**, 27
  manufacturer's default fitting, 255–256, **255**
  proprietary fittings and, 13, **14**, 15, **15**
  speech spectra, **72**
  trainable hearing aids to validate, 16–20, **17**, **19**, **20**, 257
  versions of, 55
NAL-R, 45
Newall, P., 45
99th percentile, 74
Noah software, 235, 237
Noise
  DSL v5.0 vs. NAL-NL2, 55–56
  obnoxious noise test, 165, **165**, **224**
Noise reduction. *See* Digital noise reduction
Northern, Jerry, viii
Notch approach, 247

O

Obnoxious noise test, 165, **165**, **224**
O'Brien, A., **56**
Occlusion effect, 186, 188–194
  causes of, 188, **189**, **194**
  fitting tips, 194
  gender and, **191**
  ineffective solutions for, **192**
  low-frequency gain and, **194**
  REOG and, 119
  sample findings, 192–194, **193**
  solutions for, 188–190, **192**
  test protocol, 191, **194**
Oeding, K., 22, 23
Open-ear canal fittings, 158
  FAQ, 251
  fitting tips, 161
  limitation of REAR for, **161**
  loudness measures and, **224**
  sample findings, 159, **160**, 161
  stored equalization and, 244
  test protocol, 159
Optimal audibility, **81**
OSPL90, **203**
Outcome measures, 226–242
  Client Oriented Scale of Improvement (COSI), 217, 230–231, **230**, **232**, 233, **234**, **289**
  International Outcome Inventory for Hearing Aids (IOI-HA), 230, 240, **241**, 242, **242**, **293**, **294**
  patient satisfaction, 27–31, **29–31**, 227–228, **227**, 266–267
  self-report measures, 226
  uses for, **229**
Outcomes, **228**

P

Painton, Steve, **190**
PAL. *See* Profile of Aided Loudness
Palmer, C.V., 7, 17, 233
Parkinson, A., 45
Patient counseling
  pre-fitting appointment, 197–201
  speech mapping for, 267
  test signals for, 80–82, **81**

Patient outcomes, **228**
See also Outcome measures
Patient positioning, for testing, 92–95, **93**, **94**, 102, 243–244
Patient satisfaction, 227–228, **227**
dissatisfaction as outcome, 266–267
MarkeTrak VIII study, 27–31, **29–31**
Peck, A., 11
Percent audibility, **199**
Percentile analysis, 75, **76**
Picou, E.M., 2, 5, 6, **124**
Pink noise, 68
POGO method (prescription of gain and output), 42–43, **44**, 103–104
Post-fitting testing, 226–242
Abbreviated Profile of Hearing Aid Benefit (APHAB), 21–23, 216–217, 230, 233, 235–237, **237–239**, **285–286**
Client Oriented Scale of Improvement (COSI), 217, 230–231, **230**, **232**, 233, **234**, **289**
International Outcome Inventory for Hearing Aids (IOI-HA), 230, 240, **241**, 242, **242**, **293**, **294**
Prasher, D., 24
Pre-fitting testing
loudness discomfort level testing, **43**, 201–217, **203**
Quick Speech In Noise (QuickSIN) test, 213–215, **214**, **215**
self-assessment, 215–217
Abbreviated Profile of Hearing Aid Benefit (APHAB), 21–23, 216–217, 230, 233, 235–237, **237–239**, **285–286**
Characteristics of Amplification Tool (COAT), 217
Client Oriented Scale of Improvement (COSI), 217, 230–231, **230**, **232**, 233, **234**, **289**
Expected Consequences of Hearing Aid Ownership (ECHO), 217, **287–288**
Hearing Aid Selection Profile (HASP), 217
Hearing Handicap Inventory for the Elderly/Adult (HHIE/A), 216, **283**, **284**
Profile of Aided Loudness (PAL), 217
speech-in-noise testing, 209–213
Pre-fitting tools, 197–201
Preferred dynamic range, 45
Prescriptive fitting
about, 1, 2
acceptable range for target, **131**
correction factors, 60–62
history of, 39–49
Berger method, 42
DSL methods, 47–49, **48**, **49**
FIG6 strategy, 44–45
Libby one-third method, 43, **44**, 104
Lybarger half-gain rule, 41, **42**
NAL methods, 45–46
POGO method (prescription of gain and output), 42–43, **44**, 103–104
VIOLA strategy, 43–44
loudness equalization, **47**
loudness normalization and, **46–47**, 48
manufacturer's software, **128**, 200
target verification, 67–68, 70–77
value of, 10–23
Preves, David, vii, viii, 65, 105
Probe microphone measurement
ambient noise and, 89, **90**
benefits of, 10–27
Best Practice Guidelines and, 4–7, **6**
best time for, 265–266
bilateral testing, **87**, 93
calibrating the probe tube, 89, 91–92, **92**
contralateral routing of offside signal (CROS) fittings, 182–183, **184**, 185
digital noise reduction, **77**, 81–82, 171–174
directional technology, 78, **79**, 166–171
equipment, 82–86
ethics of lack of use of, 7–8
FAQ, 243–267
equipment setup and procedures, 243–244, **245**, 246
probe tube use and placement, 246–250, **247**, **248**
unusual outcomes, 260–264, **261–263**
verification of prescriptive targets, 250–251, **252**, 253–257, **255**, **256**
verification of special features, 258–259
feedback suppression, 179–182

Probe microphone measurement *(continued)*
FM systems and, **73**
frequency lowering, 174–179
history of, vii-viii, 4, 39–49, **39**, 65–66, 103–105
loudness discomfort level testing, 201–217
methods, 62–63, **62**, **63**
FAQ, 243–267
loudspeaker placement, 93, **94**, 102, 246
patient positioning, 92–95, **93**, **94**, 102, 243–244
probe tube placement, 95–99, **96–101**, 101, **125**, **132**, **133**, 246, 263
misuse of for hearing aid fitting, **3**
open-ear canal fittings, 158–159, **160**, 161, **161**
patient behavior during test, **96**, 243–244
primary use of, ix
reasons for not using, 8–10
reflective surface and, 89, 102, 146, 243
standards, viii
terminology, viii, 2–4, 86–88, 105–106
test environment, 88–89
test setup summary, 101–102
test signals, 67–82
use statistics for, 2
wireless streaming, 185–187, **187**
See also DSL v5.0; NAL-NL2; Prescriptive fitting
Probe Microphone Measurement (Mueller, Hawkins, & Northern), viii
Probe microphone testing equipment, 82–86
loudspeaker, 82–83, **83**, 93, **94**, 102, 246
measurement microphone, 84–85
microphone system, **66**, 83–85
monitor headphones, 86
output display, 85–86, **86**
reference microphone, 83–84, **83**, **84**
signal analysis, 85
Probe-tube holder, **100**
Probe-tube microphone, 84–85
Probe-tube microphone system, vii, **44**, 66
Probe tubes, 91, **91**
calibration of, 89, 91–92, **92**
FAQ, 246–250
holders for, **100**
notch approach, 247
placement of, 95–99, **96–101**, 101, **125**, **132**, **133**, 246, 263
plugged, 248–249, **248**
use and placement, 246–250, **247**, **248**
Profile of Aided Loudness (PAL), 217, **290–292**
Project Phoenix (Nicolet), viii
Proprietary fitting, evaluation of, 10–13, **12**, **14**, 15, **15**
Pumford, J., 35

Q

Quick Speech In Noise (QuickSIN) test, 213–215, **214**, **215**

R

RadioEar, 41, **42**, 166
Raffin, M.J.M., **282**
Rasmussen, Steen, vii, 66
Rastronics CCI–10, vii, **44**, 66
REAG (real-ear aided gain), 105, **107**, 114, 122
Real-ear aided gain. *See* REAG
Real-ear aided response. *See* REAR
Real-ear aided response for 85 or 90 dB input. *See* REAR 85/90
Real ear aided-to occluded gain. *See* REAOG
Real-ear coupler difference. *See* RECD
Real-ear dial difference. *See* REDD
Real-ear insertion gain. *See* REIG
Real-ear insertion response. *See* REIR
Real-ear measurements (REM), 2
Real-ear occluded gain. *See* REOG
Real-ear occluded response. *See* REOR
Real-ear saturation response. *See* RESR
Real-ear unaided gain. *See* REUG
Real-ear unaided response. *See* REUR
REAOG (real ear aided-to occluded gain), **117**
REAR (real-ear aided response), 101, 103, **118**, 122–123, **123–126**, 125, 130, 151, 153, 253, 260–262
for assessment of audibility, 127–128
clinical applications of, 88, 129
defined, 88, **107**, 121–122
digital noise reduction and, **126**

fitting tips, 153–154, **154**
measurement of, 128–129
in open-ear canal fittings, **161**
probe placement and, 123, **125**, **132**
REIG vs., **124**
reliability of measures, 132, **133**, 134
sample findings, 152–153, **152**
test protocols for, 126–128, 151–152
REAR 85/90 (real-ear aided response for 85 or 90 dB input), 134–135, **136**, 202, 261–263, **262**, 265
clinical applications of, 88, 136
defined, 88, **107**, 134
fitting tips, 164–165, **165**
frequency lowering with, 175
measurement of, 136
sample findings, 163, **163**, 164
setting the VC for, 137
test protocol, 162
verification of MPO, 77, 78, 163, **163**, 164–165, **165**, 202, **203**
RECD (real-ear coupler difference), 62, 137–138, **139**, 140, **141**, 142, 254
ANSI standard, **138**, **139–140**
caveats for use, **138**
clinical applications of, 88, 145–146
defined, 88, 137, **203**
measurement of, **143**, 145
for open fittings, 142–145, **144**
use with children, 137–138, **139–140**, 140, **141**
REDD (real-ear dial difference), 62, 147
clinical applications of, 88, 148–149, **148**
defined, 88, 137, 146, **203**
Reference equivalent threshold in SPL. *See* RETSPL
Reference microphone, 83–84, **83**, **84**
Reflective surface, 89, 102, 146, 243
Regulating microphone, 83–84, **83**, **84**
REIG (real-ear insertion gain), 101, 103, 105, 112, 114, **118**, 122, 129–130, **131**, 153, 155, 256–257
for aided audiogram, **156**, **157**
calculation of, 134
clinical applications of, 88, 134
defined, 88, **107**, 129
favored over REAR, **124**
fitting tips, 158
placement of probe tube for, **132**, **133**
real speech and, 131–132
reliability of measures, 132, **133**, 134
sample findings, 155–156, **156**, 158
test protocol, 155
REIR (real-ear insertion response), **130**
REOG (real-ear occluded gain), 114, 115–117, 119
clinical applications of, 121
defined, **107**, 115
factors determining, 116–117
gain prediction by, 119
insertion loss and, **118**
measurement of, 120–121
occlusion effect and, 119
vent-associated resonance and, **120**, **121**
REOR (real-ear occluded response), 115, 116, **116**, 121, 260, 261, **261**, **262**
clinical applications of, 88
defined, 88, 115
REUR and, 115, **116**
RESR (real-ear saturation response), ix, 88, **107**, 134, **203**
RETSPL (reference equivalent threshold in SPL), 62, 135, 137, 147, **203**, 208–209
REUG (real-ear unaided gain), 103, 105, 106–108, **106**, **107**, **109**, 111–113, **118**, 129, 155, 164
average REUG, 106, **106**, **107**, **113**
clinical applications of, 114
defined, 106, **107**
measured REUG, **109**, 112, **113**
measurement of, 113–114
tympanic membrane perforation and, **114**
REUR (real-ear unaided response), 101, 105, 106, **110**, 111, **111**, 113, 114, 129, 130, 155, 244, **245**
average REUR, 111, **111**
clinical applications of, 88
defined, 87–88, 106
reliability of measures, **132**
REOR and, 115, **116**
test signals for, **115**
Reverberation subscale, 235
Revit, Larry, **61**, 82, **113**, 148
Ricketts, T.A., **118**, 144
Ross, D.A., 65

Ross, Mark, 47, **48**
Routine use, defined, 5–6, **6**

S

Sachs, R.M., 140
Sanders, J., 13, 15, 25, 27, 253, 254
Schroeder processing, 70
Schwartz, Dan, vii, 66
Scollie, S., 47, 50, 51, 52, 254
Seewald, R.C., 47, **48**, 142, 145
Selective amplification, 39
Self-assessment instruments
  Abbreviated Profile of Hearing Aid Benefit (APHAB), 21–23, 216–217, 230, 233, 235–237, **237–239**, **285–286**
  Characteristics of Amplification Tool (COAT), 217
  Client Oriented Scale of Improvement (COSI), 217, 230–231, **230**, **232**, 233, **234**, **289**
  Expected Consequences of Hearing Aid Ownership (ECHO), 217, **287–288**
  Hearing Aid Selection Profile (HASP), 217
  Hearing Handicap Inventory for the Elderly/Adult (HHIE/A), 216, **283**, **284**
  International Outcome Inventory for Hearing Aids (IOI-HA), 230, 240, **241**, 242, **242**, **293**, **294**
  Profile of Aided Loudness (PAL), 217, **290–292**
Shaw, E.A.G., 107
Siemens, viii
Signal-to-noise loss (SNR loss), 12–13, **12**
SII. *See* Speech intelligibility index
Sinclair, S.T., 142, 145
Smith, S., 22, 23
SNR–50, 211
SNR loss, 214
Software, 10, 27, **128**, 200
Sonotone, 166
Sound field testing, 212–213
Speech
  dynamic range of speech, 74–77
  hearing vs. understanding, **199**
  understanding, 198
Speech banana, 74, 198–199, **199**, **200**, 253, 267, **279**
Speech-in-noise testing, 209–213
  adaptive vs. fixed SNR, 211–212
  cocktail party effect, **211**
  competing noises, 211
  earphones vs. sound field testing, 212–213
  monosyllables in quiet, **210**
  presentation level, 212
  selecting tools, 210–211
Speech intelligibility index (SII), 17, 45, **49**, 265, **266**
Speech mapping, 122
  about, 3
  primary use of, ix
Speech reception threshold (SRT), 211
Speech recognition. *See* Aided speech recognition
Speech Recognition In Noise Test (SPRINT), 211
Speech signals
  ICRA signals, 70, **71**, 244
  ILTASS, **72**
  ISTS, 71–74, **72–74**, 75, 244, 259
  LTASS, 68, **68**, **69**, 70, 71, 75, 244, **245**
  testing, 70–77
Speech sounds, for frequency lowering testing, 177
Speech spectrum, 68, **69**, **72**
Speechmap(TM), 3
SPL-O-Gram, 48, **49**, 114, 122, 200–201, **201**
SPRINT. *See* Speech Recognition In Noise Test
SRT. *See* Speech reception threshold
SRT50, 211
Starkey, viii
Stelmachowicz, P.G., 137
Stoody, T.M., 13, 15
Stored equalization calibration technique, 94, 244
Storey, L., 99
Strouse, A.L., 5
Sullivan, R.F., 99
Summation, 221–222
Surr, Rauna, vii, 66
Sweetow, R.W., 132
Synthetic fricatives, 79–80, **80**

T

TD. *See* Threshold of discomfort
Telephones, wireless streaming, 185–187, **187**
Television, wireless streaming, 185–187, **187**
Test signals, 67–82, 244
choosing, 67, **67**
for demonstration or counseling purposes, 80–82, **81**
digital noise reduction and, 77, 81–82
and evaluation of specific features, 77–80, **77**, **79**, **80**
history of, 68, 70
ISTS, 71–74, **72–74**, 75, 244, 259
for prescriptive target verification, 67–68, 70–77
for REUR, **115**
signal analysis, 85
speech signals, 70–77
Thornton, A.R., **282**
Threshold of discomfort (TD), **43**, **203**
Tolstoy, Leo, 1
Tonisson, W., 45
Trainable hearing aids, to validate NAL-NL, 16–20, **17**, **19**, **20**, 257
Training, 9–10, **9**
Transcranial CROS, 185
Twain, Mark, 103
Tympanic membrane perforation, REUG and, **114**

U

Uncomfortable loudness level (UCL), **43**, **202**, **203**
Unilateral loudness testing, **223**, 246
University of Western Ontario (UWO), 78–79
Upper level of comfort (ULC), **43**, **203**

V

Valente, Michael, 9, 10, 22, 23, 105
Validation, **218**
Van Gogh, Vincent, 197
Van Tasell, D., 202
Vanderbilt Report II (1990), 4
Vent-associated resonance, REOG and, **120**, **121**
Verification
about, 1, **218**
automated real-ear verification, **104**
directional technology verification test, 78, **79**
FAQ
equipment setup and procedures, 243–244, **245**, 246
of prescriptive targets, 250–251, **252**, 253–257, **255**, **256**
probe tube use and placement, 246–250, **247**, **248**, 263
of special features, 258–259
unusual outcomes, 260–264, **261–263**
of loudness comfort, 221–222
of MPO, 225–226
room calibration, 243
Video otoscopy, **99**
VIOLA strategy (visual input-out locator algorithm), 43–44
Visually assisted positioning of probe tube, 96–97

W

Walden, Brian, vii, 66
Wallenfels, H., **206**
Weber, J.E., 13, 15, 16
Wiener, F.M., 65
Wiener filtering, 171
Wilson, R.H., 210
Wireless streaming, testing and programming, 185–187, **187**
Wu, Y.H., 11

Y

Yeend, I., **56**